MW00668735

GASTROENTEROLOGY AND HEPATOLOGY

The Comprehensive Visual Reference

GASTROENTEROLOGY AND HEPATOLOGY

The Comprehensive Visual Reference

series editor
Mark Feldman, MD

Southland Professor and Vice Chairman
Department of Internal Medicine
University of Texas Southwestern
    Medical Center at Dallas

Chief, Medical Service
Veterans Affairs Medical Center
Dallas, Texas

volume 4
Pediatric GI Problems

volume editor
Paul E. Hyman, MD

Director, Pediatric Gastrointestinal Motility Center
Children's Hospital of Orange County
Orange, California

Associate Clinical Professor of Pediatrics
University of California, Los Angeles,
    School of Medicine
Los Angeles, California

With 13 contributors

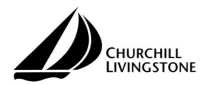

**CHURCHILL
LIVINGSTONE**

Developed by Current Medicine, Inc.
Philadelphia

Current Medicine

400 Market Street
Suite 700
Philadelphia, PA 19106

Managing Editor	*Lori J. Bainbridge*
Development Editors	*Ira D. Smiley and Raymond Lukens*
Editorial Assistant	*Scott Thomas Hurd*
Art Director	*Paul Fennessy*
Design and Layout	*Robert LeBrun*
Illustration Director	*Ann Saydlowski*
Illustrators	*Wieslawa Langenfeld, Beth Starkey,*
	Lisa Weischedel, and Gary Welch
Typesetting Supervisor	*Brian Tshudy*
Production	*David Myers and Lori Holland*
Indexer	*Maria Coughlin*

Pediatric GI problems / volume editor, Paul E. Hyman.
     p.   cm. — (Gastroenterology and hepatology : v. 4)
  Includes bibliographical references and index.
  ISBN 0-443-07852-1
    1. Pediatric gastroenterology—Diagnosis—Atlases.
2. Gastrointestinal system—Imaging—Atlases. 3. Pediatric
diagnostic imaging—Atlases.   I. Hyman, Paul E., 1949-
II. Series.
    [DNLM: 1. Gastrointestinal Diseases—in infancy & childhood—
atlases.   1997 A-754 v. 4 / WI 17 G257 1997 v.4]
RJ448.P44   1997
618.92'33—dc20
DNLM/DLC
for Library of Congress   96-23054
                                            CIP

©**Copyright 1997 by Current Medicine.** All rights reserved. No part of this publication may be reproduced, stored in a retrieval system or transmitted in any form by any means electronic, mechanical, photocopying, recording, or otherwise, without prior written consent of the publisher.

Library of Congress Cataloging-in-Publication Data
ISBN 0-443-07852-1

Printed in Singapore by Imago Productions (FE) Pte Ltd.

10 9 8 7 6 5 4 3 2 1

DISTRIBUTED WORLDWIDE BY CHURCHILL LIVINGSTONE, INC.

Although every effort has been made to ensure that drug doses and other information are presented accurately in this publication, the ultimate responsibility rests with the prescribing physician. Neither the publishers nor the authors can be held responsible for errors or for any consequences arising from the use of information contained herein. Products mentioned in this publication should be used in accordance with the prescribing information prepared by the manufacturers. No claims or endorsements are made for any drug or compound at present under clinical investigation.

At the time of publication, **cisapride** was not FDA approved for use in children. Check the package insert for any change in indications and dosage and for added warnings and precautions.

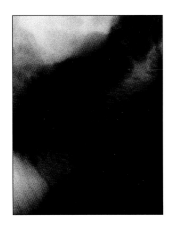

Series Preface

In recent years dramatic developments in the practice of gastro-enterology have unfolded, and the specialty has become, more than ever, a visual discipline. Advances in endoscopy, radiology, or a combination of the two, such as endoscopic retrograde cholangiopancreatography and endoscopic ultrasonography, have occurred in the past 2 decades. Because of advanced imaging technology, a gastroenterologist, like a dermatologist, is often able to directly view the pathology of a patient's organs. Moreover, practicing gastroenterologists and hepatologists can frequently diagnose disease from biopsy samples examined microscopically, often aided by an increasing number of special staining techniques. As a result of these advances, gastroenterology has grown as rapidly as any subspecialty of internal medicine.

Gastroenterology and Hepatology: The Comprehensive Visual Reference is an ambitious 8-volume collection of images that pictorially displays the gastrointestinal tract, liver, biliary tree, and pancreas in health and disease, both in children and adults. The series is comprised of 89 chapters containing nearly 4000 images accompanied by legends. The images in this collection include not only traditional photographs but also charts, tables, drawings, algorithms, and diagrams, making this collection much more than an atlas in the conventional sense. Chapters are authored by experts selected by one of the eight volume editors, who carefully reviewed each chapter within their volume.

Disorders of the gastrointestinal tract, liver, biliary tree, and pancreas are common in children and adults. *Helicobacter pylori* gastritis is the most frequent bacterial infection of humans and is a risk factor for peptic ulcer disease and gastric malignancies. Colorectal carcinoma is the second leading cause of cancer mortality in the United States, with nearly 60,000 deaths in 1990. Pancreatic cancer resulted in an additional 25,000 deaths. Liver disease is also an important cause of morbidity and mortality, with more that 25,000 deaths from cirrhosis alone in 1990. Gallstone disease is also common in our society, with increasing reliance on laparoscopic cholecystectomy in symptomatic individuals. Inflamma-tory bowel diseases (ulcerative colitis, Crohn's disease) are also widespread in all segments of the population; their causes still elude us.

The past few decades have also witnessed striking advances in the therapy of gastrointestinal disorders. Examples include "cure" of peptic ulcer disease by eradicating *H. pylori* with antimicrobial agents, healing of erosive esophagitis with proton pump inhibitor drugs, remission of chronic viral hepatitis B or C with interferon-α2b, and hepatic transplantation for patients with fulminant hepatic failure or end-stage liver disease. Therapeutic endoscopic techniques have proliferated that ameliorate the need for surgical procedures. Endoscopic advances include placement of peroral endoscopic gastrostomy tubes for nutritional support, insertion of stents in the bile duct or esophagus to relieve malignant obstruction, and the use of injection therapy, thermal coagulation, or laser therapy to treat bleeding ulcers and other lesions, including tumors. *Gastroenterology and Hepatology: The Comprehensive Visual Reference* will cover these advances and many others in the field of gastroenterology.

I wish to thank a number of people for their contributions to this series. The dedication and expertise of the other volume editors—Willis Maddrey, Rick Boland, Paul Hyman, Nick LaRusso, Roy Orlando, Larry Schiller, and Phil Toskes—was critical and most appreciated. The nearly 100 contributing authors were both creative and generous with their time and teaching materials. And special thanks to Abe Krieger, President of Current Medicine, for recruiting me for this unique project, and to his talented associates at Current Medicine.

The images contained in this 8-volume collection are available in print as well as in slide format, and the series is soon being formatted for CD-ROM use. All of us who have participated in this ambitious project hope that each of the 8 volumes, as well as the entire collection, will be useful to physicians and health professionals throughout the world involved in the diagnosis and treatment of patients of all ages who suffer from gastrointestinal disorders.

Mark Feldman, MD

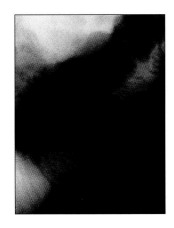

Volume Preface

Children are developing, growing organisms with special metabolic needs and stressors unfamiliar to the adult. Congenital disorders, such as glycogen storage disease and Hirschsprung's disease, and congenital malformations, such as imperforate anus and tracheoesophageal fistula, illustrate the heterogeneity of gastrointestinal pathologies important in infants but rarely encountered in adults. There are age-specific diseases, such as neonatal necrotizing enterocolitis, and functional disorders unique to children, such as toddler's diarrhea and functional fecal retention. Conditions common to adults and children, like peptic ulcer, gastroesophageal reflux, and inflammatory bowel disease, differ in phenotypes and prognoses, depending on the age of onset. In this volume, cystic fibrosis is examined not only through clinical images, but also through a succinct explanation of its genetics. In pediatric gastroenterology there is an emphasis on assuring optimal nutritional support for every child because a child's potential for growth and development must be maximized, even in the presence of digestive disease. Thus, a chapter has been devoted to nutrition; however, nutritional issues are addressed in other chapters also.

This volume was conceived not only as a visual text for pediatric gastroenterology, but also as a complementary addition to the series of organ-specific volumes on adult gastroenterology. To avoid repetition, there is emphasis on the medical, surgical, and nutritional management care of infants and children with gastrointestinal and liver disease. I am grateful to the chapter authors for producing current, authoritative, focused reviews highlighting the clinical practice of pediatric gastroenterology. It is a particular pleasure to thank each chapter author for inadvertently helping me study for the 1995 examination in pediatric gastroenterology. Editing this volume, with superb contributions from experts in every important area of pediatric gastroenterology and nutrition, may have been the best preparation I could have had for that penultimate rite of passage.

Paul E. Hyman, MD

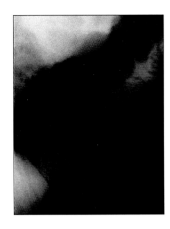

Contributors

Carol Lynn Berseth, MD
Associate Professor
Department of Pediatrics
Baylor College of Medicine
Houston, Texas

Anupama Chawla, MD, DCh
Assistant Professor of Pediatrics
Department of Pediatric Gastroenterology
Cornell University Medical College
North Shore University Hospital
Manhasset, New York

Fredric Daum, MD
Professor of Pediatrics
Department of Pediatric Gastroenterology
Cornell University Medical College
North Shore University Hospital
Manhasset, New York

Carlo Di Lorenzo, MD
Associate Professor
Department of Pediatrics
Children's Hospital of Pittsburgh
Pittsburgh, Pennsylvania

Peter R. Durie, BsC, MD, FRCPC
Head, Division of Gastroenterology and Nutrition
The Hospital for Sick Children
Toronto, Ontario, Canada

Melvin B. Heyman, MD, MPH
Professor of Pediatrics
Department of Pediatric Gastroenterology and Nutrition
University of California, San Francisco, Medical Center
San Francisco, California

Jacob C. Langer, MD
Associate Professor
St. Louis Children's Hospital
St. Louis, Missouri

Susan R. Orenstein, MD
Associate Professor
Division of Pediatric Gastroenterology
Children's Hospital of Pittsburgh
Pittsburgh, Pennsylvania

Alberto Peña, MD
Chief of Pediatric Surgery
Schneider Children's Hospital
Long Island Jewish Medical Center
New Hyde Park, New York

Philip Rosenthal, MD
Professor of Pediatrics and Surgery
University of California, San Francisco, Medical Center
San Francisco, California

Miguel Saps, MD
Pediatrician
Hospital Pereira-Rossell
Montevideo, Uruguay

Vasundhara Tolia, MD
Director, Pediatric Gastroenterology and Nutrition
Children's Hospital of Michigan
Detroit, Michigan

Jon A. Vanderhoof, MD
Professor of Pediatrics
University of Nebraska/Creighton University
Omaha, Nebraska

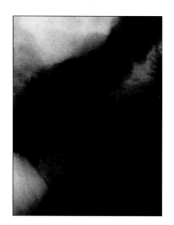

Contents

Chapter

1

The Newborn

CAROL LYNN BERSETH

The gastrointestinal tract forms early in fetal life, and it is structurally well established by mid-gestation. However, complete maturation of function does not occur until childhood. Immaturity of function is reflected in common practices concerning feeding and training for infants and children. During infancy, for example, infants are typically fed breast milk or formula because they have no teeth for masticating solids and they lack the ability to process starches. By cultural practice, fruits and cereals are introduced at 3 to 6 months, coincident with maturation of pancreatic function. Toilet training usually begins around the third year, when the child is intellectually ready to assume voluntary control of anal tone.

Because many aspects of functional maturation occur during the last trimester, immaturity of gastrointestinal function causes particular problems for infants who have been born prematurely (*ie*, before 37 weeks gestation). The ability of the newborn intestine to process and digest dietary fats, proteins, and carbohydrates is not as efficient as the adult intestine. These deficiencies are even more pronounced in the preterm infant. For example, the normal sucking mechanism is not present in many preterm infants, and these infants must be fed by orogastric tubes. In addition, specially designed infant formulas or additives for breast milk must be used to overcome deficiencies of digestive function.

A major additional concern for preterm infants is their high risk for developing necrotizing enterocolitis. Approximately 10% to 25% of preterm infants will develop signs or symptoms of this life-threatening disease. Approximately 25% of these infants will require surgery and one fourth to one half of these will die. Currently, the cause of this devastating disease is not known

A normal transient phenomenon that occurs in healthy newborn infants is the presence of clinically apparent jaundice that is accompanied by a rise in serum bilirubin. The vast majority of these infants have normal physiologic jaundice or breast milk jaundice. Neither entity is clinically life threatening. The major concern in evaluating infants who have jaundice is to identify those infants who have biliary obstruction or congenital defects from those who have normal transient physiologic or breast milk jaundice.

Another developmental phenomenon that involves gastrointestinal function is infantile colic. Although the cause of this phenomenon is multifactorial, it is frequently expressed as intense periodic crying that appears to be related to abdominal pain. Its cause is multifactional, and behavioral interventions appear to have the greatest success for treatment for those infants who do not have an underlying organic dysfunction.

■ DEVELOPMENTAL PHYSIOLOGY

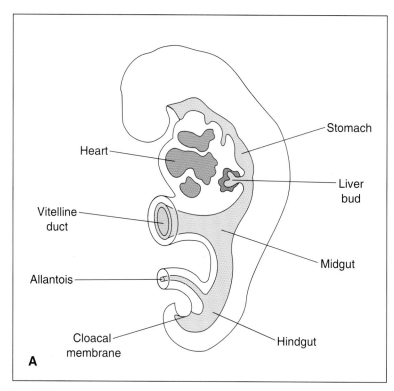 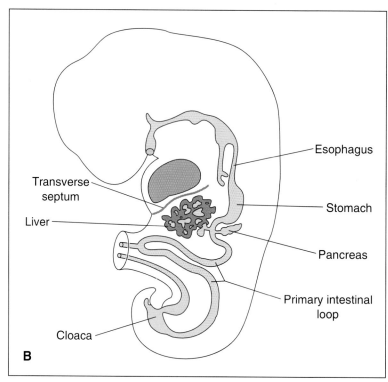

FIGURE 1-1.

The human gastrointestinal tract is initially formed as a result of the cephalocaudal flexion of the embryo (**A** and **B**). Thereafter the rupture of the buccopharyngeal and cloacal membranes provide sites of influx and reflux from the primitive gut. The liver and pancreas form as outbuddings from the premature gut.

(*continued on next page*)

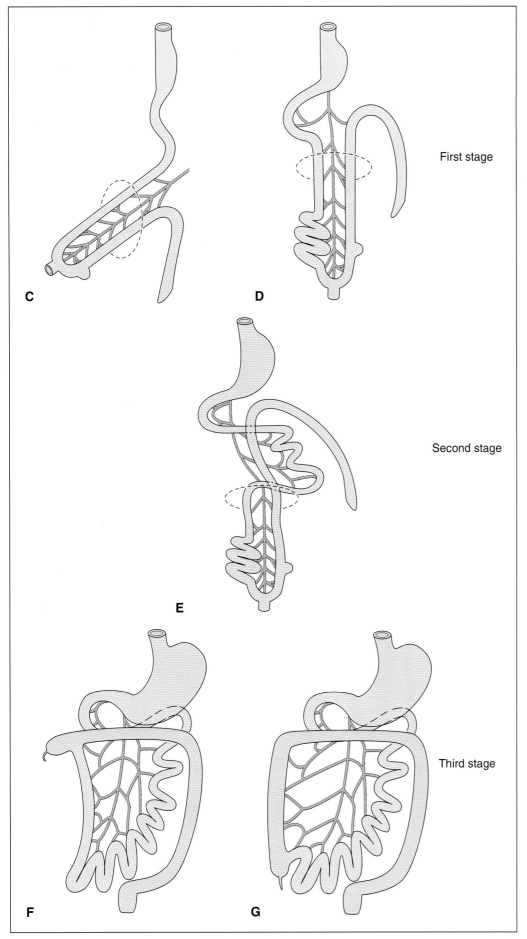

First stage

Second stage

Third stage

C

D

E

F

G

FIGURE 1-1. (CONTINUED)

At 6 weeks the primitive gut herniates into the umbilical cord as shown in **C**. On reentry to the abdominal cavity at 12 weeks, it rotates counterclockwise around the axis formed by the superior mesenteric artery (**D–F**). With the descent of the cecum (**G**) and final positioning of the large intestine, the final anatomical position of the gastrointestinal tract is completed by 20 weeks gestation [1]. (**A** and **B**, *Adapted from* Langman [2]; **C–G**, *Adapted from* Snyder and Chaffin [3].)

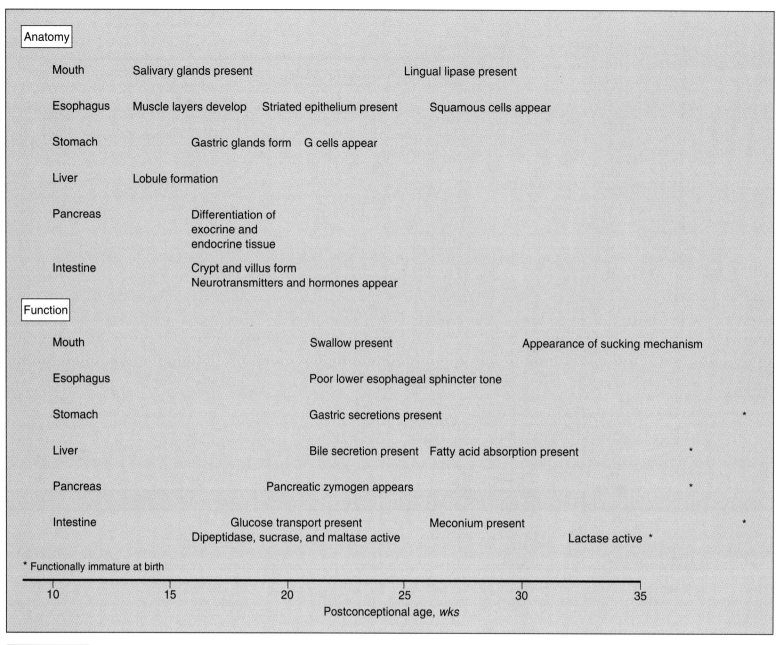

FIGURE 1-2.

Anatomical appearance of structures in the gastrointestinal tract does not necessarily correlate with the presence of functional maturation of those structures. As shown on this time line, most of the anatomic structures of the fetal intestine are present by mid gestation. Functional maturation occurs thereafter throughout the third trimester. Maturation in one organ does not occur temporally with maturation in another organ. Some aspects of function remain immature at term, and full maturation occurs during infancy or childhood. Thus, feeding practices for the preterm and term infant must be tailored for the infant's functional maturation.

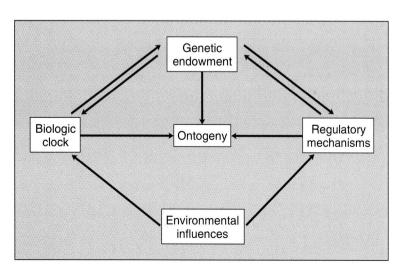

FIGURE 1-3.

Lebenthal and Lee [4] proposed four major determinants of growth and development of the human gastrointestinal tract. First, genetic endowment regulates differentiation and, in turn, may interact with the "biologic clock" and other regulatory mechanisms. The biologic clock refers to the need for certain predetermined sequential temporal events to occur within a temporal window in order for normal maturation to occur. Other regulatory mechanisms that may interact with genetic endowment are centrally mediated neurohormonal events. All three of these regulatory aspects, in turn, occur in a maternal milieu that may also influence maturational events. (*From* Lebenthal and Lee [4]; with permission.)

TABLE 1-1. REGULATION OF SMALL INTESTINAL MATURATION AND GROWTH BY HORMONES AND PEPTIDES

PEPTIDE	PLASMA LEVELS SURGE PRIOR TO FUNCTIONAL MATURATION	EARLY ADMINISTRATION INDUCES PRECOCIOUSNESS	REMOVAL OF PEPTIDE RETARDS FUNCTIONAL MATURATION
Corticosteroids	X	X	X
Thyroid	X	X	X
Insulin	X	X	X
Epidermal growth factor	X	X	X
Others (includes gastrin, enteroglucagon, IGF-I, IGF-II)	*	X	*

*Inadequately studied to date.

TABLE 1-1.

In order to demonstrate that a peptide regulates intestinal growth, maturation, or both, it should demonstrate a surge in appearance just before the natural occurrence of growth or maturation, its early administration should cause a precocious appearance of growth, maturation, or both, and its removal should result in retardation of growth, maturation, or both. Several peptides meet these characteristics and are considered to play an intimate role in regulating fetal and neonatal intestinal growth and maturation, as shown in this figure [5]. Others have been shown to have a trophic effect, but the other two criteria have not been completely met. These peptides may be of potential significance in regulating growth and maturation of neonatal intestine in the preterm infant because (1) preterm infants are often exposed to antenatal glucocorticosteroids for routine obstetrical management of preterm labor (to induce lung maturation and improve survival from preterm delivery); (2) preterm infants have abnormally low plasma T_4 concentrations; and (3) preterm delivery is a common occurrence in infants of diabetic mothers whose infants have exceedingly high circulatory plasma concentrations of insulin. High concentrations of epidermal growth factor are found in human amniotic fluid and breast milk, and the neonatal intestine is exposed to this peptide via oral ingestion. IGF—insulin-like growth factor.

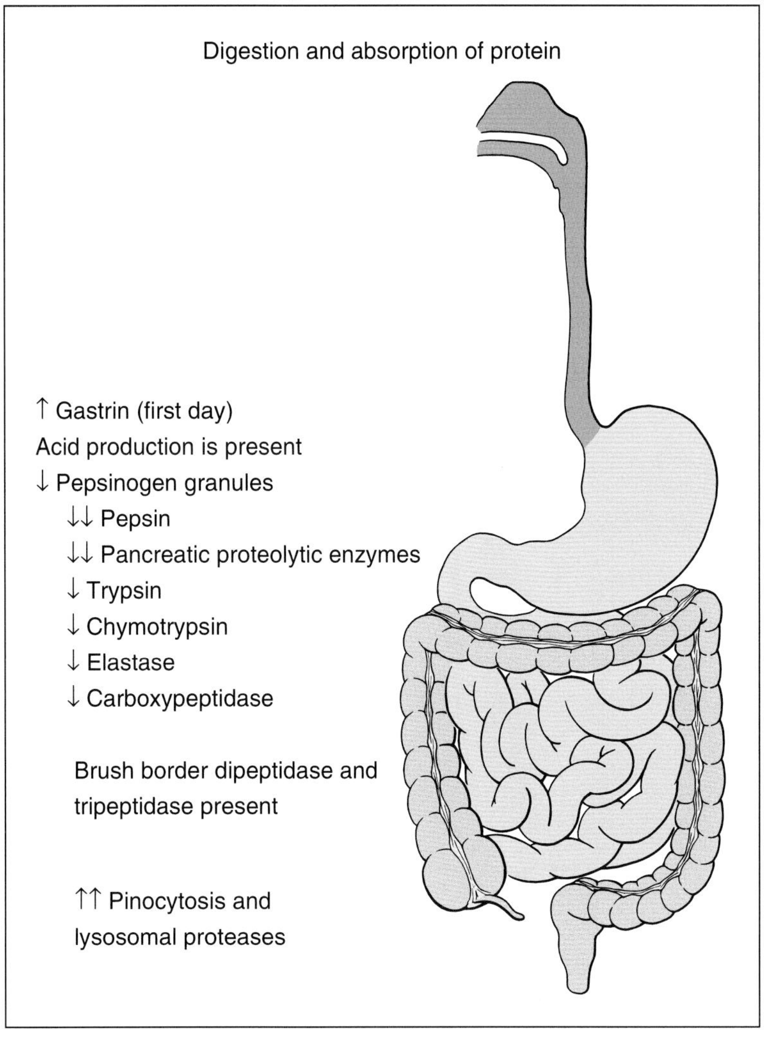

Digestion and absorption of protein

↑ Gastrin (first day)
Acid production is present
↓ Pepsinogen granules
   ↓↓ Pepsin
   ↓↓ Pancreatic proteolytic enzymes
   ↓ Trypsin
   ↓ Chymotrypsin
   ↓ Elastase
   ↓ Carboxypeptidase

Brush border dipeptidase and tripeptidase present

↑↑ Pinocytosis and lysosomal proteases

FIGURE 1-4.

In the adult, ingested protein is initially broken down to polypeptides by gastric pepsin in an acidic environment. Infants have 10% of the number of pepsin granules reported to be present in adults. However, pepsinogenic activity is present in term infants. Once protein has been processed to polypeptides, pancreatic proteolytic enzymes break these polypeptides into smaller peptides and amino acids. The release and action of these enzymes is triggered by the release of trypsin. Trypsin, as well as the other enzymes, is produced in lower concentrations in infants than in adults. Despite immaturity of these two aspects of protein processing, all of the intestinal peptides appear to be fully mature in the neonate. An additional mechanism for protein absorption is present in the neonate. Intact protein or partially digested peptides can be directly absorbed as macromolecules and further metabolized by lyzosomal proteases.

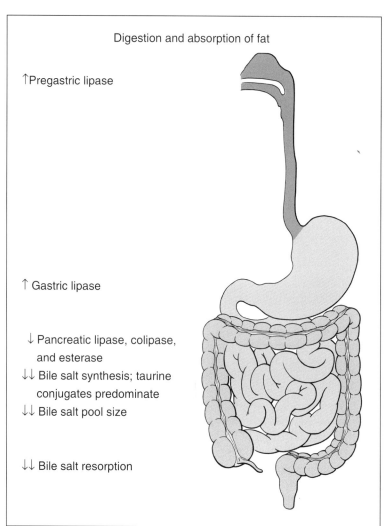

Digestion and absorption of fat

↑Pregastric lipase

↑ Gastric lipase

↓ Pancreatic lipase, colipase, and esterase

↓↓ Bile salt synthesis; taurine conjugates predominate

↓↓ Bile salt pool size

↓↓ Bile salt resorption

FIGURE 1-5.

Dietary fat constitutes half of an infant's caloric intake; however, fat is not efficiently absorbed by the neonate. In adults, fats are initially converted to free fatty acids and monoglycerides by lipases. Although pancreatic lipase is decreased in neonates, lingual and gastric lipase are increased, and may, in part, compensate for the immaturity of pancreatic lipase. In addition, breast milk contains three lipases that contribute to the gastric processing of dietary fat. In the adult, bile acids contribute to micelle formation to enhance mucosal absorption of long-chain fatty acids and monoglycerides. Several aspects of bile salt metabolism are immature in the neonate. First, bile acid synthesis in the neonate is approximately half that seen in the adult. Furthermore, the predominant salt is a taurine conjugate rather than a glycine conjugate. Secondly, bile acid pool size in the neonate is approximately half that of the adult. Finally, ileal resorption and reutilization of bile salts is inefficient in the neonate.

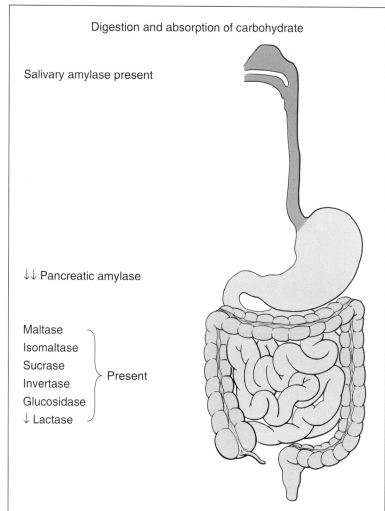

Digestion and absorption of carbohydrate

Salivary amylase present

↓↓ Pancreatic amylase

Maltase ⎫
Isomaltase ⎪
Sucrase ⎬ Present
Invertase ⎪
Glucosidase ⎪
↓ Lactase ⎭

FIGURE 1-6.

In the adult, polysaccharides are first metabolized by salivary and pancreatic amylase. Although salivary amylase is present in the neonate, pancreatic amylase levels in neonates are only 10% of the levels found in adults. Thus, neonates have a limited ability to process dietary starches. Almost all of the intestinal disaccharidases are present by term. However, lactase production is limited until 34 weeks' gestation. Thus, lactose absorption may not be complete in preterm infants.

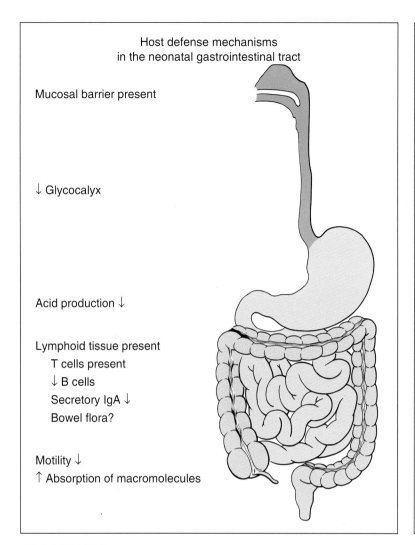

Host defense mechanisms
in the neonatal gastrointestinal tract

Mucosal barrier present

↓ Glycocalyx

Acid production ↓

Lymphoid tissue present
   T cells present
   ↓ B cells
   Secretory IgA ↓
   Bowel flora?

Motility ↓
↑ Absorption of macromolecules

FIGURE 1-7.

Host defenses in the adult are mechanical, humoral, or cellular in nature. Four *mechanical* barriers to bacterial infection are: (1) mucus, which physically bars bacteria from cell entry and traps bacteria for periodic expulsion; (2) the glycocalyx and (3) low gastric and duodenal pH, which inhibit bacterial growth; and (4) normal peristalsis, which periodically cleanses the bowel of static material and prevents bacterial overgrowth. Although the newborn produces mucus and acidifies the gastric lumen, the glycocalyx is relatively defective, and overall mouth to anal transit time is prolonged compared with adults. An additional maturational feature of the newborn intestine that is not present in the adult that contributes to weakened host defense is the ability to absorb intact macromolecules. In addition, the presence of certain bowel flora may also influence the competency of the newborn's host defenses. It is known, for example, that intestinal colonization with lactobacillus in breast-feeding infants inhibits the growth of enteric coliforms. In adults, the major humoral host defense is provided by secretory immunoglobulin A (IgA). Although B cells are present in neonates in numbers comparable with adults, secretory IgA is not present in neonatal saliva or feces during the first postnatal week. Secretory IgA appears in neonatal saliva and feces by postnatal day 20, and concentrations slowly increase during the first year of life. In adults, cellular host defense is provided by T cells. T cells are anatomically and functionally active in the neonate, as evidenced by the presence of an intact cellular response to in vivo challenges.

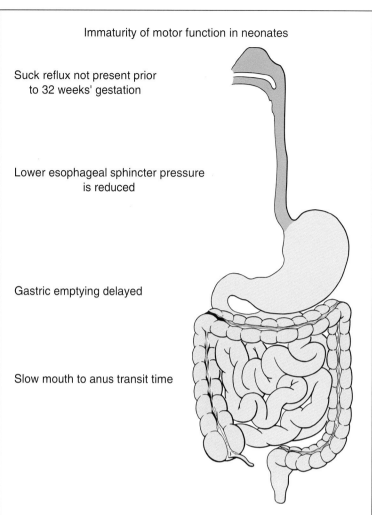

Immaturity of motor function in neonates

Suck reflux not present prior
to 32 weeks' gestation

Lower esophageal sphincter pressure
is reduced

Gastric emptying delayed

Slow mouth to anus transit time

FIGURE 1-8.

Aboral movement of nutrients is achieved by motor activity. Many aspects of motor activity are immature in the preterm infant. First, the coordinated sucking mechanism does not appear until 32 weeks' gestation. Thus, many preterm infants must be fed by tube. Secondly, lower esophageal sphincter pressure is lower in preterm infants compared with term infants, and gastric emptying is delayed in preterm infants compared with term infants. Thus, preterm infants are more prone to develop gastroesophageal reflux than term infants. Additionally, motor activity patterns in the intestine are immature in the preterm infant compared with the term infant, and this immaturity is reflected in a slower mouth to anus transit time during the first postnatal week. Regulation of motor activity is achieved by both neural and hormonal input, and many aspects of both of these major sources of regulation are immature in the infants.

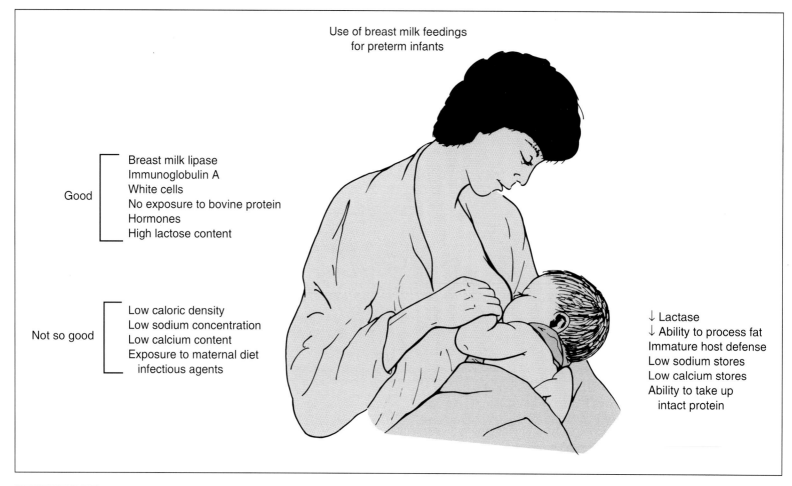

Use of breast milk feedings
for preterm infants

Good
- Breast milk lipase
- Immunoglobulin A
- White cells
- No exposure to bovine protein
- Hormones
- High lactose content

Not so good
- Low caloric density
- Low sodium concentration
- Low calcium content
- Exposure to maternal diet infectious agents

↓ Lactase
↓ Ability to process fat
Immature host defense
Low sodium stores
Low calcium stores
Ability to take up intact protein

FIGURE 1-9.

Human breast milk is nutritionally complete for the full-term infant; however, this fact is not the case for the preterm infant. Human breast milk may overcome some of the deficiencies in neonatal gastrointestinal function in preterm infants, but its use also has nutritional disadvantages. The presence of at least three forms of lipases in breast milk permits a 90% completion of hydrolysis of breast milk fats in the stomach. Although the benefit of the presence of high concentrations of immunoglobulin A and white cells in breast milk have not been shown in vivo, it is a common observation that breast-fed infants experience lower rates of infection and necrotizing enterocolitis. These immunologic benefits of breast milk are lost if the milk is frozen for storage. Breast milk also contains numerous hormones that may influence neonatal intestinal function. Because of the relatively low levels of intestinal lactase in the preterm gut, lactose may not be completely absorbed. However, the presence of nonabsorbed lactose in the gut encourages overgrowth of lactobacillus which, in turn, inhibits the growth of more aggressive enteric coliforms and thus is thought to contribute to the lower infection rates seen in breast-fed infants. Breast milk contains too little calories, calcium, and sodium to meet metabolic needs of preterm infants. Thus, breast milk must be fortified artificially for use in preterm infants. Cytomegalic virus and HIV are transmitted by breast milk as are maternal medications and cow's milk protein.

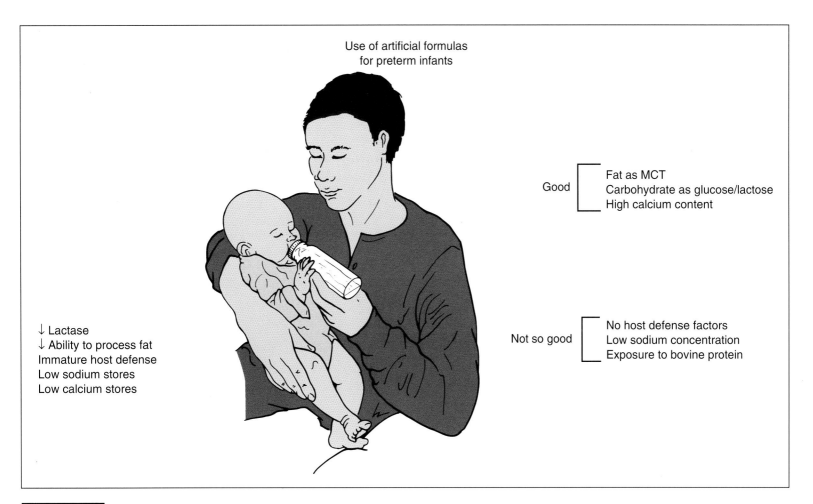

Use of artificial formulas
for preterm infants

↓ Lactase
↓ Ability to process fat
Immature host defense
Low sodium stores
Low calcium stores

Good — Fat as MCT
Carbohydrate as glucose/lactose
High calcium content

Not so good — No host defense factors
Low sodium concentration
Exposure to bovine protein

FIGURE 1-10.

Although feeding breast milk to term infants may be preferable because of its nutritional and immunologic benefits, it is not clear that its use is as beneficial in the preterm infant. Furthermore, many mothers who deliver infants prematurely may not be able to express sufficient quantities of breast milk for their infants. Other mothers may be given medications that preclude the use of their breast milk, as those medications may be transferred to the milk and, thus, to the infant. Artificial formulas for preterm infants contain nutrients that do not require a mature digestive system. Approximately half of the carbohydrate in these formulas is present in the form of glucose or glucose polymers rather than lactose to permit better carbohydrate delivery in the preterm infant who has decreased amounts of lactase. Approximately half of the fat content in these formulas is in the form of medium-chain triglycerides (MCT), and thus, does not require the presence of bile salts for intestinal absorption. These formulas also contain a high calcium content and are more capable of meeting the high calcium needs of preterm infants than are breast milk or regular formulas. However, there are disadvantages to feeding artificial formulas to preterm infants. Artificial formulas confer no host defense factors to the preterm infant, and formula-fed infants have a higher incidence of necrotizing enterocolitis. Although artificial formulas contain more sodium and calcium than breast milk, one or both of these may not be completely sufficient to meet the preterm infant's needs. There is also a concern that infants who are fed formula may absorb intact protein and later develop protein allergy.

NEC Epidemiology

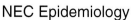

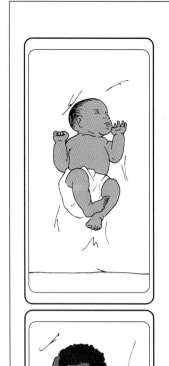

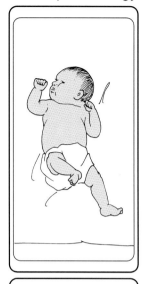

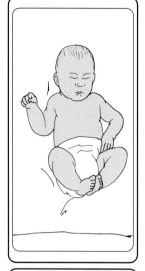

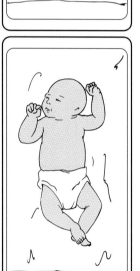

FIGURE 1-11.

The incidence of necrotizing enterocolitis (NEC) ranges from 1% to 5% of all infants admitted to the newborn intensive care unit, but NEC occurs in temporal and geographic clusters. Its incidence is highest in preterm infants, especially those with birth weights less than 1 kg, and it occurs 10 times more often in infants who have received enteral nutrition compared with those who have not. Approximately one fourth of infants who develop NEC will die, and approximately one fourth will require surgery.

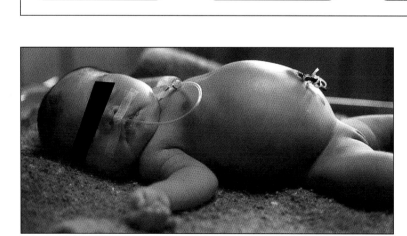

FIGURE 1-12.

Infants who are given the diagnosis of necrotizing enterocolitis present with vomiting or gastroparesis, lethargy, abdominal distention, discoloration of the abdominal wall, absent bowel sounds, abdominal tenderness to palpation, and hematochezia. Because fluid shifts may occur owing to the presence of infection, bowel perforation, or both, infants may also present with anuria, severe hypotension, poor peripheral perfusion, and bradycardia or tachycardia. Laboratory studies often reveal acid-base and electrolyte disturbances, leukocytosis or leukopenia, positive bacterial growth in blood, urine or stool specimens, and evidence of disseminated intravascular coagulopathy.

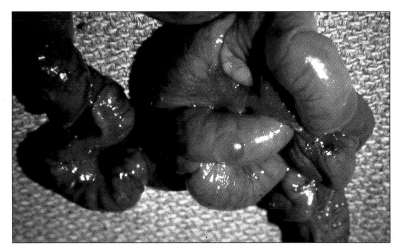

FIGURE 1-13.

Currently no single cause of necrotizing enterocolitis (NEC) has been scientifically established. The most common features of NEC are the presence of intramural bubbles of gas and large areas of necrosis. It is currently thought that the cause of NEC is multifactorial. Many infants who develop NEC have had episodes of asphyxia, hypotension, or both. Thus, poor splanchic bed perfusion may contribute to NEC. Several inflammatory mediators have been shown to be abnormal in infants who develop NEC, and many episodes of NEC are associated with specific bacteria, such as clostridia and klebsiella. Thus, bacterial gut flora may predispose an infant to developing NEC. Finally, the incidence of NEC is 10-fold higher among infants who have been fed, suggesting that the metabolic stress of feeding or specific characteristics of formulas (*ie*, osmolarity) contribute to NEC.

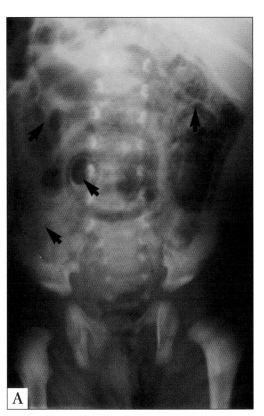

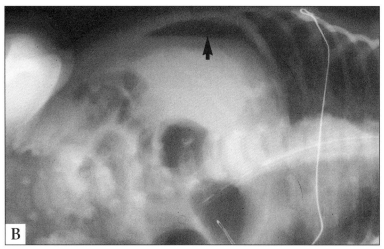

FIGURE 1-14.

Not all infants who present with symptoms of necrotizing enterocolitis (NEC) develop radiographic findings of NEC. Therefore Bell's criteria are used to designate whether an infant has Stage I (suspect), Stage II (definite), or Stage III (advanced) disease. Infants who lack radiographic findings for NEC are designated to have Stage I disease. **A,** Infants with Stage II or III disease radiographically demonstrate pneumotosis intestinalis (*arrows*) with or without air-fluid levels. **B,** In Stage III, infants are critically ill and may exhibit frank bowel perforation or presence of air tracking into the biliary tree or persistent dilation of a single bowel loop. Here there is free abdominal air (*arrow*) seen in the lateral view.

TABLE 1-2. NEC TREATMENT

Airway management

Antibiotics

Aggressive fluid management

Pressor agents

Repeated radiographic examinations

Parenteral nutrition

TABLE 1-2.

Many infants who develop abdominal distention will experience respiratory embarrassment because of the upward pressure of the peritoneal contents on the diaphragm. Thus, many infants will require endotracheal intubation and ventilator support. Although bacteria may not cause necrotizing enterocolitis (NEC), bacteria frequently invade the intestinal wall while the acute inflammatory process is occurring. Thus, broad-spectrum antibiotics are given for 10 to 14 days. Many infants experience cardiovascular collapse caused by bowel wall inflammation and swelling or frank sepsis. Moreover, acid-base and electrolyte abnormalities occur. Thus, appropriate fluids must be given early in the course of NEC and must be used aggressively during the first 24 to 72 hours. Often pressor agents must be used to maintain a normal blood pressure. The intestine will perforate in approximately one fourth to one third of infants who have NEC within the first 72 hours of the onset of the disease. Thus, abdominal radiographs should be repeated every 8 hours during the first 72 hours. Once infants recover from the acute phase of NEC, they require 10 to 14 days of parenteral nutrition to permit the intestine to heal.

TABLE 1-3. COMPLICATIONS FOLLOWING NEC

Surgical wound infection
Intra-abdominal abscess
Intestinal strictures
Short gut syndrome

TPN-related morbidity
   Cholestatic jaundice
   Sepsis
   Embolus formation
Recurrence of NEC

TABLE 1-3.

Although most infants will begin to recover from the acute phase of necrotizing enterocolitis (NEC) by 72 hours, many will develop complications 1 to 6 weeks later. Only those who have required a surgical procedure will be at risk for wound infection or short gut syndrome, but infants treated medically or surgically are at risk to develop all of the other complications listed. Approximately one third of all infants will develop intestinal strictures. Because all of these infants require parenteral nutrition, a significant number will develop morbidity related to the use of total parenteral nutrition (TPN). A small subset of infants (less than 5%) may develop recurrent disease.

BREAST MILK AND PHYSIOLOGIC JAUNDICE

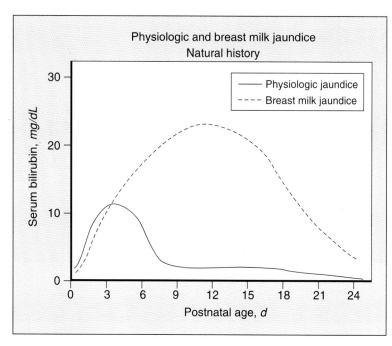

FIGURE 1-15.

Two types of nonpathologic transient jaundice occur in the newborn. Physiologic jaundice is defined as a transient increase in serum unconjugated bilirubin during the first postnatal week. Serum concentrations in the healthy newborn rise rapidly from birth to peak at a level of 7 to 10 mg/dL by postnatal day 3 to decline quickly by postnatal days 5 to 7 to a level of 2 mg/dL. This lower serum value persists for 2 weeks and then decreases to a normal adult value. Breast milk jaundice typically occurs after the third postnatal day. Serum bilirubin concentrations may increase to 20 to 25 mg/dL by the end of the second postnatal week and gradually decline over 1 to 4 months [6,7].

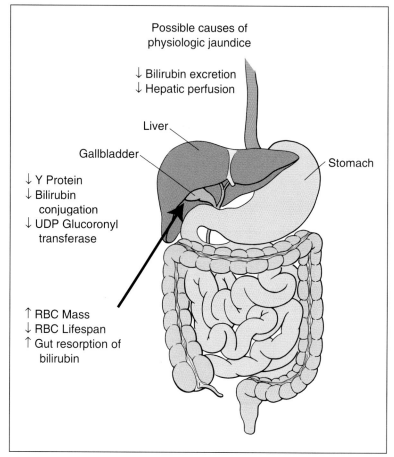

FIGURE 1-16.

The transient postnatal rise in serum bilirubin is thought to result from multiple factors. The amount of bilirubin delivered to the neonatal liver for conjugation is increased compared with that seen in the adult. This increased delivery results from the presence of an increased circulating red cell mass (normal hemoglobin in the newborn ranges 15 to 21 g/dL) and a shortened red cell life span (90 vs 120 days in the adult). There is defective uptake of bilirubin by the liver as a result of decreased levels of Y protein, and conjugation of bilirubin is decreased in that UDP-glucuronyl transferase activity is decreased in the neonate compared with the adult. Bilirubin excretion is also limited in the neonate compared with the adult. Finally, the enterohepatic circulation in the neonate is increased in the neonate, contributing to an additional increased load presented to the neonatal liver. In addition to these factors, increased bilirubin is also associated with ethnic factors, perinatal events such as birth asphyxia and maternal diseases such as diabetes. RBC—red blood cell.

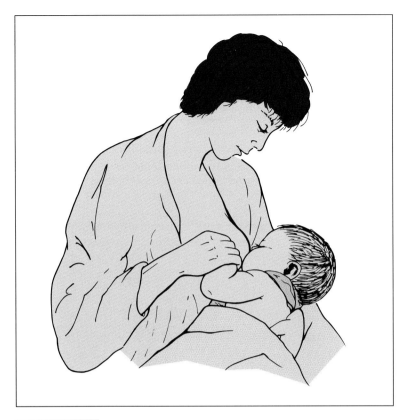

FIGURE 1-17.

The cause of breast milk jaundice has not yet been identified. The theory that breast milk contains a hormone that inhibits neonatal hepatic glucuronyl transferase activity has not been confirmed. It has also been postulated that large quantities of unsaturated fatty acids present in breast milk may inhibit bilirubin conjugation. Others have postulated that β-glucuronidase activity in breast milk may contribute to increased production and absorption of unconjugated bilirubin. An interruption in nursing will produce a rapid fall in serum bilirubin within 24 to 72 hours; however, resumption of nursing often results in a rise in bilirubin of only 2 to 3 mg/dL in most infants. If the serum bilirubin concentration rises to preinterruption levels, the physician and family can be reassured that it is because of a benign transient phenomenon. If levels do not fall with the cessation of nursing, further investigation for causes should be performed in an aggressive and timely manner.

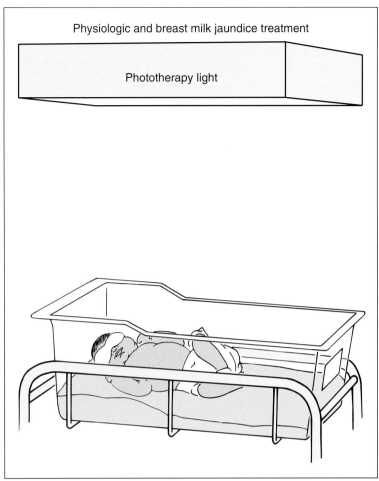

Physiologic and breast milk jaundice treatment

Phototherapy light

FIGURE 1-18.

When evaluating hyperbilirubinemia in the neonate, the first task is to discern whether it is physiologic jaundice. Maisels suggests that physiologic jaundice is a diagnosis of exclusion. The five criteria used to exclude a diagnosis of physiologic jaundice are (1) the presence of clinical jaundice in the first postnatal day, (2) the presence of a rate of rise of bilirubin that exceeds 5 mg/dL per day, (3) the presence of a serum bilirubin exceeding 13 mg/dL in a term infant and 15 mg/dL in a preterm infant, (4) the presence of a direct serum bilirubin concentration that exceeds 2 mg per day, and (5) the presence of clinical jaundice that persists greater than 1 or 2 weeks in a preterm infant [6]. When infants meet any of these criteria, the initial evaluation should include measurement of the infant's hemoglobin, reticulocyte count, blood type (as well as the mother's blood type), and a direct and indirect Coombs test. The danger of hyperbilirubinemia is the occurrence of kernicterus or the deposition of bilirubin in the central nervous system. Phototherapy is the mainstay of treatment for hyperbilirubinemia when serum bilirubin concentrations exceed 15 mg/dL. Phototherapy is most effective if applied to naked infants who have eye patches applied, as shown in the figure. Phototherapy may cause a transient skin rash, loose stools, lethargy, and abdominal distention. If the serum bilirubin concentration continues to rise despite the use of phototherapy, a double-volume exchange transfusion is used when the serum bilirubin concentration exceeds 20 mg/dL in a nonnursing infant and 25 to 30 mg/dL in a nursing infant. No case of kernicterus has been reported in a healthy nursing infant.

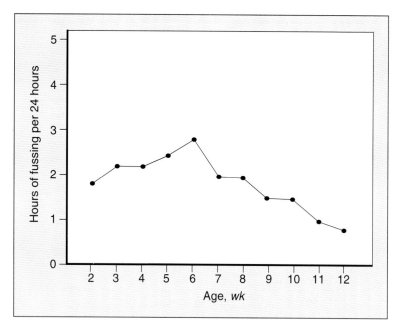

FIGURE 1-19.

There is a postnatal developmental pattern for infant crying as demonstrated in this figure [8]. The overall daily duration gradually increases from birth to 6 weeks to peak at approximately 3 hours per day. In addition, 60% to 70% of crying in the healthy newborn typically clusters in the evening hours. Colic is described to be excessive crying that is paroxysmal in nature, is accompanied by physical signs of hypertonia, and is inconsolable in an otherwise healthy, thriving infant. The Wessel criteria (or the rule of threes) for the diagnosis of colic include the presence of paroxysm of crying in an otherwise healthy infant occurring for more than 3 hours per day for 3 days per week persisting for 3 weeks [9]. (*Adapted from* Brazelton [8].)

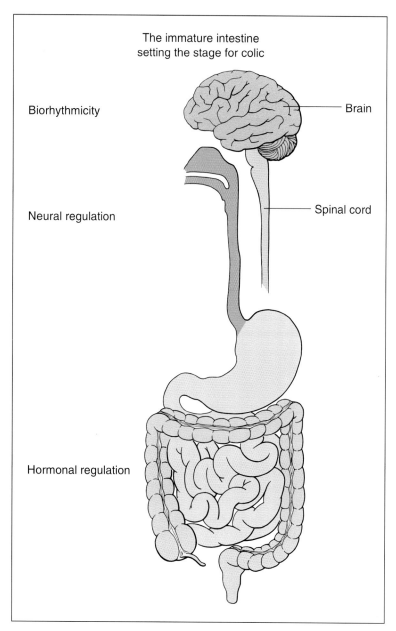

The immature intestine setting the stage for colic

Biorhythmicity

Neural regulation

Hormonal regulation

Brain

Spinal cord

FIGURE 1-20.

Motor activity is responsible for the aboral movement of nutrients. Motor activity is regulated by a complex interaction of neural input from the central nervous system, autonomic nervous system (ANS), and a separate component of the ANS called the enteric nervous system (ENS) as well as a variety of peptides that may have endocrine, paracrine, or neurocrine functions. Although neither neural nor peptide regulation of motor activity has been extensively studied in neonates, multiple aspects of both regulatory systems are immature. The presence of diurnal rhythms and organized sleep stages, both of which appear to regulate lower esophageal sphincter and colonic pressures in adults, are absent or immature in the newborn. Diurnal rhythms as expressed by heart rate and body temperature are absent at birth, and they gradually emerge by 3 to 6 months. Sleep and awake cycles are disorganized at birth and become more distinct at 3 to 6 months. Both parasympathetic and sympathetic aspects of the ANS are immature at birth and establish adult patterns by 3 to 6 months postnatal age. Although maturation of the ENS has not been studied, studies in various animal models have shown that many of the functional aspects of ENS are established postnatally. The release of numerous peptides are immature in the neonate, and the cyclic release of serotonin and motilin, two peptides that regulate intestinal motor activity, is not present at birth. Thus, regulation of gastrointestinal motility in the neonate is complex, precarious, and vulnerable to very small changes in the neonatal milieu. Current studies have not established whether colic is actually caused by dysfunction of these regulatory systems or if colic is a response to environmental and behavioral events.

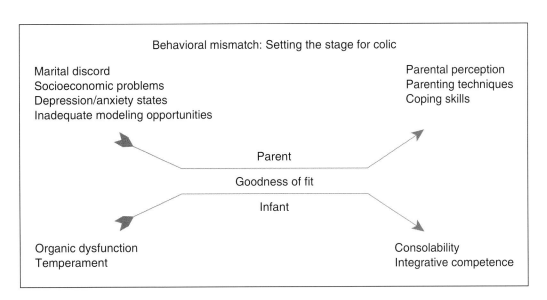

Behavioral mismatch: Setting the stage for colic

Marital discord
Socioeconomic problems
Depression/anxiety states
Inadequate modeling opportunities

Parental perception
Parenting techniques
Coping skills

Parent

Goodness of fit

Infant

Organic dysfunction
Temperament

Consolability
Integrative competence

FIGURE 1-21.

The interactions that occur between the newborn and a parent represent a composite of complex interrelationships of processes occurring within the parent, processes occurring with the infant, and the interactions between the infant and the parent [10]. Both the parent and the infant arrive at the point of their interaction with predisposing characteristics. For the parent, the presence of marital discord, psychiatric issues such as depression, distraction by socioeconomic issues, or lack of adequate modeling for parenting behavior may alter parental perceptions, attentiveness, or coping abilities. In turn, infants may bring temperament-related problems, real organic disease, or normal physiologic development to the interaction. In addition, parental deficiencies and skills must match infant deficiencies and skills to optimize the interaction. All of the determinants shown in this figure have been studied in families whose infants have colic, and all have been shown to play a contributing role to colic, but none has been shown to have an independent causal relationship [10].

TABLE 1-4. COLIC: TREATMENT STRATEGIES

PARENTAL DIRECTED	INFANT DIRECTED
Perception	Exclusion of dietary bovine protein
Parenting techniques	? Dietary manipulation
Reassurance	? Pharmacologic manipulation

TABLE 1-4.

Most treatment strategies for colic are focused on the parent. This is not to say that the cause of colic necessarily resides in the parent, and it is important that the physician alleviate the parent of unnecessary guilt and feelings of inadequacy of parenting skills [11]. Some parents may require additional education concerning the natural history of crying and the transient nature of colic. They also require reassurance that they did not cause their baby's colic and empathetic support for coping with a difficult situation. Strategies often employ redefinitions for parents in an attempt to alter their perception or threshold for excessive crying and encouragement to have respite from caring for the infant. Parents may need advice or observe actual role modeling to be taught appropriate coping strategies. A small number of infants may have bovine protein sensitivity, and exclusion of that protein from the nursing mother's diet or the formula-fed diet may alleviate symptoms. Numerous trials have shown little effectiveness for multiple changes in the formula fed to the infant or the use of medications.

REFERENCES

1. Motil KJ: Development of the gastrointestinal tract. In *Pediatric Gastrointestinal Disease*. Edited by Wyllie R, Hyams JS; Philadelphia: WB Saunders; 1993.

2. Langman J: *Medical Embryology*. Baltimore: Williams & Wilkens; 1969.

3. Snyder WH Jr, Chaffin L: Embryology of the intestinal tract. *Ann Surg* 1954, 140:368–380.

4. Lebenthal E, Lee PC: Concepts in gastrointestinal development. In *Textbook of Gastroenterology and Nutrition*. Edited by Lebenthal E. New York: Raven Press; 1987.

5. Henning SJ, Rubin DC, Shulman RJ: *Ontogeny of the Intestinal Mucosa Physiology of the Gastrointestinal Tract*, edn 3. Edited by Johnson LR. New York: Raven Press; 1994.

6. Gardner LM, Auerbach KG: Breast milk and breastfeeding jaundice. *Adv Pediatr* 1987, 34:249.

7. Oski FA: Disorders of bilirubin metabolism. In *Diseases of the Newborn*. Edited by Taeusch HW, Ballard RA, Avery ME. Philadelphia: WB Saunders; 1991.

8. Brazelton TB: Crying in infancy. *Pediatrics* 1962, 29:579.

9. Wesel MA, Cobb JC, Jackson EB, *et al.*: Paroxysmal fussing in infancy, sometimes called "colic." *Pediatrics* 1954, 14:421.

10. Popoulsek H, Papoulsek M: Biological basis of social interactions: Implications of research for an understanding of behavioral deviance. *J Child Psychol and Psychiatry* 1983, 24:117–29.

11. Weissbluth M: Colic. In *Current Pediatric Therapy*. Edited by Gellis SS, Kagan BM. Philadelphia: WB Saunders; 1993:233–236.

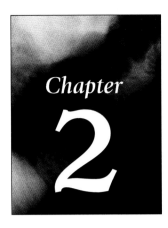

Chapter

2

Nutrition

MIGUEL SAPS
MELVIN B. HEYMAN

In 1967, Dudrick and coworkers demonstrated, first in beagle puppies and then in a human infant, positive nitrogen balance and growth, development, and restoration of weight loss with total parenteral nutrition (TPN) [1,2]. Their report, using a safe and efficient delivery system for a hypertonic nutrient solution, popularized the use of central venous catheters to administer TPN solutions. By 1974, Bistrian and associates' report of a substantial prevalence of severe malnutrition in surgical patients at Boston City Hospital [3], and a similar report 2 years later in medical patients [4] provided the catalyst for explosive growth and interest in parenteral and enteral nutrition support. Economic incentives in the 1970s led to a successful transfer of parenteral nutrition management from the hospital to the home [5]. Finally TPN provided a means to achieve an adequate caloric intake and even restore weight loss in patients whose gastrointestinal tracts were unavailable for use because of ileus or injury in a variety of clinical situations.

At the same time parenteral nutrition became the standard of community care, enteral tube feeding, although used in clinical medicine for over 100 years, still involved the use of large intranasal or enterostomy tubes (often used for other purposes, such as bladder drainage) for infusion of blenderized food or homemade diets which were often nutritionally inadequate. Since the early 1970s, the concept of "tube" feeding has been replaced by "fine-catheter feeding" and "enteral hyperalimentation" [6]. Today, new specialized feeding catheters and many formula diets are commercially available.

MALNUTRITION

TABLE 2-1. RISK FACTORS FOR PRIMARY PROTEIN-ENERGY MALNUTRITION IN CHILDREN

Small for gestational age	Medical neglect
Poor growth in early life	Family poverty
Twins or other multiple births	Maternal illiteracy, especially in areas where most people are literate
Large family	
Short interval between births	
Short breast-feeding period (early weaning)	Teenage mother
Multiple episodes of infection	Recent immigration
Poor prenatal care	Single caretaker
	War or famine

TABLE 2-1.

The objectives of nutritional assessments and interventions are to prevent, identify, and treat protein energy malnutrition (PEM). PEM is an acronym that refers to a broad spectrum of clinical conditions, ranging from moderate growth failure to severe malnutrition. PEM develops under circumstances where a host does not receive (or does not ingest or absorb) adequate and appropriate nutriture. The widespread prevalence of PEM in hospitalized patients was recognized in adults in the United States over 20 years ago [3,4]. In a nutritional survey based on weight-for-height of hospitalized pediatric patients in the United States, almost one third of the patients were classified as undernourished [7]. This is significant because lower weight-for-height indices, but not stunting, are associated with wound dehiscence, prolonged hospital stay, and compromised host defenses, all of which contribute to infections and increased morbidity and mortality from respiratory compromise [7–9].

Primary malnutrition results from inadequate intake resulting from economic, cultural, social, political, or religious reasons, including aberrations in mother-child interactions, lower sociocultural and economic strata, restricted (sometimes hypoallergenic) diets, and extremes of food faddism. Population migration, wartime periods, restricted or alternative diets, and nutrition policies influence nutrition status, growth, and development [10–14]. Secondary malnutrition appears when diseases involving appetite, digestion, or absorption interfere with the assimilation of food; it may be the consequence of any chronic disorder involving a major organ system, such as liver, kidney, lung, heart, or gastrointestinal tract, congenital malformations, intrauterine growth retardation, infection, AIDS, burns, trauma, cancer and its treatment, anorexia nervosa, and alteration in the metabolism of nutrients resulting from drug or nutrient interactions.

TABLE 2-2. MARASMUS: TYPICAL FINDINGS

HISTORY
Decreased caloric intake over months to years

PHYSICAL EXAMINATION
Impression: cachectic, severely ill, "little old man"; irritable, apathetic, hungry

Underweight, growth retardation

Hair sparse

Corneal opacity

Poor skin turgor

Nails fragile and thin

Loss of subcutaneous tissue

Muscle wasting

Vital signs: hypothermia, hypotension, bradycardia

ANTHROPOMETRY
Wasting or stunting; weight for height or height for age is less than 65% of the mean average

FIGURE 2-1 AND TABLE 2-2.

Patients with marasmus have "balanced starvation," an inadequate intake of both energy and protein for an extended period accompanied by weight loss and fat store depletion. The tendency towards preservation of protein stores, shifting the metabolic processes away from loss of visceral proteins, explains the maintenance of serum albumin and other protein markers at nearly normal levels.

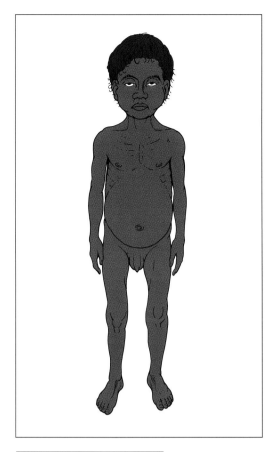

TABLE 2-3. KWASHIORKOR: TYPICAL FINDINGS

HISTORY
Decreased calorie intake over weeks to months

PHYSICAL EXAMINATION
May look well nourished, even "fat"; apathetic, irritable, anorexic

Moon facies, pitting edema

Overall fatness

Thin upper arms

Flaking paint rash, pellagrous lesions, fissures, ulcerations

Mucosal thinness, mild anemia

Lifeless, thin, pale, weak, or dry hair

Fragile and thin nails

Hepatomegaly (steatosis)

Vital signs: hypothermia, hypotension

ANTHROPOMETRY
Usually underweight; occasional fat appearance

FIGURE 2-2 AND TABLE 2-3.

Kwashiorkor is seen most often in children from 1 to 3 years of age. These children, also known as "sugar babies," usually look miserable, apathetic, have no appetite, and are difficult to feed. This condition has the classical signs of edema, hepatomegaly, and skin lesions, with a low or normal weight for height secondary to hypoalbuminemia and edema. Swelling is almost always present, mainly on the feet and lower legs, and the child may appear "moon-faced." The child may look fat because of edema, skin may be pale, and the child is usually anemic. The hair often turns brown, red, or gray, and is straight, sparse, and easy to pull out. More subcutaneous fat remains compared with children with marasmus. Kwashiorkor is a consequence of deficient protein intake or an inability to synthesize protein with normal or near normal energy balance. Hypoalbuminemia affects gastrointestinal function promoting gastric stasis, prolonged small-bowel transit time, diminished absorptive capacity for food and drugs, altered colonic water and electrolyte reabsorption, and impaired immunity.

TABLE 2-4. CLINICAL AND LABORATORY MEASUREMENTS IN MARASMUS AND KWASHIORKOR

PARAMETER	MARASMUS	KWASHIORKOR
Weight	↓	NL, ↓, or ↑
Skinfold/arm circumference	↓	NL to ↑
Albumin	NL to slightly ↓	↓
Prealbumin	Slightly ↓	↓
Transferrin	Slightly ↓	↓
Retinol-binding protein	Slightly ↓	↓
24-hour urine creatinine and urea excretion	Slightly ↓	↓
Blood urea nitrogen	NL to slightly ↓	↓
Glucose	↓	NL to ↓
Lipids	↓	↓
Cell-mediated immunity	NL	↓
Leukocyte count	NL	↓
Hemoglobin	NL	↓
Platelet count	NL	NL to ↓
Vitamin A level	↓	↓

TABLE 2-4.

Comparison of objective clinical and laboratory measurements in marasmus and kwashiorkor. Severe protein energy malnutrition is divided into three classical types: marasmus, kwashiorkor or severe protein deficiency, and a mixed form (marasmic kwashiorkor). Marasmus is characterized by a hungry and remarkably emaciated child with poor skin turgor [15] and height for their age, and weight for height under the fifth percentile. The child with marasmus is usually under 1 year of age with little or no subcutaneous fat and with loose skin that seems to be too big for the body. Muscles are flabby in sites where they are usually thick and strong. Edema and hair color changes are uncommon. Vitamin and mineral deficiencies may be clinically evident.

Most physiologic functions examined in severe protein energy malnutrition have been found to be altered, particularly in children with kwashiorkor and marasmic kwashiorkor. In contrast with kwashiorkor, marasmus has little effect on length of hospitalization, nosocomial infection, sepsis, and mortality rate [16], but complications superimposed on an unstable patient may provoke the progression to a mixed type of undernutrition (marasmic kwashiorkor). NL—normal.

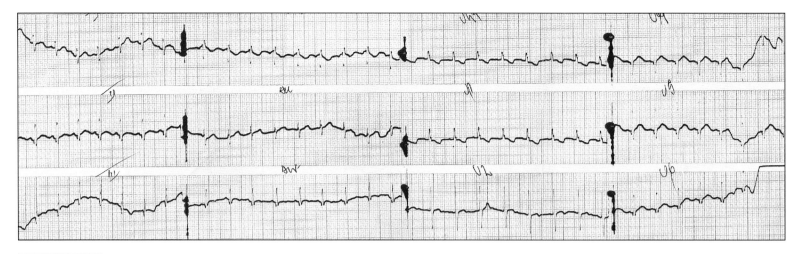

FIGURE 2-3.

Physiologic effects of undernutrition: cardiopulmonary effects. This reading is from a 4-month-old boy from Uruguay who was fed cow's milk for 3.5 months. His birthweight was 3250 g; weight at 4 months was 3000 g. Electrocardiographic changes included diminished voltage (<2.5 mm) and prolonged QT intervals (>0.10 sec). Protein energy malnutrition (PEM) morphologic effects on the cardiovascular system are characterized by a decreased cardiac mass, myofibrillar atrophy, and interstitial edema. Cardiovascular dysfunction includes decreased cardiac index, blood pressure, pulse, and ventricular contractility. Impaired cardiorespiratory function may lead to cardiac failure when PEM is complicated with severe anemia, overhydration, rapid expansion of circulatory volume, hypermetabolic states, and pulmonary infections.

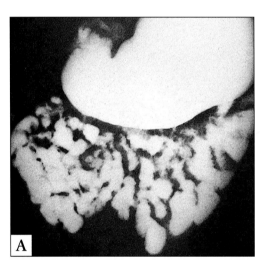

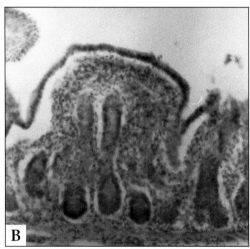

FIGURE 2-4.

Physiologic effects of undernutrition: gastrointestinal effects. **A,** Marasmic infant with massive gastric dilatation and edematous small intestine with separation of bowel loops. Acute gastric dilatation has also been observed upon refeeding undernourished children [17]. **B,** Histologic features of the small intestine (jejunum) in malnutrition. Villus flattening and mucosal atrophy as seen here are typical findings.

Protein energy malnutrition (PEM) is associated with small intestinal villus and submucosal atrophy. Findings include decreased mitotic activity and cellularity, edema, and lymphocytic infiltration. Regeneration time is delayed. Brush border disaccharidases are deficient and glucose absorption is impaired by enterocyte damage. PEM causes pancreatic acinar atrophy and creates scarcity of zymogen granules. Pancreatic digestive enzymes are decreased and pancreatic insufficiency persists, even months after resolution of malnutrition. Pancreatic endocrine function can also be affected. (**B,** Hematoxylin and eosin stain, original magnification × 100; *Courtesy of* Dr. C. Gutierrez, Uruguay.)

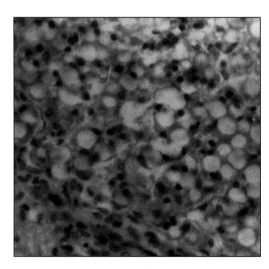

FIGURE 2-5.

Physiologic effects of undernutrition on the liver. Fatty liver in kwashiorkor. Most of the hepatocytes contain fat vacuoles, some of which have coalesced. Liver fat synthesis is increased, but inadequate synthesis of transport proteins, including lipoproteins, results in retention of lipids in the liver. Fatty liver and hypertriglyceridemia develop, especially with gram-negative infections. (Needle biopsy, hematoxylin and eosin stain, original magnification × 100.) (*Courtesy of* Dr. C. Gutierrez, Uruguay).

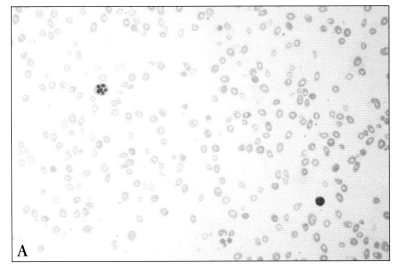

A

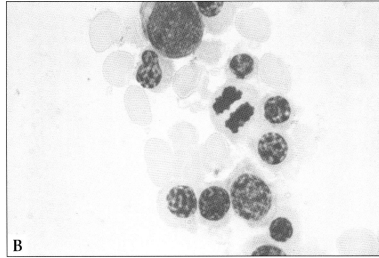

B

FIGURE 2-6.

Megaloblastic anemia. Megaloblastic anemia associated with hyper-segmented neutrophils (**A**) and nucleated erythrocyte precursors (**B**) is caused by vitamin B_{12} or folic acid deficiency. Intrinsic factor secretion is usually preserved except in the most severe protein energy malnutrition. Dietary folate deprivation leads to anemia in 18 to 20 weeks [18]. Folate deficiency also impairs delayed hypersensitivity skin response and lymphocyte proliferation [19]. (**A**, original magnification × 40; **B**, original magnification × 100). (*Courtesy of* Dr. Susan Atwater, San Francisco.)

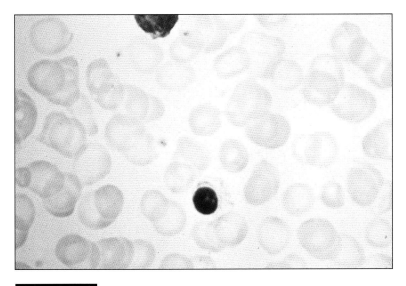

FIGURE 2-7.

Hypochromic microcytic anemia. Hypochromic microcytic anemia is usually caused by iron deficiency resulting from either inadequate intake, gastrointestinal blood, or iron loss. Decline of serum ferritin levels, transferrin saturation, and elevation of erythrocyte protoporphyrin helps identify iron deficiency before the onset of anemia.

Iron deficiency is associated with impaired macrophage function and bactericidal capacity, reduced lymphocyte proliferation, low total lymphocyte blood counts, and delayed hypersensitivity skin response [20–22]. A reduction in the number of immunocompetent cells and activity of iron-dependent and iron-containing enzymes explains the impaired immune response. Copper functions as a cofactor to many enzymes (metalloenzymes, serum amino-oxidase, and superoxide dismutase) is required for the detoxification of oxygen radicals. Copper is absorbed in the proximal intestine; in plasma it binds to ceruloplasmin, albumin, and metallothionein. Clinically significant deficits are uncommon despite low content of copper in the usual diet in the United States, but are occasionally found in premature infants, patients receiving total parenteral nutrition, and patients with Menkes' disease, a rare congenital X-linked disease characterized by defective copper transport. Clinical manifestations of copper deficiency include hyperlipidemia, hypercholesterolemia, leukopenia, bone demineralization, hypochromic, sometimes microcytic, anemia, and neural demyelinization. Copper deficiency is associated with altered cell-mediated immunity; T- and B-cell numbers are normal or in the low-normal range. Pyridoxine and vitamin C deficiencies have also been reported to be associated with microcytic anemia. (Original magnification × 100). (*Courtesy of* Dr. Susan Atwater, San Francisco.)

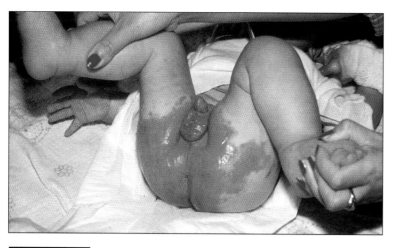

FIGURE 2-8.

Zinc deficiency in a 3-month-old child with severe diarrhea. Zinc is a normal constituent of many enzymes, including carbonic acid anhydrase, alkaline phosphatase, and superoxide dismutase. Zinc is an essential cofactor of thymulin (epithelial thymic hormone) and a potent mitogen of B cells. Body zinc status influences protein turnover rates [23]. Diets poor in zinc or containing high amounts of zinc-binding substances interfering with its absorption, chronic

diarrhea, and excessive gastrointestinal losses from ostomies increase the risk of zinc deficiency [24,25]. Zinc requirements increase during pregnancy, lactation, rapid growth periods and during post-operative periods [26]. Zinc deficiency is common in patients with AIDS, malabsorptive syndromes, sickle-cell disease, chronic renal and hepatic disease, and acrodermatitis enteropathica [19]. Deficit manifestations include failure to thrive, hypogonadism, anemia, lethargy, hepatosplenomegaly, chronic diarrhea, ulcerations of the skin in the extremities, mouth, and anus, impaired wound healing, deficient cell-mediated immunity, anorexia, and impaired taste acuity [27–31]. Acrodermatitis enteropathica is a congenital autosomal recessive disorder of zinc transport across the intestinal mucosa characterized by growth failure, skin ulcers, alopecia, diarrhea, and frequent severe viral, bacterial, and fungal infections. Symptomatic correction and diagnostic confirmation are achieved with therapeutic doses of oral zinc (1 to 2 mg/kg/day) [32].

Zinc deficiency may be detected by measuring plasma zinc levels. Low zinc concentrations in the hair reflect chronic suboptimal status. A low level of alkaline phosphatase, a zinc-dependent enzyme, may indicate zinc deficiency, although this finding is nonspecific. However, the lack of a single sensitive and specific biochemical test to determine mild zinc deficiency in children makes a positive response of linear growth to zinc supplementation the most reliable method [33].

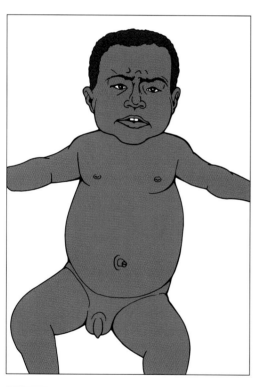

FIGURE 2-9.

Hypothyroidism (cretinism). Iodine deficiency will lead to hypothyroidism and cretinism. Hypothyroidism caused by protein energy malnutrition in older infants and toddlers causes myxedema of the subcutaneous tissues and tongue, difficulty in swallowing, and a hoarse cry. Eventually, hypotonia, constipation, protuberant abdomen with an umbilical hernia, and diminished cardiovascular function (bradycardia, low pulse pressures, low voltage electrocardiogram, and mottling) develop. Congenital hypothyroidism may be subtle until the infants are 3 to 6 months old. Neonatal screening is an effective method for detecting these infants. Prenatal iodine deficiency may also lead to abnormal neural development [34]. Furthermore, specific maternal nutritional deficiencies, such as those of folic acid [35] and zinc [36], can impair central nervous system development by a possible role in the pathogenesis of neural-tube defects.

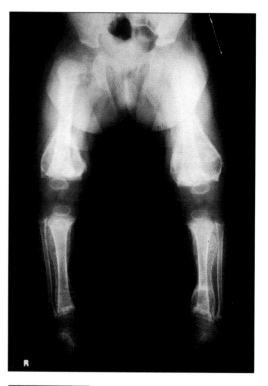

FIGURE 2-10.

Rickets and scurvy caused by nutritional deprivation. Rickets is occasionally observed among undernourished pediatric patients, especially among infants with low birth weight and in third-world countries [37,38]. Vitamin C deficiency (scurvy) is rare with current world health policies and supplementation programs [39]. Radiography in this undernourished toddler living in rural Uruguay demonstrates features of both, with splaying and irregular metaphyses (vitamin D deficiency) and cloaking of metaphyses and epiphyses by calcified subperiosteal hemorrhages (vitamin C deficiency). Vitamin C deficiency may initially lead to leukopenia before any other clinical signs appear.

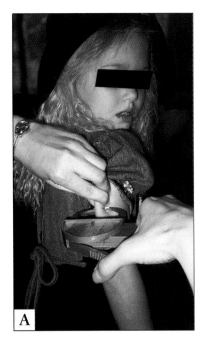
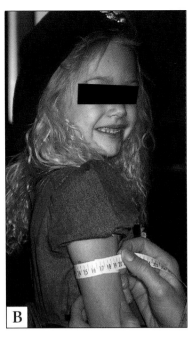

A **B**

FIGURE 2-11.

Anthropometric measurements: triceps skinfold (**A**) and mid-arm circumference (**B**) measurements. Based on the assumption that the thickness of subcutaneous adipose tissue reflects total body fat, anthropometric methods, in addition to weight, height, and head circumference, are often used to determine the presence of malnutrition. The most commonly used methods are skinfolds to assess fat stores. The most common site to measure skinfolds is the triceps. The accuracy of this method is limited because fat distribution is not uniform, varies with the age and sex, and measurement is difficult in edematous and obese patients. Skinfold thickness is a poor predictor of total body fat in infants [40], although it can be used in the individual patient to follow the response to nutritional therapy.

Combining the triceps skinfold and mid-arm circumference measurements provides an estimate of lean body (somatic or muscle protein) mass. (Mid-arm muscle circumference=mid-arm circumference – [0.314 × triceps skinfold]). (*Courtesy of* Maria Melko, RD, San Francisco, CA.)

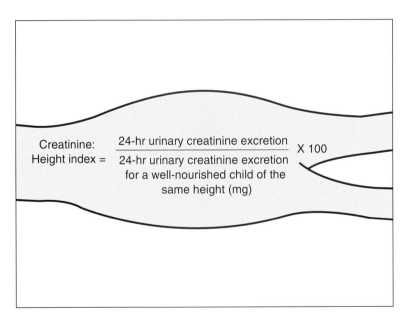

$$\text{Creatinine: Height index} = \frac{\text{24-hr urinary creatinine excretion}}{\substack{\text{24-hr urinary creatinine excretion} \\ \text{for a well-nourished child of the} \\ \text{same height (mg)}}} \times 100$$

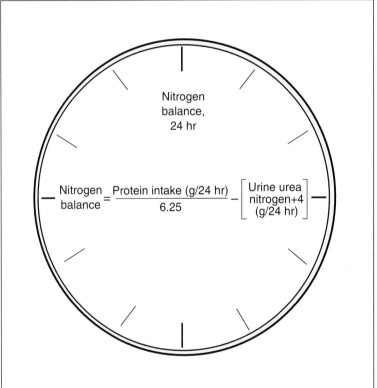

Nitrogen balance, 24 hr

$$\frac{\text{Nitrogen}}{\text{balance}} = \frac{\text{Protein intake (g/24 hr)}}{6.25} - \left[\substack{\text{Urine urea} \\ \text{nitrogen+4} \\ \text{(g/24 hr)}}\right]$$

FIGURE 2-12.

Creatinine height index. Creatinine is produced from creatine catabolism and is excreted by the kidney. Twenty-four-hour urinary excretion reflects muscle mass breakdown, and consequently, lean body mass. Effects of renal function, hematuria, hydration, protein intake, bed rest, age, fever, infection, trauma, stress, and surgery limit its accuracy and usefulness [41]. Therefore, the ratio of 24-hour urinary creatinine excretion to height is used to create a more accurate index of body muscle reserve. The index requires a 24-hour urine collection. A patient with an index under 40% is considered as suffering a severe protein depletion; between 40% and 60% is moderate depletion, and 60% to 80% is mild depletion.

FIGURE 2-13.

Nitrogen balance. Nitrogen balance is calculated from the difference between 24-hour intake and excretion. A constant excretion of 4 g/day is assumed to estimate nitrogen losses other than urine (skin, stool, etc.). The constant of 6.25 is used to estimate the nitrogen content of the protein intake. Nitrogen balance yields no information about protein reserve or nutritional status and reflects only recent intake and short-term protein metabolism. The determination is also limited by liver and renal diseases, drugs, and abnormal hydration states. Blood urea nitrogen levels tend to decrease with starvation; however, in patients in whom water intake is restricted, the serum value may actually be elevated.

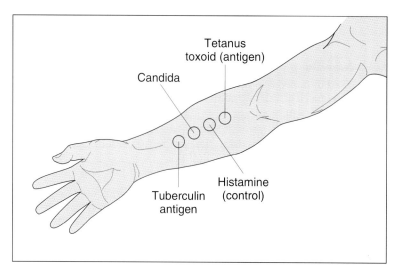

FIGURE 2-14.

Delayed hypersensitivity tests. Skin tests of delayed hypersensitivity reactions are based on the activation of sensitized circulating lymphocytes against a foreign antigen that results in the release of mediators to produce an inflammatory response. Protein energy malnutrition is associated with defective skin test responsiveness (anergy) that correlates with the severity of weight loss [42]. Cellular immune function may also be compromised by specific nutrient deficiencies including vitamin A, pyridoxine, biotin, zinc, selenium, copper, and iron [43]. Anergy may also be induced by infection, trauma, and other stresses that are associated with release of cell mediators [44] and by medications such as corticosteroids that inhibit the immune response. Other immunologic findings during undernutrition include declines in total lymphocyte number, T-cell number, phagocyte and lymphocyte function, and in vitro changes of the lymphocyte response to phytohemagglutinin stimulation [45].

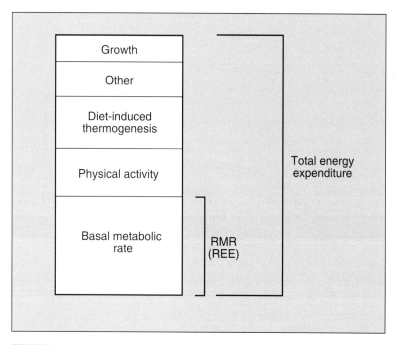

FIGURE 2-15.

Measurement of energy expenditure. Basal metabolic rate is the quantity of energy expended in a thermoneutral environment in a resting (recently awakened) supine subject after 12 hours of fasting. Resting energy expenditure (REE) is the metabolic rate obtained in patients at rest, preferably fasted, but in the hospitalized patient may include some form of continuous nutritional intake. When nutrition support (such as tube feedings, parenteral nutrition, or a meal) is included in the measurement of energy expenditure, inclusion of the thermic effect of the food increases approximately 5% to 10% above REE. Metabolic rate increases as temperature rises. Energy expenditure will be altered by underlying conditions, including sepsis, neurologic injuries, dialysis, mechanical ventilation, and surgery. When measured REE exceeds predicted REE by 10% or more, the patient is considered to be in a hypermetabolic state, whereas if measured REE is 10% or more below predicted REE, the patient is considered to be hypometabolic. Total energy expenditure should be considered in many of these situations. Because expenditure measurement is usually taken during resting state, approximately 5% should be added in mechanically ventilated patients whereas active ones should add 10% to 20%.

After a goal of energy requirement for nutritional support is determined, quantities of each nutrient of the formula or solution should be calculated to meet these estimated requirements. RMR—resting metabolic rate.

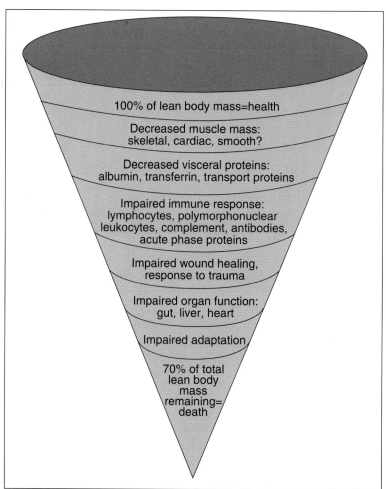

FIGURE 2-16.

Effects of undernutrition related to severity of nitrogen depletion. Hypothesis: loss of lean body mass leads to death. Preservation of lean body mass is essential for normal body functions. As somatic protein stores (muscle mass) becomes significantly depleted, visceral proteins are eventually lost, and patients develop immune dysfunction (with impaired wound healing and increased susceptibility to infections) and organ failure. (*Adapted from* Steffee [46].)

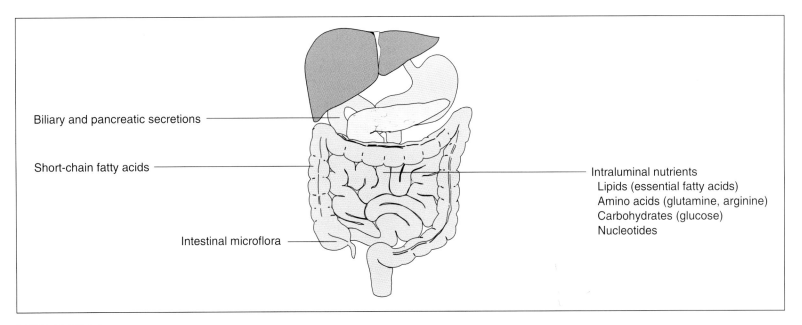

Biliary and pancreatic secretions

Short-chain fatty acids

Intestinal microflora

Intraluminal nutrients
  Lipids (essential fatty acids)
  Amino acids (glutamine, arginine)
  Carbohydrates (glucose)
  Nucleotides

FIGURE 2-17.

Adaptive response to enteral nutrient stimulation. Intraluminal nutrition appears to be critical to maintain intestinal structure and function [47]. Elimination of enteral intake leads to intestinal mucosal atrophy with decreased enterocyte proliferation and migration, a process reversible by refeeding. Small-bowel resection is followed by increased nutrient transport rate. The presence of nutrients in the lumen stimulates adaptation of remaining intestine following small intestinal resection [48,49].

Different components of enteral diets in the early postoperative period have various effects on gut function and mass, unrelated to its consistency and total calorie and protein content [50]. The use of dipeptides and tripeptides rather than intact protein may enhance protein absorption and trophic stimulation of the intestine [50–52]. Glutamine (a preferred metabolic energy source used by the enterocyte) added to enteral diets in the setting of intestinal injury results in preservation of gut mass with improved nitrogen retention, protection against bacteremia following endotoxin challenge, hepatic protection, higher survival rates in chemically induced enterocolitis, and possibly diminished bacterial translocation [53–55].

Carbohydrates (primary fiber and starch) are metabolized by colonic bacteria in the cecum to short-chain fatty acids. Short-chain fatty acids, particularly butyrate, are key energy substrates for colonocytes that contribute to the trophic effect on the intestinal mucosa [56]. Short-chain fatty acids (acetic, propionic, and butyric acids) are rapidly absorbed from the lumen [57,58]. Parenteral short-chain fatty acids also prevent mucosal atrophy in the colon. Pectin (a water soluble fiber) supplementation to enteral diets enhances intestinal mucosal growth [59].

Secretion of insulin, gastrin, and enteroglucagon is stimulated by enteral feeds and has an indirect effect of maintaining mucosal structure and function. Other hormones, including glucagon, prolactin, epinephrine, and androgenic and estrogenic steroids, may play a role in gut adaptation. Pancreatic and biliary secretions also influence mucosal recovery. The sympathetic nervous system may stimulate crypt turnover. Growth factors (*eg*, epidermal growth factor and insulin growth factor-1) may be important in intestinal stimulation towards adaptation.

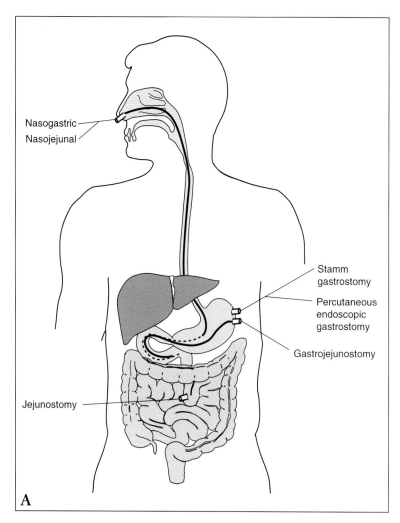

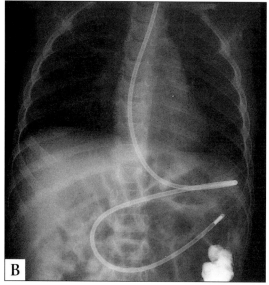

FIGURE 2-18.

Enteral tube feeding routes. **A,** Selection of the route of gastro-intestinal access depends on the indication, physiologic, and anatomic availability for feeding at different gastrointestinal sites, and planned duration, potential complications, and the feasibility to be an operative candidate. **B,** Transpyloric feeding tube placement can be documented radiographically by demonstrating the feeding tube to progress through the duodenum (on the right side of the spine) and cross back over the spine to the left side of the abdomen. The size and position of the stomach must be considered when evaluating these radiographs, and occasionally a lateral film is helpful to document posterior passage of the tube into the duodenum.

FIGURE 2-19.

Nutrient absorption: sites of absorption of major nutrients. Note that absorption of vitamin B_{12} and bile acids is facilitated by specific receptors in the ileum. Loss of this section of the intestine results in permanent loss of ability to absorb vitamin B_{12}, which will necessitate parenteral vitamin B_{12} supplementation. Bile acid loss may result in significant steatorrhea and bile acid-induced colonic fluid loss (choleretic diarrhea) that will respond to cholestyramine therapy.

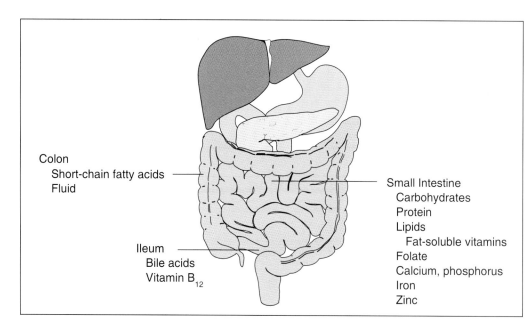

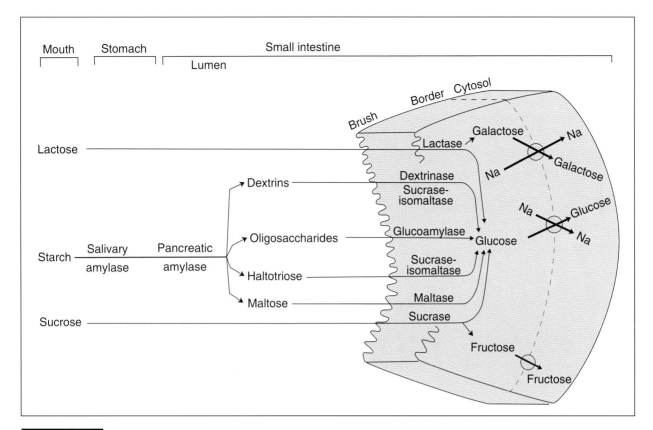

FIGURE 2-20.

Carbohydrate digestion and absorption. Digestion and absorption of carbohydrates occur in the intestinal lumen, at the epithelial cell surface, and within the apical membrane of the absorptive cells. In specialized nutritional support, most energy is derived from carbohydrates. Commercial formulas contain different and some unique carbohydrates. Oligosaccharides are commonly used in formulas because of their low osmolarity and a slower transit time compared with monosaccharides and disaccharides. They are readily hydrolyzed at the brush border; absorption of oligosaccharides is sometimes better tolerated and can lead to improved calcium, magnesium, and zinc retention compared with glucose. Lactase deficiency is common among children with intestinal disorders requiring nutritional support. Na—sodium.

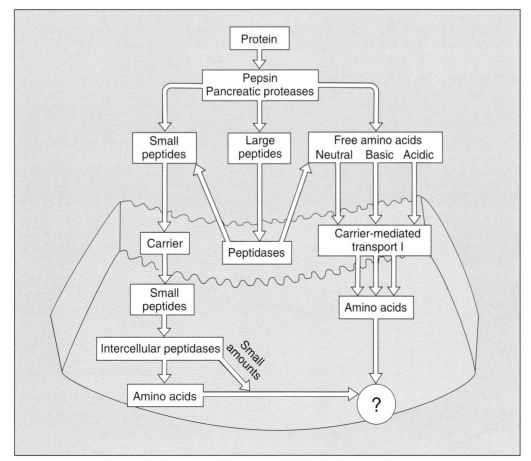

FIGURE 2-21.

Digestion and absorption of protein in the small bowel. The nitrogen content and source vary among the nutritional formulas used for enteral nutrition support. Exogenous nitrogen is provided in enteral products as whole protein, enzyme hydrolysates, defined amino acids (either all free amino acids or combinations of dipeptides, tripeptides, and small polypeptides), or as any combination of these. The more simple the protein (*ie*, the more "elemental"), the more expensive the formula.

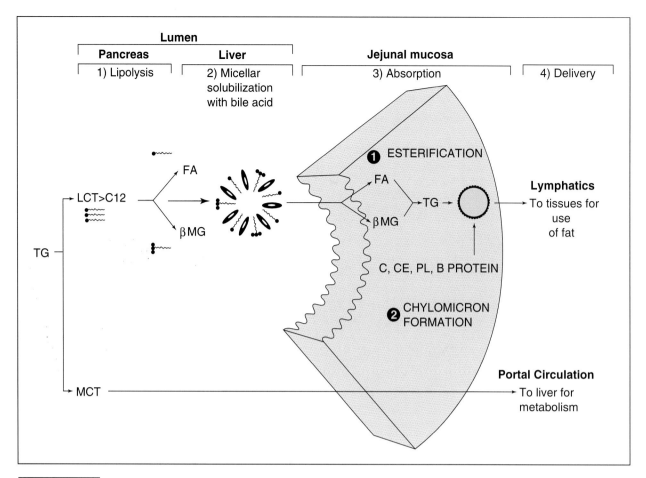

FIGURE 2-22.

Digestion and absorption of lipids in the small bowel. Dietary lipids are mostly triglycerides derived from plant oils or animal fats. Nutrient formulas contain vegetable oils rather than animal fats. The digestive process for lipids begins with luminal lipase, with six types of lipases having now been identified. The predominant preduodenal lipase is gastric lipase, accounting for 10% to 40% of the process. In artificial feeding at the intestinal level, lipolysis results from the combination of the pancreatic lipase, phosphorylase A2, and a nonspecific lipase. Pancreatic lipase acting with a cofactor lipase is responsible for the greatest proportion of triglyceride hydrolysis [60]. Short- and medium-chain tryglycerides can still be absorbed in the absence of bile acids because of immaturity or hepatobiliary diseases as they do not require bile salts to form micelles and do not undergo acylation to carnitine to enter the mitochondria for beta-oxidation. B protein—apoprotein B; C—cholesterol; CE—cholesterol ester; FA—fatty acid; LCT—long-chain triglycerides; MCT—medium-chain triglycerides; MG—monoglyceride; PL—phospholipid; TG-triglycerides.

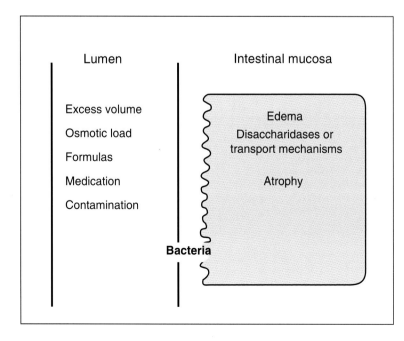

FIGURE 2-23.

Causes of diarrhea in enteral nutrition. Gastrointestinal side effects account for 50% of enteral feeding complications, the most common of which are diarrhea and delayed gastric emptying [61]. Others include nausea, vomiting, constipation, and fat malabsorption. The mechanism causing diarrhea in these patients may involve hypertonic nutrition overload of the gut that will result in a sudden increase of water flow into the lumen, provoking distension, rapid transit time, malabsorption of carbohydrates, and production of bile. In the colon the carbohydrate excess is metabolized to lactic acid, which, in addition to the diarrheagenic effect of the bile salts, exacerbates the problem. Osmotic diarrhea is usually explosive and presents with low pH and lactic acid in the stools that irritates the perianal region. Diarrhea is more frequent in critically ill patients, correlating inversely to albumin levels [62].

Bacterial contamination of enteral diets is usually exogenous [63]. As higher-risk patients are being managed with enteral nutrition, bacterial contamination of the diet and delivery systems are assuming increasing importance.

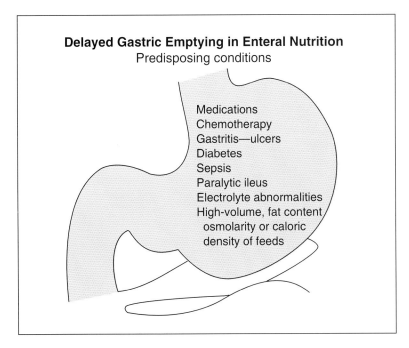

Delayed Gastric Emptying in Enteral Nutrition
Predisposing conditions

Medications
Chemotherapy
Gastritis—ulcers
Diabetes
Sepsis
Paralytic ileus
Electrolyte abnormalities
High-volume, fat content
  osmolarity or caloric
  density of feeds

FIGURE 2-24.

Delayed gastric emptying in enteral nutrition. Disease and many medications are associated with delayed gastric emptying. Diagnostic confirmation is usually obtained by physical examination, residual volume measurement, records of fluid balance, and radiographic and radioisotopic studies. Gastric retention may lead to gastroesophageal reflux. The incidence of pulmonary aspiration in tube-fed patients is also increased [64]. Despite the widely publicized reports of complications of enteral feeding, it continues to be a relatively safe feeding route [65]. Pulmonary aspiration episodes are generally benign, preventable, and occur with neutral pH solutions [65–67].

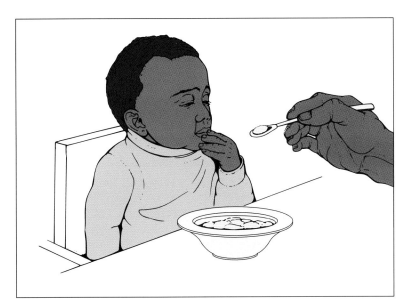

FIGURE 2-25.

Feeding aversion. Food aversion with distinct oral defensive behaviors may develop in children excluded from oral feeding stimulation for long periods. The feeding aversion appears to be a consequence of impaired development or loss of oral sensitivity, lack of hunger-satiety cycle because of around-the-clock feedings, and resultant lack of interest by this child, all of which, either by themselves or in combination with parents' insecurity, make the transition from tube to oral feeds long and difficult [68,69].

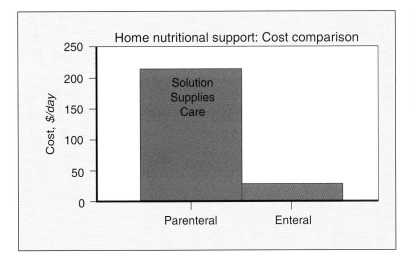

Home nutritional support: Cost comparison

Solution
Supplies
Care

FIGURE 2-26.

Home nutrition support: cost comparison. Home enteral tube feeding improves the cost-effectiveness of nutritional therapy. Careful consideration of the indications for parenteral versus enteral nutrition management is an important issue for medical, logistic, and economic reasons.

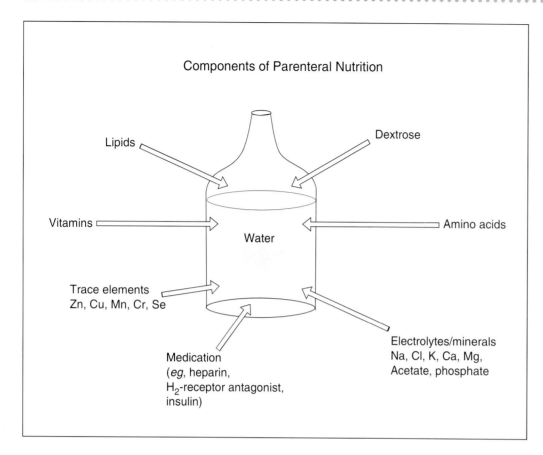

FIGURE 2-27.

Components of parenteral nutrition (PN). PN solutions are complex formulations designed to meet the unique requirements of each patient. Fluid requirements depend on hydration status, body habitus, age, environmental factors, and underlying diseases. The major sources of nonprotein calories in PN are dextrose and lipids. A PN solution with a balance of carbohydrate and fat is usually prescribed to avoid metabolic complications [70]. Electrolytes, minerals, trace elements, and vitamins are added to meet the ongoing daily requirements of these nutrients. Medications may be added if compatible with the solution.

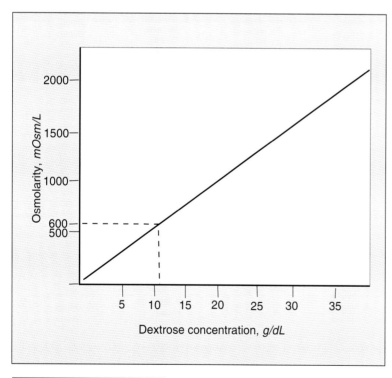

TABLE 2-5. GLUCOSE CONCENTRATION AND SOLUTION OSMOLARITY

DEXTROSE CONCENTRATION, G/DL	OSMOLARITY, MOSM/L
2.5	126
5	252
10	505
20	1010
25	1262
30	1515
35	1767
40	2020
50	2525
60	3030
70	3535

FIGURE 2-28 AND TABLE 2-5.

Glucose concentration and solution osmolarity. Glucose provides 3.4 kcal/g when in solution (as a glucose-monohydrate). Aliquots from a stock solution of 70% glucose are added to other parenteral nutrition components to achieve the final glucose concentration.

The osmolarity of parenteral solutions primarily depends on the glucose concentration. Initiation of carbohydrate infusions should be slow enough to allow adaptation of the insulin response to prevent hyperglycemia, glucosuria, and osmotic diuresis.

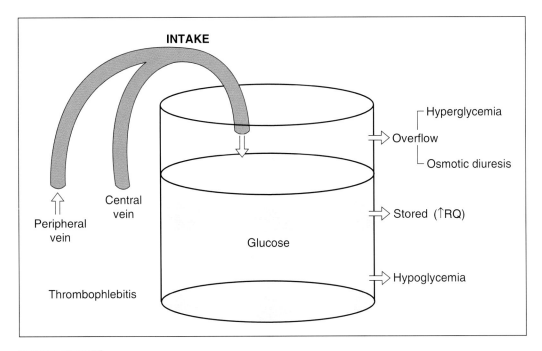

FIGURE 2-29.

Complications associated with glucose infusions. Glucose administration in concentrations greater than 10% (osmolarity >600 mOsm/L; *see* Fig. 2-28) by a peripheral vein increases the risk of phlebitis as a result of its high osmolarity and should be delivered through a central vein.

Excessive carbohydrate administration to patients with decreased ventilatory reserve may precipitate ventilatory failure or impair "weaning" from mechanical ventilation [71,72]. Glucose provided in excess of metabolic requirements results in lipid synthesis, in turn leading to a respiratory quotient (RQ) greater than 1.0 and excessive carbon dioxide production. Excessive glucose infusion can lead to hyperglycemia and an osmotic diuresis, resulting in dehydration, hypotension, hyperosmolar nonketotic coma, ketoacidosis, or metabolic acidosis. Infusion of parenteral nutrition solutions containing more than 20% glucose at 150 mL/kg/day has been associated with hepatic steatosis [73].

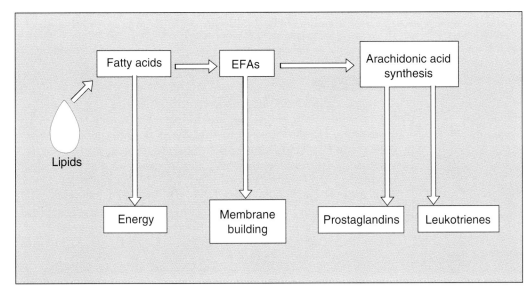

FIGURE 2-30.

Role of lipids in parenteral nutrition. Fat is an important source of energy, and essential fatty acids (EFAs) (*ie*, linoleic, linolenic, and arachidonic acids) are necessary for normal nervous system development and somatic growth. At least 1% to 2% of total calories should be linoleic acid to prevent essential fatty acid deficiency [74]. The use of lipid infusions as a source of calories permits a decrease in glucose concentration.

The respiratory quotient from fat metabolism is 0.69, compared with 1.0 from carbohydrates. In particular, this factor makes lipids attractive as a calorie source in patients with compromised pulmonary status.

Fat emulsions have either a soy or a safflower oil base, both of which are high in omega-6-polyunsaturated fatty acids, well tolerated, and able to serve as a precursor for arachidonic acid. Fat may be provided as a continuous or intermittent infusion or as part of a three-in-one (glucose, protein, and lipid) admixture.

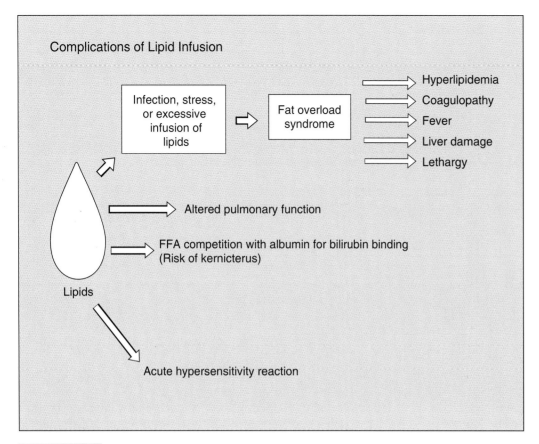

FIGURE 2-31.

Complications associated with lipid infusions. Hyperlipidemia may appear in situations where excessive (>4 g/kg/day) lipid is infused or in specific conditions, such as prematurity, infection, and stress, when lipid-clearing mechanisms are insufficient. Hyperlipidemia may place the patient at risk for hyperbilirubinemia and kernicterus (because of the competition of the free fatty acids (FFA) with albumin for the bilirubin binding), altered pulmonary function, acute hypersensitivity reactions, and fat overload syndrome. The fat overload syndrome is characterized by the acute onset of fever, irritability, jaundice, spontaneous hemorrhage, and hyperlipemia [75]. Hyperlipidemia may be avoided by limiting the rate of infusion of lipid emulsions to 4 or less g/kg/day.

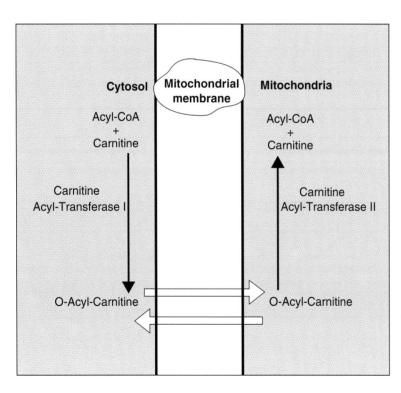

FIGURE 2-32.

Carnitine-facilitated lipid transport. Carnitine is a quaternary amine synthesized in the liver and kidney or absorbed from the gastrointestinal tract [76]. Carnitine is necessary for the transfer of long-chain fatty acids into mitochondria for oxidation. This small, water-soluble molecule also facilitates branched-chain α-ketoacid oxidation [77]. Total parenteral nutrition (TPN)–related deficiency may appear in premature infants on carnitine-free TPN and in pediatric or adult patients receiving long-term parenteral nutrition [78]. The clinical relevance of the biochemical deficiency state under these circumstances remains to be clarified.

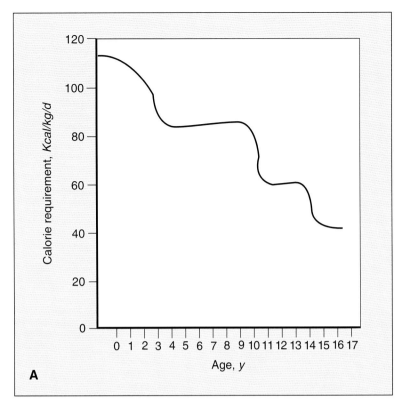

A

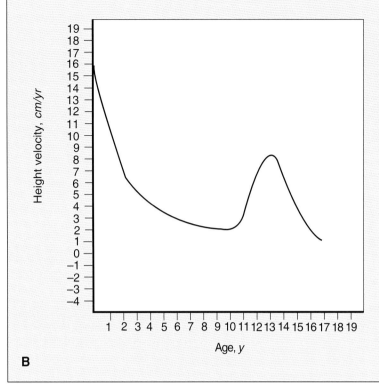

B

FIGURE 2-33.

Nonprotein calorie requirements. Calorie requirements (**A**) and growth velocity (**B**) vary according to age. Energy requirements are highest in premature neonates (~120 kcal/kg body weight), when growth rate is greatest, and decline with age and decreasing growth velocity. Term newborns and young infants require 90 to 120 kcal/kg/day, compared with 30 to 40 kcal/kg/day in adults. Energy intake must be adjusted to account for excess losses (*eg*, fecal or urinary nutrient losses) and increased metabolic needs (*eg*, due to fever, infection, wound healing). The pubertal growth spurt, when energy requirements increase slightly, occurs later in boys compared with girls.

Essential Amino Acids

Arginine

Taurine | Tyrosine | Cysteine

Valine | Isoleucine | Leucine | Threonine

Phenylalanine | Tryptophan | Histidine | Lysine | Methionine

▱ Essential in neonates
and premature infants

FIGURE 2-34.

Essential amino acids. Parenteral amino acid products are mixtures of essential and nonessential amino acids. Pediatric formulations have added taurine and higher concentrations of histidine and tyrosine compared with standard formulas. Parenteral nutrition should be started with 0.5 g protein/kg/day in neonates and 1.0 g protein/kg/day in infants and children, increasing by 0.5 g protein/kg/day until the goal is attained. For efficient protein anabolism, the nonprotein calorie (kcal) to nitrogen (g) ratio should be 150 to 200:1. One gram of nitrogen is equivalent to approximately 6.25 g of protein, so for every gram of protein infused, 24 to 32 non-nitrogen calories must be supplied.

TABLE 2-6. RECOMMENDED INTAKE OF TRACE ELEMENTS FOR INTRAVENOUS INFUSION

	PRETERM AND TERM INFANTS AND CHILDREN, μG/KG/D	MAXIMUM INTAKE, μG/KG/D
Zinc*	50–400	5000
Copper	20	300
Selenium	2	30
Chromium	0.2	5
Manganese	1	50
Molybdenum	0.25	5
Iodide	1	1

*Zinc requirements decrease with age, from 400 μg/kg/d in preterm infants to 50 μg/kg/d in children.

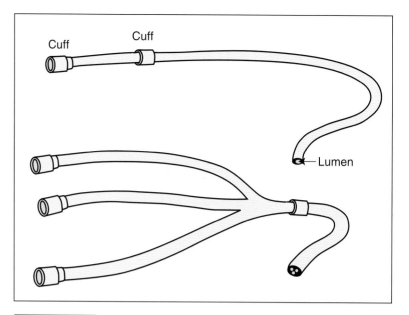

FIGURE 2-35.

TABLE 2-6.

Recommended intake of trace elements for intravenous infusion. Iron, zinc, copper, selenium, chromium, manganese, and molybdenum deficiency syndromes have been reported in humans. Predisposing factors include reduced intake, malabsorption, increased losses, and excessive metabolic demand. Extra zinc may be required to replace diarrheal losses. Under certain conditions, some trace elements may accumulate and should be withheld from infusion. For example, copper and manganese, which are excreted in bile, should be limited in patients with cholestasis, and selenium, chromium, and molybdenum should not be administered to patients with renal failure. Topical agents used for wound and catheter care appear to provide adequate amounts of iodide. Iron is provided enterally if possible or by intravenous bolus infusion of iron dextran as needed. Fluoride may be indicated in infants and children with developing teeth, particularly if they have no other source of fluids containing fluoride. (*Adapted from* Green et al. [78a].)

Right atrial Silastic catheter. The primary determining factors for selecting the route for parenteral nutritional support are the caloric and fluid requirements. To achieve safe, intravenous, high caloric infusions, a hyperosomolar solution should be delivered through a central, large vein to reduce the risk of thrombosis and phlebitis.

Several types of long-term indwelling right atrial Silastic catheters are available to achieve access. Cuffed, silicon elastomer (Silastic) tunneled catheters decrease infections and provide stability through a polyethylene terephthalate (Dacron) cuff attached to the distal internal (subcutaneous) portion. The cuff stimulates formation of fibrous adhesions that anchor the catheter and create a barrier against ascending bacteria.

Catheters of single and multiple lumen can be used, depending on the size of the patient and the therapy planned. Multilumen catheters permit the simultaneous infusion of incompatible solutions or medications. However, the additional lumens allow additional sites for infectious and thrombotic complications.

Nutrition solution, blood product and chemotherapeutic agent administration, and obtaining of blood samples can all be accomplished through these catheters.

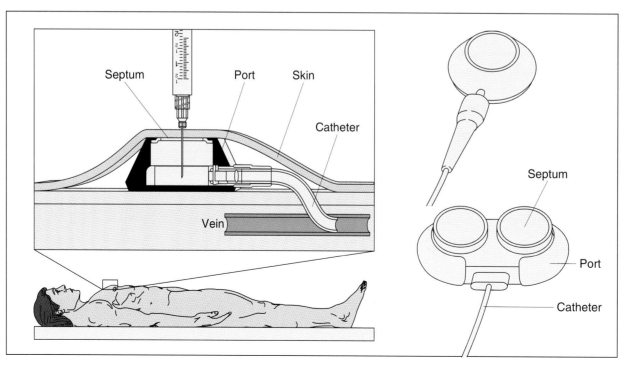

FIGURE 2-36.

Subcutaneous vascular access systems. Various single and dual lumen access ports are available for patients who prefer subcutaneous venous lines. These are usually deployed in patients who do not require daily intravenous access and are not used routinely in patients on long-term parenteral nutrition infusions.

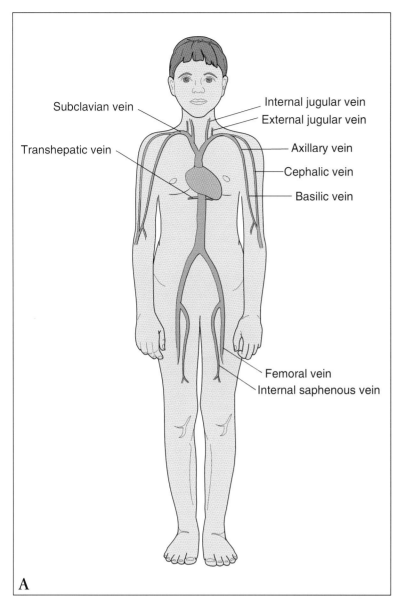

Subclavian vein
Transhepatic vein
Internal jugular vein
External jugular vein
Axillary vein
Cephalic vein
Basilic vein
Femoral vein
Internal saphenous vein

A

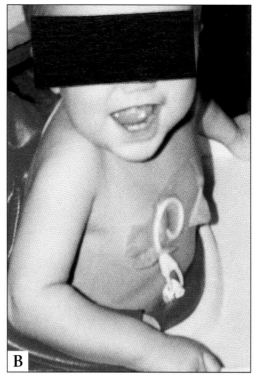

B

FIGURE 2-37.

Central venous catheter sites. **A**, Access to the central venous circulation may be achieved by several veins. **B**, Indwelling catheters for long-term parenteral nutrition are usually inserted by cephalic cutdown and tunneled through subcutaneous tissues to exit the skin. Thus, nutrients infused directly into the vena cava are not subjected to the first-pass effect through the liver, as are the enteral nutrients. In some situations it may become necessary to insert the catheter through the femoral or saphenous vein into the inferior vena cava. Catheter placement in the lower limb with an abdominal exit site does not necessarily have a greater risk of infection [79]. Recently, percutaneous long ("spaghetti") peripheral catheters have also been used for short-term inpatient and home parenteral nutrition infusion.

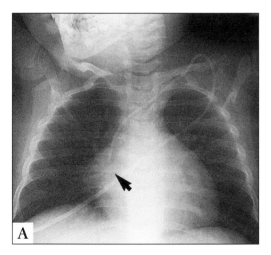

A

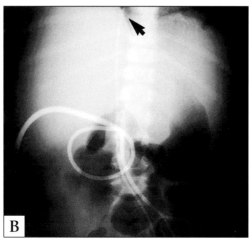

B

FIGURE 2-38.

Complications of central venous lines: location. Catheter-related complications can be minimized with application of careful technique. Prior to initiating any infusion, line location must be documented. **A**, Optimal location in the superior vena cava just proximal to the right atrium (*arrow*). **B**, Alternative location in the inferior vena cava ("femoral line") in a patient whose superior vena cava was thrombosed (*arrow*).

(*continued on next page*)

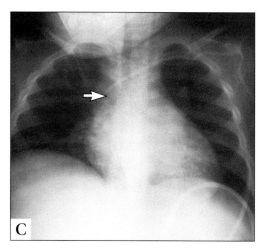

C

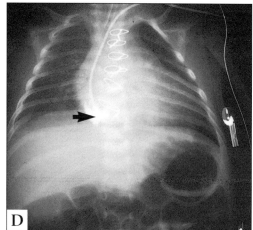

D

FIGURE 2-38. (CONTINUED)

C, Catheter placed too proximal in the left innominate vein (*arrow*). D, Extravasation of dye in a catheter that passed into the right pleural cavity (*arrow*).

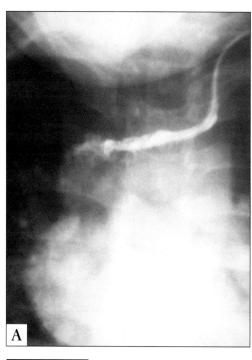

A

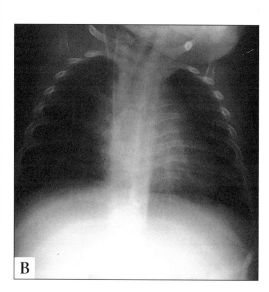

B

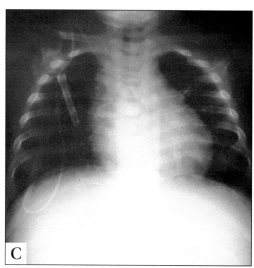

C

FIGURE 2-39.

Complications of central venous lines. Thrombosis is a common complication that can lead to secondary complications, including superior vena cava syndrome and embolic episodes. A 3-year-old boy dependent on total parenteral nutrition (TPN) with chronic intestinal pseudo-obstruction developed swelling on the left side of his neck and face associated with pump occlusion. A, A catheter dye study demonstrates a thrombus formed around the catheter tip. The dye migrates back along the catheter and around the thrombus before finally diffusing into the venous blood flow.

Another 18-month-old child had a right atrial Silastic catheter since the neonatal period for treatment of necrotizing enterocolitis and eventually adapted to enteral feedings. B, A calcified thrombus is present at the catheter tip. C, The catheter was removed, but the thrombus was dislodged and wedged in the pulmonary artery. (B and C *courtesy of* Dr. Paul Hyman, Orange County, CA.)

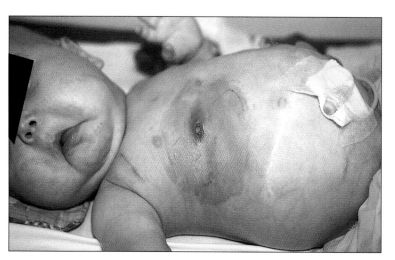

FIGURE 2-40.

Complications of central venous lines. Infectious complications are minimized by proper aseptic technique and avoiding unnecessary catheter intrusion, particularly by inexperienced and untrained personnel. Localized skin infections can lead to dislodgment of a catheter if the infection spreads into the catheter tunnel and affects the cuff that anchors a "permanent" Silastic catheter. Patients must be monitored compulsively for symptoms and signs of bacteremia and sepsis that should all be treated as serious, potentially life-threatening events. This figure also shows formation of granulation tissue at the catheter exit site, a benign but troublesome problem.

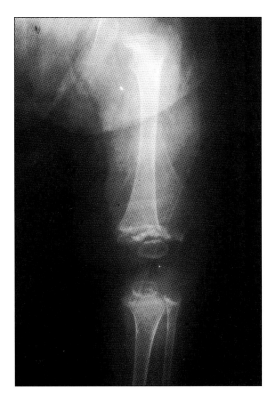

FIGURE 2-41.

Complications associated with minerals and trace elements. Rickets may be a consequence of the underlying medical problem (malabsorption) or a complication of prolonged parenteral nutrition [80]. Signs of rickets seen in this figure include a cupping and fraying of the epiphyses and slipped capital femoral epiphysis, with interruption of Shenton's line.

Metabolic bone disease resulting from parenteral nutrition is caused by the inability to provide adequate parenteral mineral supplementation (specifically phosphorus and calcium) for normal bone mineral accretion and may be diagnosed as early as 2 months in small preterm infants with birth weight under 1.5 kg [81,82]. Radiographic manifestations of parenteral nutrition–related bone disease in infants, including osteopenia, rickets, and fractures, are often late evidence of an underlying silent process [81].

A

B

r = −0.70
p < 0.003
● Casein hydrolysate
○ Amino acids

Bone formation rate, μ^2/mm^2 tissue area/day

Stainable bone aluminum, mm/mm^2 surface

FIGURE 2-42.

Complications associated with minerals and trace elements. Aluminum has been noted as a contaminant of parenteral solutions and has been implicated in the development of metabolic bone disease and hepatotoxicity, although a definitive role for aluminum in these problems remains to be demonstrated. **A**, Goldner's trichrome stain of the iliac crest in a patient on long-term total parenteral nutrition (TPN) demonstrates aluminum accumulation (dark line) at the mineralization front, where new bone forms. **B**, Bone formation rate as a function of stainable bone aluminum in TPN patients receiving either aluminum-contaminated casein hydrolysate or low aluminum-containing crystalline amino acid solutions. The dotted line indicates the lower limit of normal for bone formation rate [80]. (**A**, *Courtesy of* Dr. Gordon Klein, University of Texas, Galveston, TX; **B**, *Adapted from* Vargas *et al.* [83].)

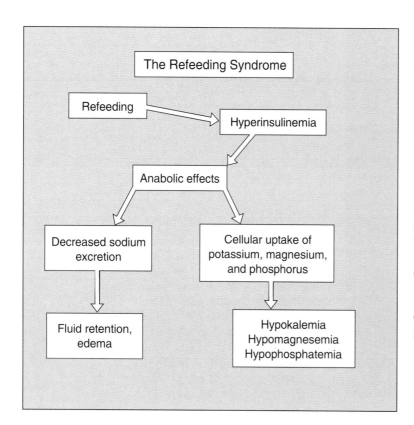

FIGURE 2-43.

Complications associated with minerals and trace elements: the refeeding syndrome. Refeeding starved and undernourished catabolic patients can lead to significant shifts in intracellular and extracellular fluids and minerals, which can sometimes place patients at serious risk for complications [84]. During refeeding, anabolic hormones, including insulin, causes intracellular uptake of ions including especially phosphorus, potassium, and magnesium that can lead to significant decline in extracellular (serum) concentrations. Particularly dangerous is severe hypophosphatemia, which may result in central nervous system abnormalities, muscle weakness, and depression of cardiac, respiratory, renal, and hepatic functions. Close monitoring and appropriate supplementation avoids these complications.

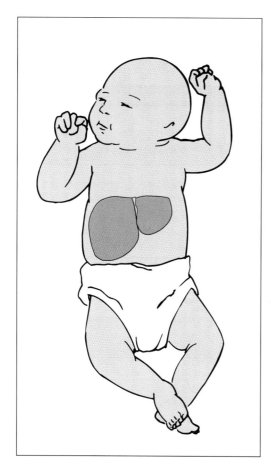

TABLE 2-7. PARENTERAL NUTRITION–ASSOCIATED HEPATOTOXICITY: RISK FACTORS

Prematurity

Lack of enteral stimulation

Sepsis

Hepatic copper accumulation

Medication (*eg*, furosemide)

Other potential contributing factors

Dextrose or amino acid solution

Contaminants (*eg*, aluminum)

Oxidant stress (*eg*, glutathione deficiency)

FIGURE 2-44 AND TABLE 2-7.

Parenteral nutrition–associated hepatotoxicity: risk factors. Hepatotoxicity in patients receiving parental nutrition is most common and severe in neonates and infants. Approximately 20% to 30% of these patients will develop significant cholestasis if they are sustained on prolonged (>2 weeks) parental nutrition. The most important risk factors for the development of parental nutrition-associated hepatotoxicity in infants are prematurity, sepsis, and surgical procedures on the gastrointestinal tract.

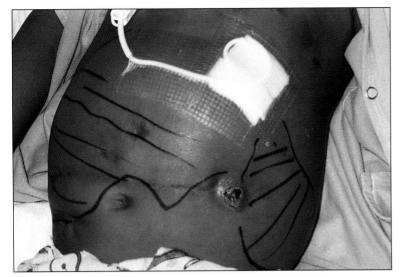

FIGURE 2-45.

Parenteral nutrition–associated hepatotoxicity. This 5-year-old child with short-bowel syndrome has severe chronic liver disease with jaundice, portal hypertension, and secondary hypersplenism (all associated with total parenteral nutrition [TPN]); the liver and spleen are outlined. As a last possible life-saving measure, he is awaiting a combined small intestine–liver transplant.

Abnormalities of liver enzymes and cholestasis are found in 30% to 90% of patients after 2 weeks of TPN, especially in neonates and young infants. Predisposing conditions include sepsis, prematurity, gastrointestinal surgery, and prolonged requirements for TPN. The cause remains unclear, although several possible mechanisms are proposed, including lack of oral intake, malnutrition, excessive caloric infusion, excess of dextrose, amino acid imbalance, hepatotoxic products of tryptophan conversion, choline, carnitine and glutathione deficiencies, essential fatty acid deficiency, excess lipids, and bacterial translocation [83–94].

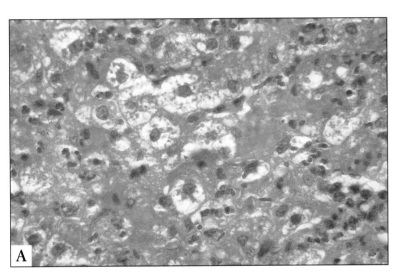

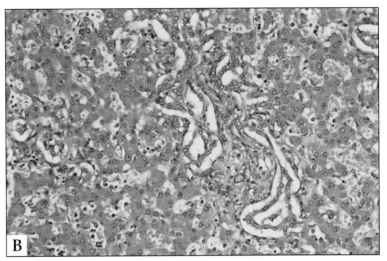

FIGURE 2-46.

Parenteral nutrition–associated hepatotoxicity. Parenteral nutrition may cause simple steatosis or lead to significant cholestasis, fibrosis, and eventually (when the fibrosis is irreversible) cirrhosis. **A,** Cholestasis and necrosis of cells are evident; both are reversible if the parenteral nutrition can be discontinued shortly. **B,** Bile duct proliferation, early fibrosis, and mild cholestasis are evident. In young infants, the biopsy may resemble that of extrahepatic biliary atresia. The degree of fibrosis is a helpful distinguishing feature because patients with biliary atresia by 2 months of age have severe and mature fibrotic changes whereas the parenteral nutrition-associated scarring is only starting to form and is much less prominent. **C,** Severe cirrhosis, now irreversible, has become established and the patient will develop chronic liver failure. Steatosis is also evident and can be seen at any time during parenteral nutrition administration. It usually is reversible by reducing the calories infused into the child. (*Courtesy of* Dr. Linda Ferrell, San Francisco, CA.)

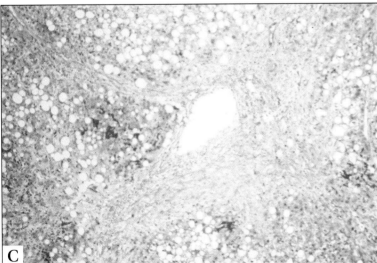

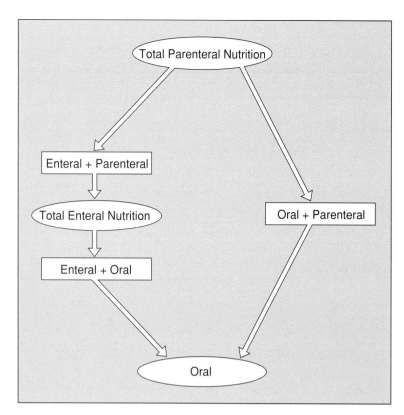

FIGURE 2-47.

Progression of weaning pediatric patients from nutrition support. The optimal and ultimate goal of complete oral feeding is achieved at differing rates, and success depends on underlying disease and gastrointestinal tract function. Enteral feedings are more physiologic, have fewer adverse reactions and complications, and are less costly than parenteral nutrition. Similarly, oral feedings do not require enteral tube access and other equipment, and sometimes costly formulas are necessary for enteral support. Some patients, for example a child receiving parenteral nutrition for bowel rest for treatment of Crohn's disease, may progress directly from total parenteral nutrition to oral diet.

■ REFERENCES

1. Dudrick SJ, Wilmore DW, Vars HM, Rhoads JE: Can intravenous feeding as the sole means of nutrition support growth in the child and restore weight loss in an adult? An affirmative answer. *Ann Surg* 1969, 169:974–984.

2. Dudrick SJ, Wilmore DW, Vars HM, Rhoads JE: Long term parenteral nutrition with growth, development and positive nitrogen balance. *Surgery* 1968, 64:134–142.

3. Bistrian BR, Blackburn GL, Hallowell E, Heddle R: Protein status of general surgical patients. *JAMA* 1974, 230:858–860.

4. Bistrian BR, Blackburn GL, Vitale J, *et al.*: Prevalence of malnutrition in general medical patients. *JAMA* 1976, 235:1567–1570.

5. Scribner BH, Cole JJ, Christopher TG, *et al.*: Long term total parenteral nutrition. The concept of an artificial gut. *JAMA* 1970, 212:457–463.

6. Heymsfield SB, Bethel RA, Ansley JD, *et al.*: Enteral hyperalimentation: an alternative to central venous hyperalimentation. *Ann Int Med* 1979, 90:63–71.

7. Merritt RJ, Suskind RM: Nutritional survey of hospitalized pediatric patients. *Am J Clin Nutr* 1979, 32:1320–1325.

8. Long CL, Schiller WR, Blakemore WS, *et al.*: Muscle protein catabolism in the septic patient as measured by 3-methylhistidine excretion. *Am J Clin Nutr* 1977, 30:1349–1352.

9. Murray MJ, Marsh HM, Wochos DN, *et al.*: Nutritional assessment of intensive care unit patients. *Mayo Clin Proc* 1988, 63:1106–1115.

10. Dagnelie PC, van Staveren WA: Macrobiotic nutrition and child health: Results of a population based, mixed-longitudinal cohort study in the Netherlands. *Am J Clin Nutr* 1994, 59(suppl 5):1187S–1196S.

11. Waterlow JC: Introduction. Causes and mechanisms of linear growth retardation (stunting). *Eur J Clin Nutr* 1994, 48(suppl 1):S1–S4.

12. Egan MC: Public health nutrition: a historical perspective. *J Am Diet Assoc* 1994, 94:298–304.

13. Kanaka C, Schultz B, Zuppinger KA: Risks of alternative nutrition in infancy: a case report of severe iodine and carnitine deficiency. *Eur J Pediatr* 1992, 151:786–788.

14. Speckter BL: Nutritional concerns of lactating women consuming vegetarian diets. *Am J Clin Nutr* 1994, 59(suppl 5):1182S–1186S.

15. Grant JP: *Handbook of Total Parenteral Nutrition.* Philadelphia: WB Saunders, 1975:15.

16. McClave SA, Mitoraj TE, Thielmeier KA, Greenburg RA: Differentiating subtypes (hypoalbuminemic vs. marasmic) of protein-caloric malnutrition: incidence and clinical significance in a university hospital setting. *JPEN J Parenter Enteral Nutr* 1992, 16:337–342.

17. Shulman BH, Evans HE, Manvar D, Flicker S: Acute gastric dilatation following feeding of nutritionally abused children. *Clin Pediatr* 1984, 23:108.

18. Herbert V: Experimental nutritional folate deficiency in man. *Trans Assoc Am Physicians* 1962, 75:307–320.

19. Lewinter-Suskind L, Suskind K, Murphy KK, Suskind RM: The malnourished child. In *Textbook of Pediatric Nutrition*, edn 2. Edited by Suskind RM, Lewinter-Suskind L. New York: Raven Press; 1993:127–160.

20. Krantman HJ, Young SR, Ank BJ, *et al.*: Immune function in pure iron deficiency. *Am J Dis Child* 1982, 136:840–844.

21. Walter T, Arredondo S, Avevalo M, Stekel A: Effects of iron therapy on phagocytosis and bactericidal activity in neutrophils of iron-deficient infants. *Am J Clin Nutr* 1986, 44:877–882.

22. Kuvibidila S, Wade S: Macrophage function as studied by the clearance of 125I-labeled polyvinylpyrrolidone in iron-deficient and iron-replete mice. *J Nutr* 1987, 117:170–176.

23. Giugliano R, Millward DJ: Growth and zinc homeostasis in the severely Zn-deficient rat. *Br J Nutr* 1984, 52:545–560.

24. O'Dell BL: Effect of dietary components upon zinc availability. A review with original data. *Am J Clin Nutr* 1969, 22:1315–1322.

25. World Health Organization: *Measuring Change in Nutritional Status, Guidelines for Assessing the Nutritional Impact of Supplementary Feeding Programmes for Vulnerable Groups.* Geneva: World Health Organization, 1983.

26. Ronaghy HA, Reinhold JG, Mahloudji M, *et al.*: Zinc supplementation of malnourished schoolboys in Iran: increased growth and other effects. *Am J Clin Nutr* 1974, 27:112–121.

27. Walravens PA, Krebs NF, Habidge KM: Linear growth of low income preschool children receiving a zinc supplement. *Am J Clin Nutr* 1983, 38:195–201.

28. Hambidge KM, Hambidge C, Jacobs M, Baum JD: Low levels of zinc in hair, anorexia, poor growth, and hypogeusia in children. *Pediatr Res* 1972, 6:868–874.

29. Barrett DE, Radke-Yarrow M: Effects of nutritional supplementation on children's responses to novel, frustrating, and competitive situations. *Am J Clin Nutr* 1985, 42:102–120.

30. Golden MHN, Golden BE, Harland PSEG, Jackson AA: Zinc and immunocompetence in protein energy malnutrition. *Lancet* 1978, 1:1226–1228.

31. Cavan KR, Gibson RS, Grazioso CF, *et al.*: Growth and body composition of periurban Guatemalan children in relation to zinc status: a cross sectional study. *Am J Clin Nutr* 1993, 57:334–343.

32. Chandra RK: Trace element and immune response. *Clin Nutr* 1987, 6:118–125.

33. Cavan KR, Gibson RS, Grazioso CF, *et al.*: Growth and body composition of periurban Guatemalan children in relation to zinc status: A logitudinal zinc interventional trial. *Am J Clin Nutr* 1993, 57:344–352.

34. DeLong GR: Effects of nutrition on brain development in humans. *Am J Clin Nutr* 1993, 57(suppl):286S–290S.

35. Laurence KM, James N, Miller M, *et al.*: Double blind randomized controlled trial of folate treatment before conception to prevent recurrence of neural tube defects. *Br Med J* 1981, 282:1509–1511.

36. Nevin NC: Prevention of neural tube defects in an area of high incidence. In *Prevention of Spina Bifida and Other Neural Tube Defects.* Edited by Dobbing J. London: Academic Press; 1983:127–154.

37. Bhattacharyya AK, Chattopadhyay PS, Paladhi PK, *et al.*: Kwashiorkor and marasmus: changing hospital incidence of syndromic presentation (1957-88). *Indian Pediatr* 1990, 27:1191–1198.

38. Neu J, Valentine C, Meetze W: Scientifically-based strategies for nutrition of the high-risk low birth weight infant. *Eur J Pediatr* 1990, 150:2–13.

39. Scrimshaw NS: Nutrition: prospects for the 1990s. *Ann Rev Public Health* 1990, 11:53–68.

40. Kabir N, Forsum E: Estimation of total body fat and subcutaneous adipose tissue in full-term infants less than 3 months old. *Pediatr Res* 1993, 34:448–454.

41. Benjamin DR: Laboratory tests and nutritional assessment: protein-energy status. *Pediatr Clin North Am* 1989, 36:139–161.

42. McMurray DN, Yetley EA, Burch T: Effects of malnutrition and BCG vaccination on macrophage activation in guinea pigs. *Nutr Res* 1981, 1:373–384.

43. McMurray DN: Cell-mediated immunity in nutritional deficiency. *Prog Food Nutr Sci* 1984, 8:193–228.

44. McLoughlin GA, Wu AV, Saporoschetz I, *et al.*: Correlation between anergy and a circulating immunosuppressive factor following major surgical trauma. *Ann Surg* 1979, 190:297–304.

45. Chandra RK: Immunocompetence as a functional index of nutritional status. *Br Med Bull* 1981, 37:89–94.

46. Steffee WP: Malnutrition in hospitalized patients. *JAMA* 1980, 244:2630–2635.

47. Lo CW, Walker WA: Changes in the gastrointestinal tract during enteral or parenteral feeding. *Nutr Rev* 1989, 47:193–198.

48. Jacobs LR, Lupton JR: Effect of dietary fibers on rat large bowel mucosal growth and cell proliferation. *Am J Physiol* 1984, 246:G378–385.

49. Dowling RH, Booth CC: Structural and functional changes following small intestinal resection in the rat. *Clin Sci* 1967, 32:139–149.

50. Zaloga GP, Black KW, Prielipp R: Effect of rate of enteral nutrient supply on gut mass. *JPEN J Parenteral Enteral Nutr* 1992, 16:39–42.

51. Viall C, Porcelli K, Teran C, *et al.*: A double-blind clinical trial comparing the gastrointestinal side effects of two enteral feeding formulas. *JPEN J Parenter Enteral Nutr* 1990, 14:265–269.

52. Matthews DM, Abibi SA: Peptide absorption. *Gastroenterology* 1976, 71:151–161.

53. Souba WW, Smith RJ, Wilmore J: Glutamine metabolism by the intestinal tract. *JPEN J Parenter Enteral Nutr* 1985, 9:608–617.

54. Fox AD, Kripke SA, De Paula J, *et al.*: Effect of a glutamine-supplemented enteral diet on methotrexate-induced enterocolitis. *JPEN J Parenter Enter Nutr* 1988, 12:325–331.

55. Barber AE, Jones WG, Minei JP, *et al.*: Glutamine or fiber supplementation of a defined formula diet: impact on bacterial translocation, tissue composition, and response to endotoxin. *JPEN J Parenter Enteral Nutr* 1990, 14:335–343.

56. Scheppach W, Bartram P, Richter A, *et al.*: Effect of short chain fatty acids on the human colonic mucosa in vitro. *JPEN J Parenter Enteral Nutr* 1992, 16:43–48.

57. Cummings JH: Colonic absorption: The importance of short-chain fatty acids in man. *Scand J Gastroenterol* 1984, 19(suppl 93):89–99.

58. Ruppin H, Bar-Meir S, Soergel KH, *et al.*: Absorption of short-chain fatty acids by the colon. *Gastroenterology* 1980, 78:1500–1507.

59. Koruda MJ, Rolandelli RH, Settle RG, *et al.*: The effect of a pectin supplemented elemental diet on intestinal adaptation to massive small bowel resection. *JPEN J Parenter Enteral Nutr* 1986, 10:343–350.

60. Boehm G, Bierbach U, Senger H, *et al.*: Activities of lipase and trypsin in duodenal juice of infants small for gestational age. *J Pediatric Gastroenterol Nutr* 1991, 12:324–327.

61. Cataldi-Betcher EL, Seltzer MH, Slocum BA, *et al.*: Complications occurring during enteral nutrition support. A prospective study. *JPEN J Parenter Enteral Nutr* 1983, 7:546–552.

62. Brinson RR, Kobts BE: Hypoalbuminemia as an indicator of diarrhea incidence in critically ill patients. *Crit Care Med* 1981, 15:506–509.

63. Anderson A: Microbiological aspects of the preparation and administration of nasogastric and nasoenteric tube feeds in hospitals—a review. *Hum Nutr Appl Nutr* 1983, 37A:426–440.

64. Olivares L, Segovia A, Revuelta R: Tube feeding and lethal aspiration in neurological patients: A review of 720 autopsy cases. *Stroke* 1974, 5:654–657.

65. Mullan H, Roubenoff RA, Roubenoff R: Risk of pulmonary aspiration among patients receiving enteral nutrition support. *JPEN J Parenter Enteral Nutr* 1992, 16:160–164.

66. LeFrock JL, Clark TS, Davies B, Klainer AS: Aspiration pneumonia: A ten year review. *Am Surgeon* 1979, 45:305–313.

67. Young LS: Formulas. In *Enteral and Tube Feeding.* Edited by Rombeau JL, Caldwell MD. Philadelphia: WB Saunders; 1984:187.

68. Reeves-Garcia J, Heyman MB: A survey of complications of pediatric home enteral tube feedings and discussion of developmental and psychological issues. *Nutrition* 1988, 4:375–379.

69. Palmer MM, Heyman MB: Assessment and treatment of sensory versus motor-based feeding problems in infants and young children. *Inf Young Children* 1993, 6:67–73.

70. Nose O, Tipton JR, Ament ME, Yabuuchi H: Effect of the energy source on changes in energy expenditure, respiratory quotient, and nitrogen balance during total parenteral nutrition in children. *Pediatr Res* 1987, 21:538–541.

71. Berger R, Adams L: Nutritional support in the critical care setting (part 2). *Chest* 1989, 96:372–380.

72. Askanazi J, Carpentier YA, Elwyn DH, *et al.*: Influence of total parenteral nutrition on fuel utilization in injury and sepsis. *Ann Surg* 1980, 191:40–46.

73. Committee on Nutrition, American Academy of Pediatrics: Commentary on parenteral nutrition. *Pediatrics* 1983, 71:547–552.

74. Pollack MM: Nutritional support of children in the intensive care unit. In *Textbook of Pediatric Nutrition*, edn 2. Edited by Suskind RM, Lewinter-Suskind L. New York: Raven Press; 1993:127–160.

75. Heyman MB, Storch S, Ament ME: The fat overload syndrome: a case report and review of the literature. *Am J Dis Child* 1981, 135:628–630.

76. Bremer J: Carnitine-metabolism and functions. *Physiol Rev* 1983, 63:1420–1480.

77. Pons R, De Vivo DC: Primary and secondary carnitine deficiency syndromes. *J Child Neurol* 1995, 10(suppl):S8–S24.

78. Schmidt-Sommerfeld E, Penn D, Wolf H: Carnitine deficiency in premature infants receiving total parenteral nutrition: Effect of L-carnitine supplementation. *J Pediatr* 1983, 102:931–935.

78a. Green HL, Hambridge KM, Schanler R, *et al.*: Guidelines for the use of vitamins, trace elements, calcium, magnesium, and phosphorus in infants and children receiving total parenteral nutrition: Report of the Subcommittee on Clinical Practice Issues of The American Society for Clinical Nutrition. *Am J Clin Nutr* 1988, 48:1324–1342.

79. Moukarzel AA, Haddad I, Ament ME, *et al.*: 230 patient years of experience with home long-term parenteral nutrition in childhood: natural history and life of central venous catheters. *J Pediatr Surg* 1994, 29:1323–1327.

80. Cannon RA, Byrne WJ, Ament ME, *et al.*: Home parenteral nutrition in infants. *J Pediatr* 1980, 96:1098–1104.

81. Koo WWK: Parenteral nutrition-related bone disease. *JPEN J Parenter Enteral Nutr* 1992, 16:386–394.

82. Koo WWK Tsang RC, Succop P, *et al.*: Minimal vitamin D and high calcium and phosphorus needs of preterm infants receiving parenteral nutrition. *J Pediatr Gastroenterol Nutr* 1989, 8:225–233.

83. Vargas JH, Klein GL, Ament ME, *et al.*: Metabolic bone disease of total parenteral nutrition: course after changing from casein to amino acids in parenteral solutions with reduced aluminum content. *Am J Clin Nutr* 1988, 48:1070–1078.

84. Solomon SM, Kirby DF: The refeeding syndrome: a review. *JPEN J Parenter Enteral Nutr* 1990, 14:90–97.

85. Leaseburge LA, Winn NJ, Schloerb PR: Liver test alterations with total parenteral nutrition and nutritional status. *JPEN J Parenter Enteral Nutr* 1992, 16:348–352.

86. Manginello FP, Javitt NB: Parenteral nutrition and neonatal cholestasis. *J Pediatr* 1979, 94:296–298.

87. Postuma R, Trevenen CL: Liver disease in infants receiving total parenteral nutrition. *Pediatrics* 1979, 63:110–115.

88. Sheldon GF, Peterson SR, Sanders R: Hepatic dysfunction during hyperalimentation. *Arch Surg* 1978, 113:504–508.

89. Sondheimer JM, Bryan H, Andrews W, Forstner GG: Cholestatic tendencies in premature infants on and off parenteral nutrition. *Pediatrics* 1978, 62:984–989.

90. Heyman MB, Tseng H-C, Thaler MM: Total parenteral nutrition (TPN) decreases hepatic glutathione (GSH) concentrations in weanling rats (abst). *Hepatology* 1984, 4:1049.

91. Touloukian RJ, Seashore JH: Hepatic secretory obstruction with total parenteral nutrition in the infant. *J Pediatr Surg* 1975, 10:353–360.

92. Freund HR, Muggia-Sullam M, LaFrance R, *et al.*: A possible beneficial effect of metronidazole in reducing TPN-associated liver function derangements. *J Surg Res* 1985, 38:356–363.

93. Merritt RJ: Cholestasis associated with total parenteral nutrition. *J Pediatr Gastroenterol Nutr* 1986, 5:9–22.

94. Cohen C, Olsen MM: Pediatric total parenteral nutrition. Liver histopathology. *Arch Path Lab Med* 1981, 105:152–156.

Chapter 3

Neonatal Surgery and the Acute Abdomen

JACOB C. LANGER

The most common reason for surgery in the newborn is the presence of a congenital anomaly. In some cases, the anomaly may interfere with normal growth and development in utero, and the diagnosis may be made prenatally using ultrasound. Examples include polyhydramnios due to high intestinal obstruction, elevated maternal serum α-fetoprotein from gastroschisis, and mediastinal shift in a fetus with a diaphragmatic hernia. In other infants, such as those with an imperforate anus, Hirschsprung's disease, or tracheoesophageal fistula, the diagnosis may not be made until the newborn period. In all cases, the first priority is resuscitation of the infant, ensuring adequate ventilation, fluid status, and temperature stability. The urgency of surgical repair depends on the pathophysiology of the condition, the risk of infection, and the severity of associated conditions, such as other organ malformations, prematurity, and chromosomal anomalies. This chapter outlines the wide range of neonatal surgical problems, providing a brief description of each problem and an approach to its management.

The term *acute abdomen* refers to the presence of peritonitis, defined as inflammation of the peritoneal surfaces. In children, peritonitis can be caused by a multitude of disease processes. In this chapter I have concentrated on the most common processes, particularly appendicitis, and tried to stress the special problems of making the diagnosis of peritonitis and arriving at a correct diagnosis in the pediatric population. The two most common causes of acute abdomen in the neonate, necrotizing enterocolitis and midgut volvulus, are included in the neonatal surgery section. Finally, although gastroesophageal reflux is neither a strictly neonatal problem nor a cause of peritonitis, fundoplication is a common surgical procedure in children and has therefore been included at the end of this chapter.

NEONATAL SURGERY

General principles

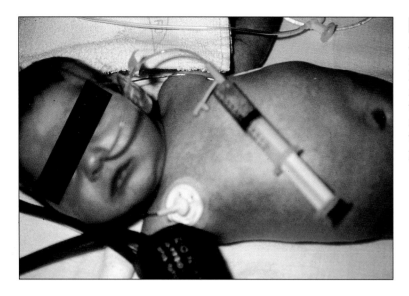

FIGURE 3-1.

Surgical neonates are at high risk for temperature instability and fluid loss. Therefore, such children must be kept warm and well-hydrated through a reliable intravenous line. Management of most neonatal surgical emergencies requires decompression of the gastrointestinal tract, which should be accomplished by using as large a gauge of nasogastric tube as feasible. A soft, sump-type tube, such as a Repogle tube, is preferable, using an 8-Fr tube in preterm infants and a 10-Fr tube in most infants carried to term.

TABLE 3-1.

Many surgical conditions are associated with other structural or chromosomal abnormalities that may be missed if a high index of suspicion is not maintained. This table outlines anomalies frequently associated with some of the more common neonatal surgical conditions.

TABLE 3-1. SURGICAL CONDITIONS ASSOCIATED WITH STRUCTURAL AND CHROMOSOMAL ABNORMALITIES

SURGICAL CONDITION	ASSOCIATED ANOMALIES
Esophageal atresia	Trisomy 13, 18, 21 VACTERL* Duodenal atresia
Duodenal atresia	Trisomy 21 Esophageal atresia
Jejunoileal atresia	Other intestinal atresias
Hirschsprung's disease	Trisomy 21
Malrotation	Duodenal atresia and stenosis Biliary atresia
Imperforate anus	VACTERL OISE† Caudal regression syndrome
Omphalocele	Trisomy 13, 18, 21 Cardiac anomalies Genitourinary anomalies Pentalogy of Cantrell‡ Beckwith-Weideman syndrome
Gastroschisis	Jejunoileal atresia

*Vertebral, anorectal, cardiac, tracheoesophageal, renal, limb.
†Omphalocele, cloacal exstrophy, imperforate anus, spinal deformities.
‡Omphalocele, Morgagni diaphragmatic hernia, periardial defect, sternal defect, intrinsic cardiac defect.

Esophageal atresia and tracheoesophageal fistula

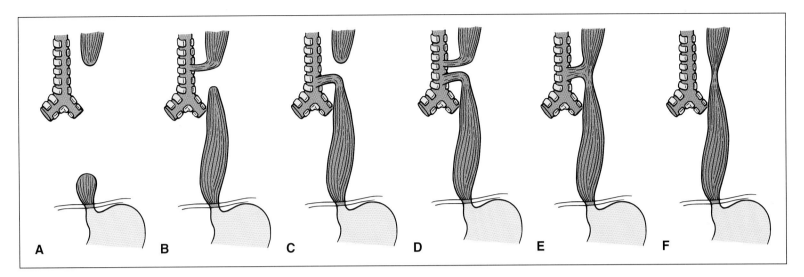

FIGURE 3-2.

Tracheoesophageal malformations can be divided into six classifications (A–F), although esophageal atresia with a distal type tracheoesophageal fistula (TEF) (type C) accounts for almost 90% of cases. Diagnosis is usually made in the neonatal period, except for infants with an H-type TEF (type E), who may present in the first few months because of recurrent aspiration pneumonia. (*From* Gross [1]; with permission.)

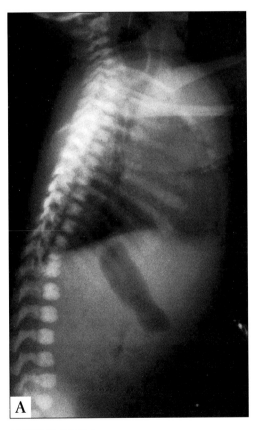
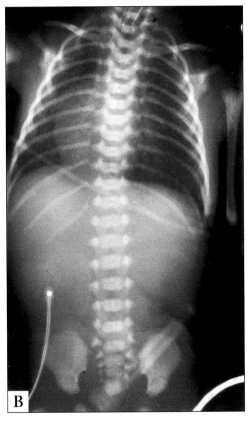

FIGURE 3-3.

Preoperative radiographs of an infant with esophageal atresia with tracheoesophageal fistula (TEF) (A) and without a distal TEF (B). Note the absence of intestinal gas with pure esophageal atresia.

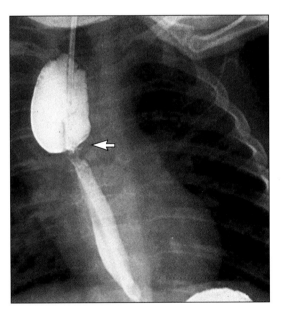

FIGURE 3-4.

Postoperative contrast study following surgical repair. Note the narrowing at the level of the anastomosis (*arrow*). The infant had poor esophageal motility and gastroesophageal reflux. These findings are common in this group of patients.

Congenital diaphragmatic hernia

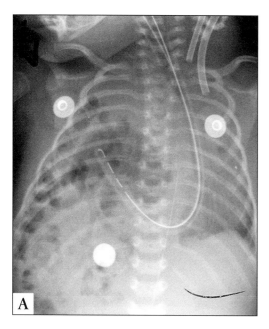

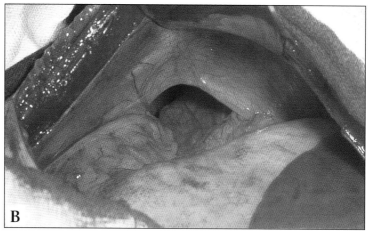

sion. Stabilization with mechanical ventilation and occasionally extracorporeal membrane oxygenation may be necessary before surgical repair is contemplated. **B,** Intraoperative photograph of a left-sided congenital diaphragmatic hernia. The defect is usually in the posterolateral aspect of the diaphragm (Bochdalek's foramen).

FIGURE 3-5.

A, Radiograph of an infant with a left-sided congenital diaphragmatic hernia. These infants usually present with severe respiratory distress due to pulmonary hypoplasia and associated pulmonary hyperten-

Duodenal atresia

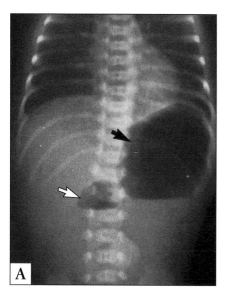

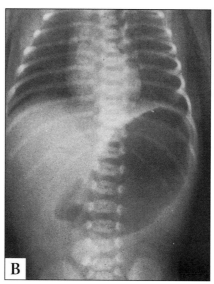

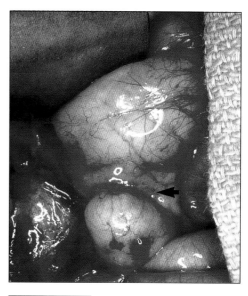

FIGURE 3-6.

A–B, The typical "double-bubble" effect seen with complete duodenal obstruction. The smaller bubble represents the proximal, dilated duodenum (*open arrow*); the larger bubble represents the stomach (*closed arrow*). This effect can be seen with duodenal atresia, duodenal web, annular pancreas, and preduodenal portal vein. It can also be seen, less commonly, with complete duodenal obstruction from Ladd's bands in a patient with malrotation.

FIGURE 3-7.

Intraoperative photograph of duodenal atresia. The pancreas can be seen between the two blind ends of the duodenum (*arrow*). Surgical repair usually involves a side-to-side anastomosis, although a duodenojejunostomy can also be done if technically easier. Return of function often takes 1 to 2 weeks because of poor motility of the proximal duodenum.

TABLE 3-2. DIFFERENTIAL DIAGNOSIS OF NEONATAL DUODENAL OBSTRUCTION

Complete obstruction
  Duodenal atresia
  Complete duodenal web
  Preduodenal portal vein

Partial obstruction
  Duodenal stenosis
  Incomplete duodenal web
  Annular pancreas
  Preduodenal portal vein
  Malrotation with Ladd's bands

TABLE 3-2.

Differential diagnosis of neonatal duodenal obstruction. Neonatal duodenal obstruction may be partial or complete, determined by the presence of gas in the distal bowel on abdominal radiograph. In patients with partial obstruction, urgent upper GI study should be done to rule out malrotation, which is a surgical emergency.

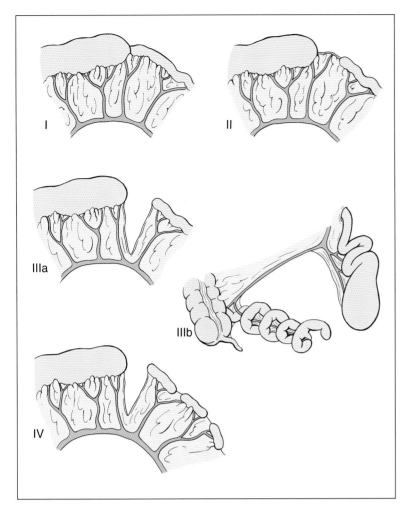

FIGURE 3-8.

Classification of jejunoileal atresia according to Grosfeld [2]. In type IIIb ("apple peel" or "Christmas tree" atresia), most of the mesentery is absent. The distal small bowel lives off the marginal artery. Infants with this type are at risk for ischemia and for necrosis of the small bowel. (*From* Grosfeld [2]; with permission.)

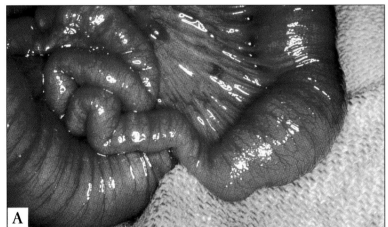

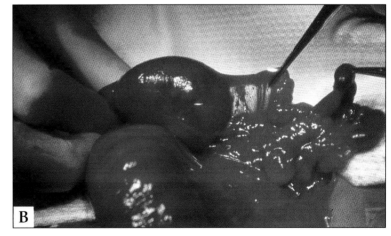

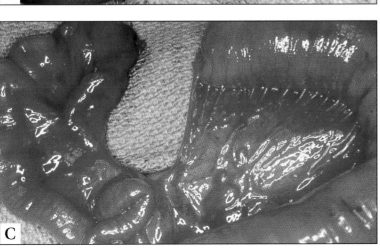

FIGURE 3-9.

Intraoperative photographs of various types of jejunoileal atresia. A, Type I; B, type II; and C, type IIIa.

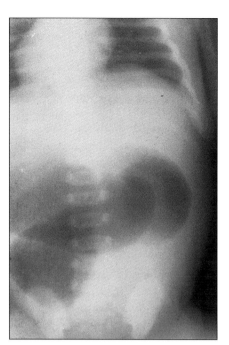

FIGURE 3-10.

Radiograph of an infant with proximal jejunal atresia. Large dilated loops are seen in the upper abdomen with no distal gas. It is impossible to determine which type of atresia is involved until the time of laparotomy. Contrast studies are unnecessary in most cases.

Distal bowel obstruction

TABLE 3-3. COMMON CAUSES OF DISTAL INTESTINAL OBSTRUCTION IN THE NEONATE

Distal ileal atresia

Meconium ileus (usually in infants with cystic fibrosis)

Hirschsprung's disease

Small left colon syndrome (usually in infants from a diabetic mother)

Meconium plug syndrome (usually in premature infants)

Imperforate anus (diagnosed by physical examination)

Incarcerated inguinal hernia (diagnosed by physical examination)

TABLE 3-3.

Common causes of distal intestinal obstruction in the neonate. It is important to determine the diagnosis in a timely fashion because appropriate management options differ considerably among these conditions.

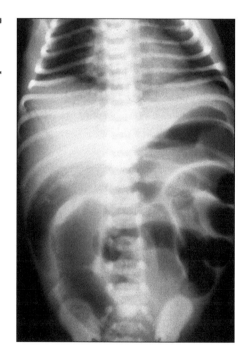

FIGURE 3-11.

Radiograph of a distal bowel obstruction. It is impossible to distinguish the small bowel from the colon in neonates. In such cases, it is best to proceed using a water-soluble contrast enema. In infants with meconium plug, small left colon, and meconium ileus, the obstruction may be relieved by enema, without any need for surgical intervention. In infants with Hirschsprung's disease or ileal atresia, the contrast study may provide the means for a diagnosis.

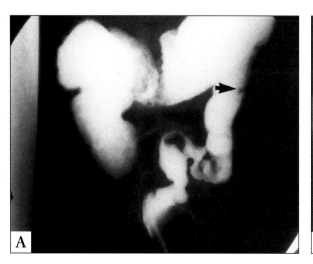

A

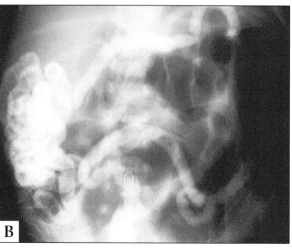

B

FIGURE 3-12.

A, Contrast enema in an infant with Hirschsprung's disease. Note the transition zone in the mid-descending colon (*arrow*). Approximately half of all newborns with Hirschsprung's disease have an obvious transition zone. A rectal biopsy is diagnostic, even after a negative contrast enema. **B,** Contrast enema in an infant with meconium ileus.

(*continued on next page*)

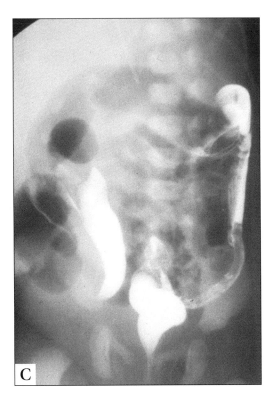

FIGURE 3-12. (CONTINUED)

In approximately 50% of patients, the hypertonic contrast material will break up the inspissated meconium and avoid the need for laparotomy. True meconium ileus is almost always caused by cystic fibrosis. Therefore, sweat chloride concentrations must be measured in children with meconium ileus. **C,** Contrast enema in an infant with small left colon syndrome. The contrast study usually stimulates colonic motility; surgery is usually unnecessary.

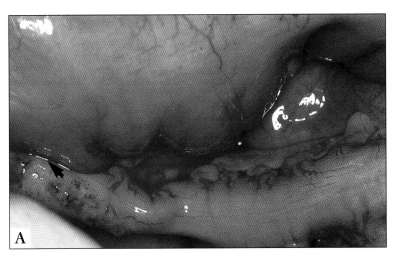

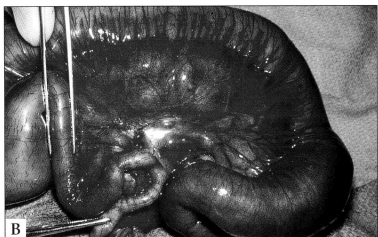

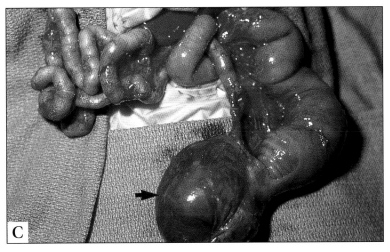

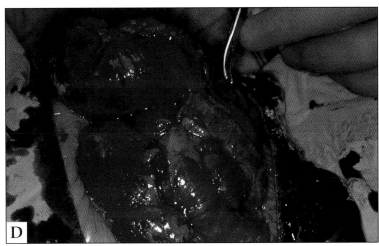

FIGURE 3-13.

A, Intraoperative photograph of Hirschsprung's disease. The transition zone between agangionic (narrow) and normally innervated (dilated) bowel is clearly seen (*arrow*). **B,** Intraoperative photograph of meconium ileus. The dilated proximal bowel narrows gradually because of inspissated intraluminal meconium. **C,** Patient with meconium ileus and in utero perforation. The intraperitoneal meconium has been walled off and has formed a meconium cyst (*arrow*). **D,** Another patient who has suffered in utero perforation secondary to ileal atresia. In this case, the meconium did not form a cyst, and there is meconium peritonitis.

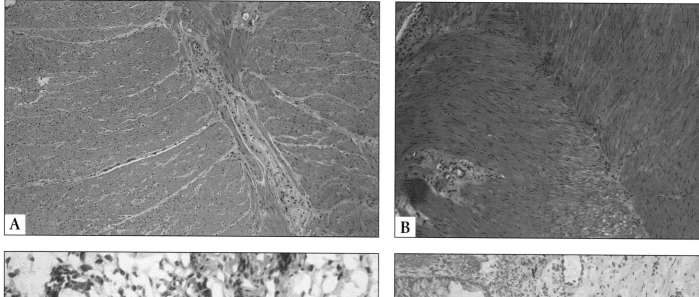

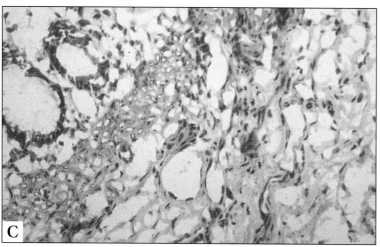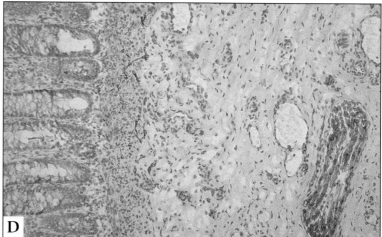

FIGURE 3-14.

Histopathologic findings in an infant with Hirschsprung's disease. **A**, Hematoxylin-and-eosin (H and E)– stained photomicrograph of normal colon. Ganglion cells (neuron cell bodies) are evident in the myenteric plexus. **B**, H and E–stained photomicrograph of aganglionic colon. No ganglion cells are seen, and large nerve trunks are present. **C**, Cholinesterase-stained photomicrograph of normal colon. No staining is seen in the submucosal layer. **D**, Cholinesterase-stained photomicrograph of aganglionic colon. Significant staining is seen in the submucosal layer.

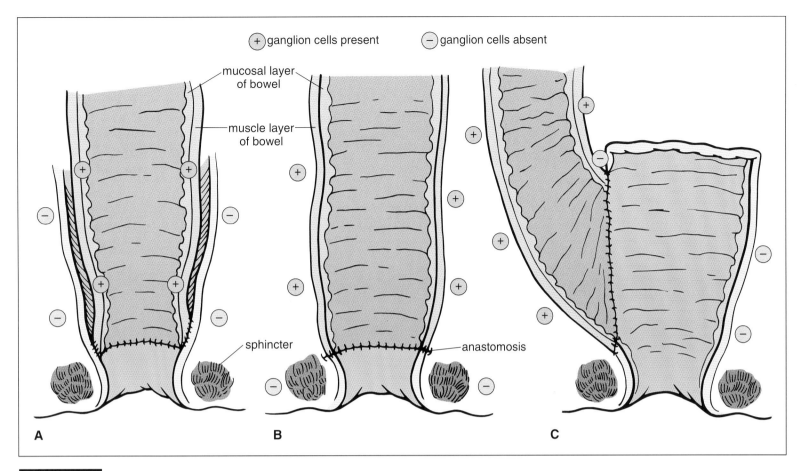

FIGURE 3-15.

Three common operations for Hirschsprung's disease. Some surgeons choose to do a colostomy initially and perform more definitive surgery in a second stage. More recently, however, some surgeons have begun to perform the definitive procedure in a single stage without colostomy. **A,** Soave procedure in which the mucosa is stripped from the aganglionic distal bowel and the normally innervated bowel is anastomosed to the anus. **B,** Swenson procedure in which the aganglionic bowel is resected down the sphincters and an end-to-end anastomosis is done. **C,** Duhamel procedure. The normally innervated bowel is anastomosed end-to-side to the aganglionic rectum above the sphincter.

Malrotation

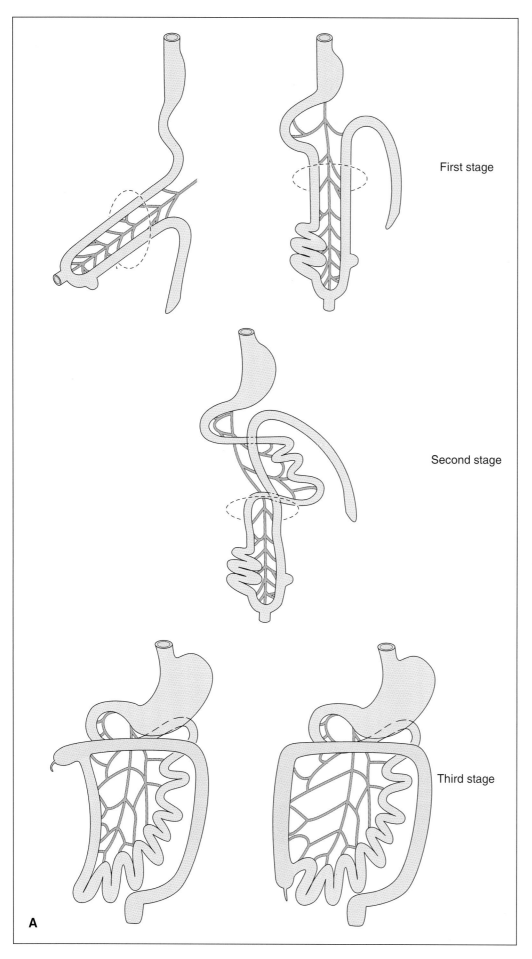

First stage

Second stage

Third stage

A

FIGURE 3-16.

A, Embryology of malrotation. Both the duodenum and the cecum rotate counter-clockwise around the superior mesenteric artery. Malrotation occurs if this process is incomplete.

(*continued on next page*)

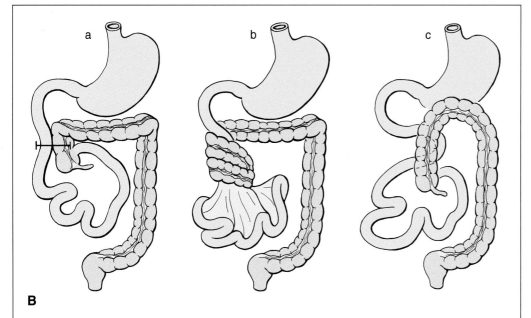

FIGURE 3-16. (CONTINUED)

B, Risk of midgut volvulus results from the close approximation of Treitz's ligament and the ileocecal junction, which creates a narrow-based mesentery. (*Adapted from* Filston and Kirks [3] and Snyder and Chaffin [3a].)

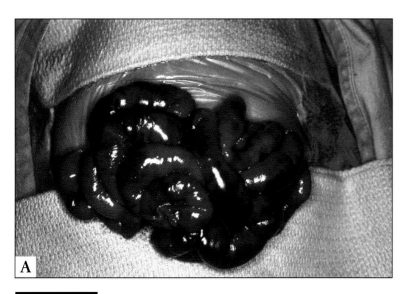

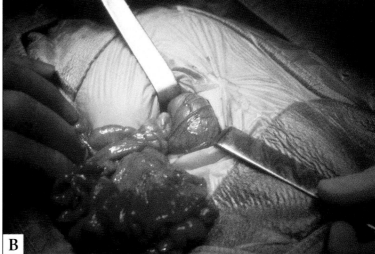

FIGURE 3-17.

Midgut volvulus with ischemia (**A**) and without ischemia (**B**). This condition can occur in children at any age who were previously well. The bowel (and the patient) can be salvaged only by immediate recognition, laparotomy, and detorsion. For this reason, immediate surgical consultation should be obtained in all children who present with bilious or protracted vomiting.

Imperforate anus

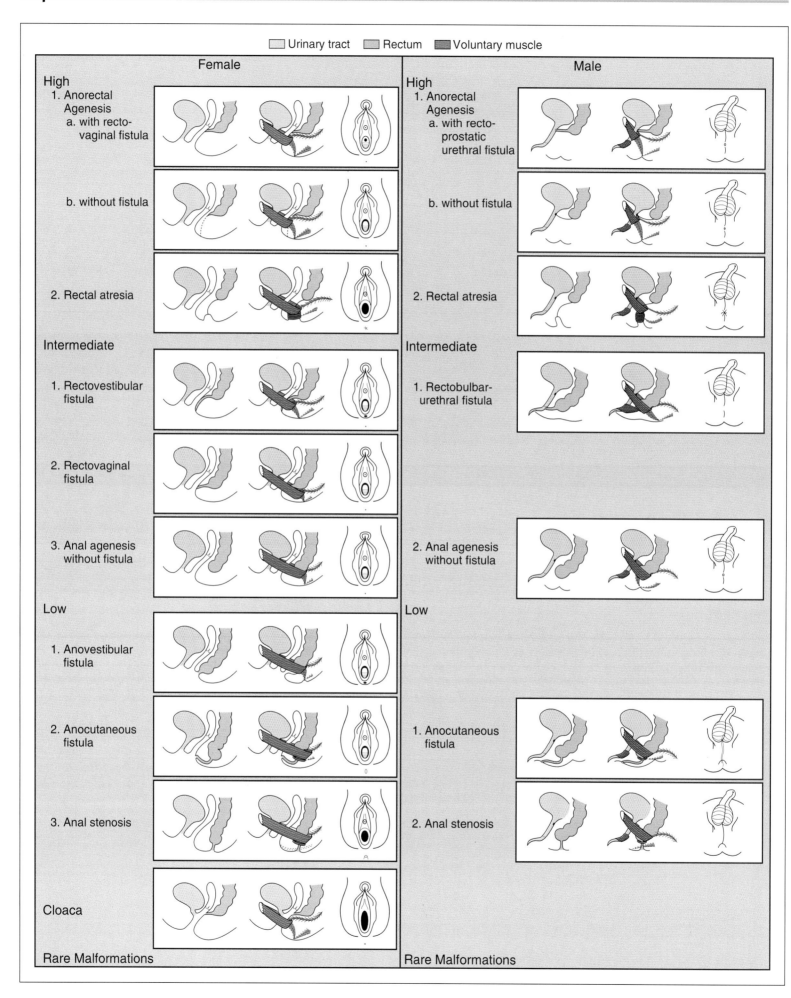

Urinary tract   Rectum   Voluntary muscle

Female

High
1. Anorectal Agenesis
   a. with recto-vaginal fistula
   b. without fistula
2. Rectal atresia

Intermediate
1. Rectovestibular fistula
2. Rectovaginal fistula
3. Anal agenesis without fistula

Low
1. Anovestibular fistula
2. Anocutaneous fistula
3. Anal stenosis

Cloaca

Rare Malformations

Male

High
1. Anorectal Agenesis
   a. with recto-prostatic urethral fistula
   b. without fistula
2. Rectal atresia

Intermediate
1. Rectobulbar-urethral fistula
2. Anal agenesis without fistula

Low
1. Anocutaneous fistula
2. Anal stenosis

Rare Malformations

FIGURE 3-18. (**ON FACING PAGE**)

"Wingspread" classification of anorectal anomalies. This classification was developed during a consensus conference held at the Wingspread center. Boys and girls are dealt with separately. Anomalies are divided into three groups, which are based on the relationship of the rectum to the levator sling. The classification is significant for deciding on the surgical approach and predicting the chance of normal fecal continence. (*From* Raffensperger [4]; with permission.)

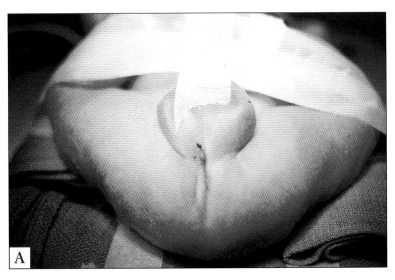

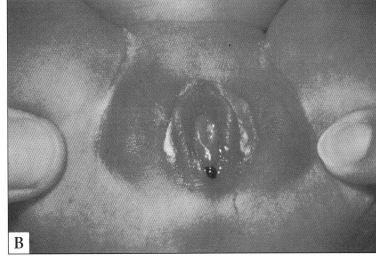

FIGURE 3-19.

A, Low imperforate anus in a boy. Note the anterior position of the anus at the base of the scrotum. **B,** Low imperforate anus in a girl. Note the anal opening in the posterior vaginal forchette. Both of these conditions can be managed using a local cutback or transposition procedure, usually without a colostomy. In very mild cases, anal dilatation may be sufficient with no need for a surgical procedure. Because the rectum extends through the puborectalis sling, the most important component of the external sphincter mechanism, children with low imperforate anus should have completely normal continence.

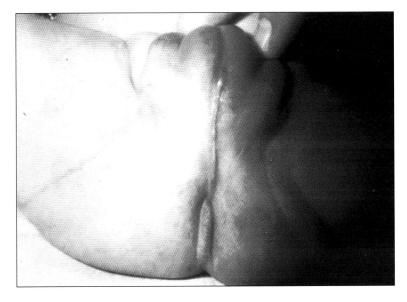

FIGURE 3-20.

High imperforate anus in a boy. These children may pass meconium or air per urethra due to a rectourethral fistula. Note the typical "bucket handle" appearance in the perineum. High imperforate anus in both boys and girls is usually treated by colostomy at birth with the definitive pull-through done between 3 and 9 months of age. Because the rectum usually ends above the puborectalis sling, children with high imperforate anus almost always have some degree of incontinence.

TABLE 3-4. DIFFERENCES BETWEEN GASTROSCHISIS AND OMPHALOCELE

	GASTROSCHISIS	OMPHALOCELE
Maternal age	Younger	Older
Associated anomalies	10% (usually intestinal atresia)	50% (structural and chromosomal)
Sac covering abdominal contents	No	Yes
Liver out through abdominal wall defect	No	Often
Intestinal dysfunction (hypomotility and malabsorption)	Yes	No

TABLE 3-4.

Differences between gastroschisis and omphalocele. Omphalocele and gastroschisis represent the two most common forms of congenital abdominal wall defect. Omphalocele is caused by delayed return of the abdominal viscera from the umbilical cord during the tenth postconceptual week. Although gastroschisis was thought to be a ruptured omphalocele, it is now recognized as a distinct entity that consists of uncovered intestinal loops protruding through a defect to the right of the umbilicus.

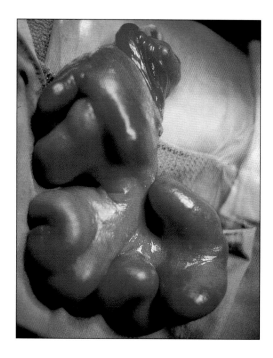

FIGURE 3-21.

Infant with gastroschisis. The bowel is thickened, dilated, and has a shortened mesentery. Infants with gastroschisis frequently suffer from digestive problems and often require total parenteral nutrition for several weeks to months until bowel function returns.

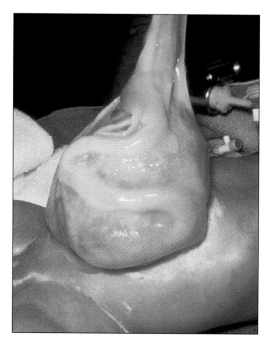

FIGURE 3-22.

Infant with omphalocele. The liver and bowel are herniated into the umbilical cord and are thereby covered by a sac composed of Wharton's jelly. The most common cause of mortality in these infants is associated anomalies, particularly lethal chromosomal abnormalities, cardiac defects, and renal problems.

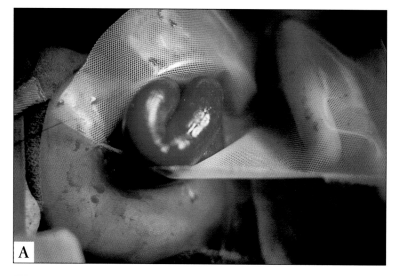

A

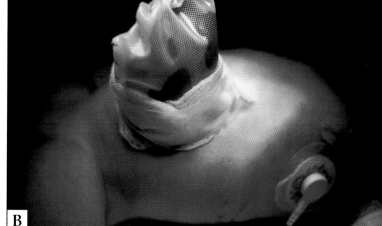

B

FIGURE 3-23.

Staged repair of an abdominal wall defect. In patients in whom the viscera cannot be returned to the abdomen without undue intra-abdominal pressure, a reinforced silastic sheet is sewn around the defect (**A**). The viscera are slowly reduced into the abdomen over the next 3 to 7 days (**B**).

(*continued on next page*)

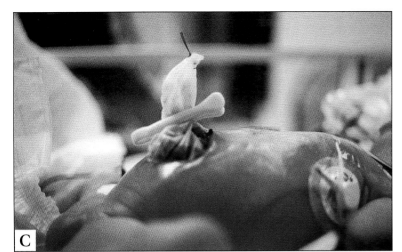

FIGURE 3-23. (CONTINUED)

The fascia is then closed during a second procedure (C).

C

Intestinal duplication

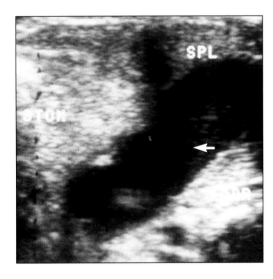

FIGURE 3-24.

Prenatal sonogram of a fetus with gastric duplication. A large fluid-filled sac is seen in the midabdomen adjacent to the stomach (*arrow*).

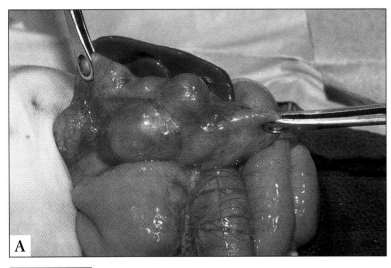

A

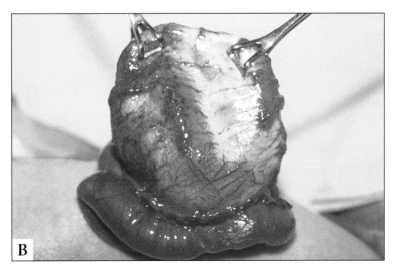

B

FIGURE 3-25.

A, Intraoperative appearance of gastric duplication. The cyst lies along the greater curvature of the stomach and does not communicate with the lumen. B, Intraoperative appearance of jejunal duplication. The duplication is found between the leaves of the mesentery and can present with an abdominal mass, intestinal obstruction, bleeding resulting from ectopic gastric mucosa in the duplication, or may be discovered serendipitously by an ultrasound test done for other reasons.

Necrotizing enterocolitis

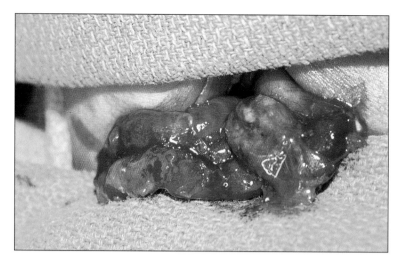

FIGURE 3-26.

Intraoperative appearance of necrotizing enterocolitis. The bowel is inflamed and necrotic, with multiple areas of perforation. Clinically, this disease is most common in preterm infants who present after the first few days of life with sepsis, abdominal distension, ileus, and peritonitis.

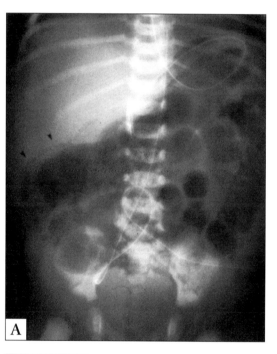

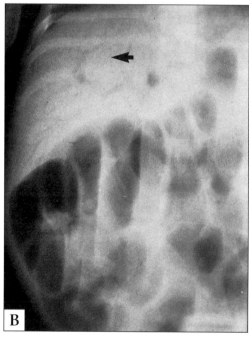

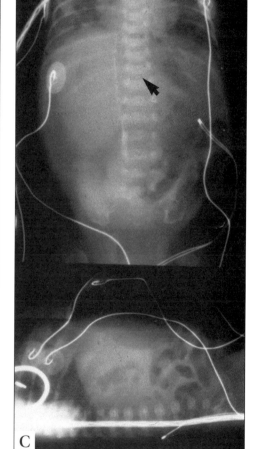

FIGURE 3-27.

Radiologic features of necrotizing enterocolitis. **A,** Pneumatosis intestinalis, which is pathognomonic of this disease in the newborn (*arrowheads*). **B,** Portal vein gas, considered to be a very poor prognostic sign (*arrow*). **C,** Free intraperitoneal air. This may be a subtle finding on a film taken with the patient lying supine, where it appears as the "football sign," a midabdominal lucency with the "laces" formed by the falciform ligament in the midline (*arrow*).

Principles of peritonitis

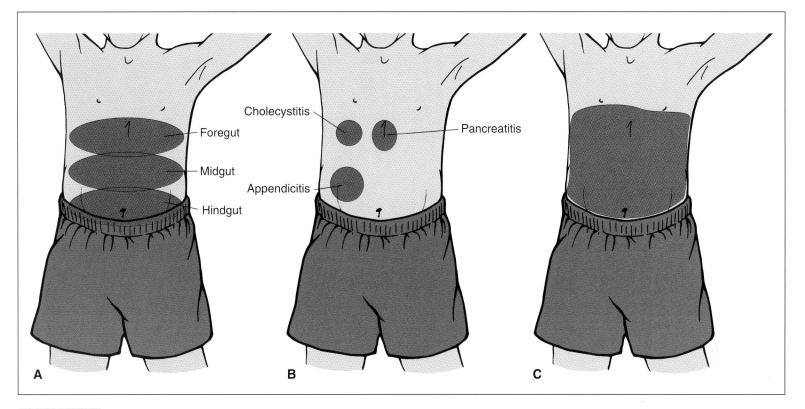

FIGURE 3-28.

Patterns of acute pain in the abdomen. **A**, Visceral pain due to distension, spasm, or ischemia is poorly localized in the midabdomen: foregut pain in the epigastrium, midgut pain in the periumbilical region, and hindgut pain in the hypogastrium. **B**, Somatic pain due to localized peritoneal inflammation is severe and localized. These differences explain the natural progression of appendicitis, in which the initial periumbilical pain is due to appendiceal obstruction and distension, and the subsequent right lower quadrant pain is due to local peritoneal inflammation. **C**, Somatic pain due to diffuse peritoneal inflammation, such as seen with a freely perforated appendicitis, is felt throughout the abdomen with widespread involuntary guarding and rigidity. Because newborns breathe primarily through their diaphragms, respirations become shallow and rapid.

TABLE 3-5. CAUSES OF PERITONITIS IN CHILDHOOD

Gastrointestinal	Genitourinary	Other
Appendicitis	Pyelonephritis	Trauma
Gastroenteritis	Ovarian cyst	Rectus hematoma
Inflammatory bowel disease	rupture	Primary bacterial peritonitis
Meckel's diverticulitis	torsion	Sickle cell crisis
Torsion of omental cyst	hemorrhage	Porphyria
Intestinal obstruction with ischemic bowel	Ovarian tumor with torsion	Henoch-Schönlein purpura
Midgut volvulus	Mittelschmerz	Familial Mediterranean fever
Acute cholecystitis	Pelvic inflammatory disease	
Pancreatitis		
Necrotizing enterocolitis		
Intestinal perforation		

TABLE 3-5.

Causes of peritonitis in childhood. Peritonitis may be caused by a large number of disease processes involving several different organ systems.

TABLE 3-6. STRATEGIES FOR DIAGNOSING PERITONITIS IN CHILDHOOD

Establish rapport from a distance before beginning examination

Use diversionary tactics

Watch facial expression and body position

Assess for percussion tenderness before starting to palpate

Use surreptitious palpation with a stethoscope or the patient's own hand

TABLE 3-6.

Strategies for diagnosing peritonitis in children. Peritonitis may be very difficult to diagnose in children because of characteristically atypical presentation, problems with communication, anxiety, and lack of cooperation during the physical examination. A number of strategies may be helpful in differentiating true peritonitis from voluntary guarding in children.

Appendicitis

TABLE 3-7. DIAGNOSTIC CRITERIA FOR APPENDICITIS

History
- Periumbilical pain migrating to the right lower quadrant
- Nonbilious vomiting
- Anorexia
- Pain on walking, jumping, and driving over bumps

Physical examination
- Flushed face
- Low-grade fever (fever usually higher with perforation)
- Lies on side with hips flexed
- Localized peritoneal signs in right lower quadrant (may have diffuse peritonitis if perforated)
- Referred rebound tenderness to right lower quadrant

Laboratory
- Mild elevation in leukocyte count, usually higher with perforation
- May have mild hematuria or pyuria from bladder or ureteral irritation

Radiologic
- Local ileus in right lower quadrant (may have diffuse ileus if perforated)
- Appendicolith in right lower quadrant
- Scoliosis to right side
- Loss of psoas shadow on right side

Ultrasound
- Noncompressable, thick-walled tubular structure with localized tenderness
- May see appendicolith with acoustic shadow
- No evidence of ovarian pathology to explain symptoms

Computerized tomography
- Thick-walled structure with surrounding inflammation in right lower abdomen
- May show localized appendiceal abscess if perforated

TABLE 3-7.

Diagnostic criteria for appendicitis. The diagnosis is made clinically, and not all these criteria need to be satisfied. It is important to remember that "not every child with appendicitis has read the textbook."

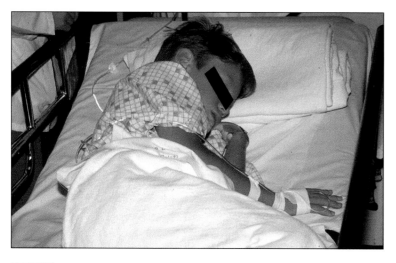

FIGURE 3-29.

Typical position of a child with appendicitis. The child lies quietly with hips flexed. The clinician should also note the facial flushing.

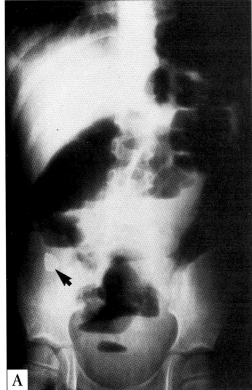

A

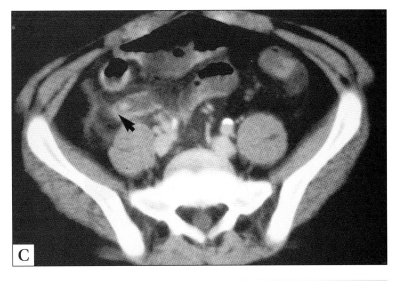

C

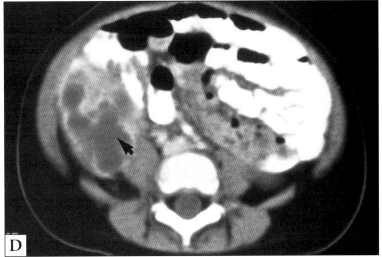

D

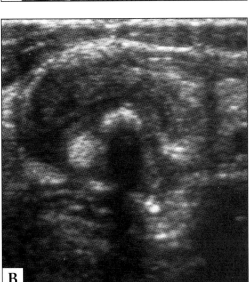

B

FIGURE 3-30.

Radiologic studies in the diagnosis of acute appendicitis. **A**, Abdominal radiograph showing appendicolith (*arrow*) and local ileus in lower abdomen. **B**, Ultrasound showing cross-section of a noncompressible, thick-walled tubular structure with acoustic shadowing from an appendicolith. **C**, Computed tomographic (CT) scan showing thick-walled structure with surrounding inflammation in right lower abdomen (*arrow*). **D**, CT scan showing localized appendiceal abscess in right lower abdomen (*arrow*). (*Courtesy of* Dr. M. Siegel, St. Louis, MO.)

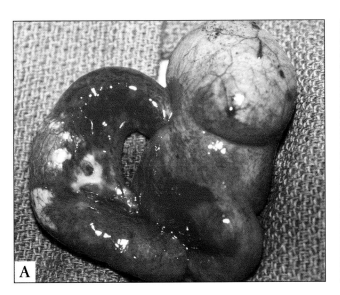

A

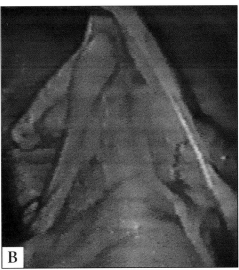

B

FIGURE 3-31.

Intraoperative photograph of an inflamed appendix during open appendectomy (**A**) and laparoscopic appendectomy (**B**). It remains controversial whether laparoscopic appendectomy results in a shorter hospital stay, fewer wound infections, or faster return to normal activity than open appendectomy. In the pediatric population we currently reserve the laparoscopic approach for adolescents, particularly girls in whom ovarian pathology may be causing the problem.

Other causes of acute abdomen

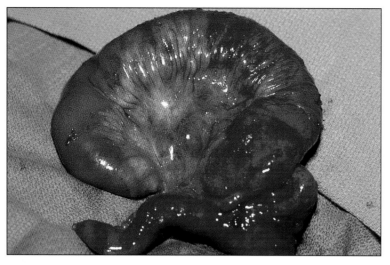

FIGURE 3-32.

Intraoperative photograph of ileitis resulting from *Yersinia* infection. This may be misdiagnosed preoperatively as appendicitis or Crohn's disease. In most cases, no resection is done. If the appendix and cecum are uninflamed, the appendix should be removed; however, where appendiceal or cecal inflammation is present (as shown in this patient), no appendectomy should be done.

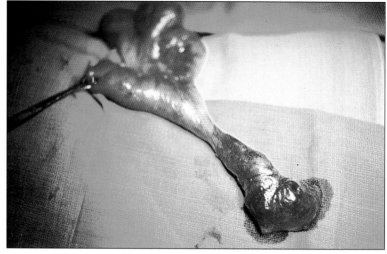

FIGURE 3-33.

Intraoperative photograph of Meckel's diverticulitis. Ectopic gastric mucosa leads to chronic ulceration at the base of the diverticulum, which causes obstruction and inflammation. Treatment is resection of the Meckel's diverticulum.

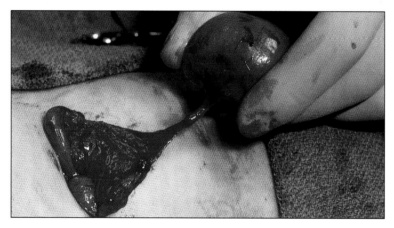

FIGURE 3-34.

Intraoperative photograph of an omental cyst that has undergone torsion. This was treated by resection.

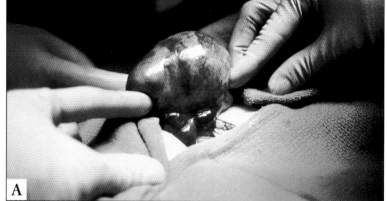

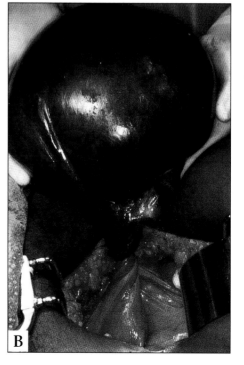

FIGURE 3-35.

Intraoperative photograph of ovarian torsion resulting from a large teratoma in a 7-year-old girl (**A**) and a hemorrhagic corpus luteum cyst in a 14-year-old girl (**B**).

Fundoplication

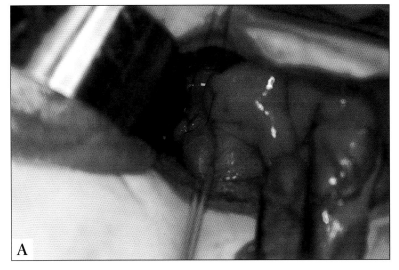
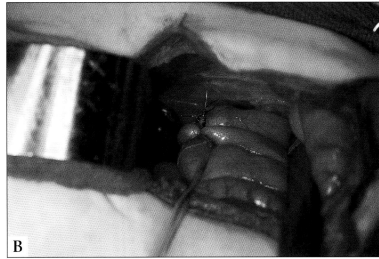

FIGURE 3-36.

Open Nissen fundoplication in an infant. **A,** The blue vessel loop is seen around the gastroesophageal junction. A stitch has been placed from the anterior fundus to the esophagus and to the posterior fundus, which has been wrapped around the back of the esophagus. **B,** The completed wrap.

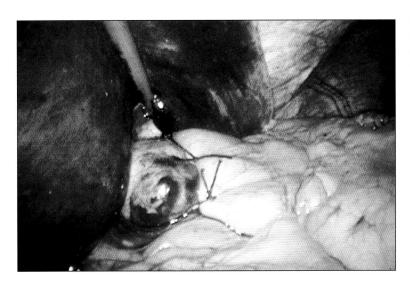

FIGURE 3-37.

Laparoscopic Nissen fundoplication in an older child. The abdomen is insufflated with carbon dioxide; the liver is being retracted anteriorly. (*Courtesy of* Dr. M. Anvari, Hamilton, Ontario, Canada.)

▌REFERENCES

1. Gross RE: *Surgery of Infancy and Childhood.* Philadelphia, WB Saunders; 1952:74.

2. Grosfeld J: Jejunoileal atresia and stenosis. In *Pediatric Surgery.* Edited by Welch KJ, *et al.* Chicago: Year Book Medical Publishing; 1986:843.

3. Filston HC, Kirks DR: Malrotation—the ubiquitous anomaly. *J Pediatr Surg* 1981, 16:614–620.

3a. Snyder WH, Chaffin L: Embryology and pathology of the intestinal tract: Presentation of 48 cases of malrotation. *Ann Surg* 1954, 140:368–380.

4. Rattensperger JG: *Swenson's Pediatric Surgery,* edn. 5. New York: Appleton and Lange; 1990.

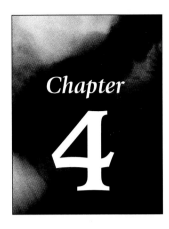

Chapter 4

Gastroesophageal Reflux

Gastroesophageal reflux is an important disorder in children because of its frequency and the morbidity that it can cause. During recent years its importance has become clearer; efforts to understand its pathophysiology have begun to yield results. Concurrently, the variety of symptomatic presentations of gastroesophageal reflux disease particularly in children, has been illuminated. Diverse tests have been applied to its diagnosis. Therapy has been improved, so that continuing morbidity and surgery are usually avoidable.

SUSAN R. ORENSTEIN

At the time of publication, **cisapride** was not FDA approved for use in children. Check the package insert for any change in indications and dosage and for added warnings and precautions.

Reflux episodes

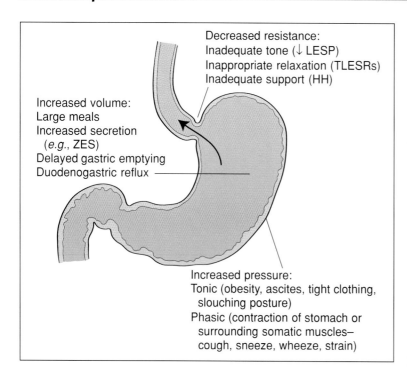

FIGURE 4-1.

Occurrence of gastroesophageal reflux episodes (frequency). Gastroesophageal reflux episodes are normal physiologic events that may accompany relaxation of the lower esophageal sphincter (LES) during swallowing or during gastric venting by belching. These events are increased in frequency by conditions that decrease resistance to reflux, those that increase gastric volume, or those that increase intragastric pressure. Resistance to reflux at the gastroesophageal junction is produced by the LES and supporting structures [1]. The LES pressure (LESP) may be low tonically (particularly when esophagitis is present) or may lower with inappropriate frequency ("transient LES relaxations" [TLESRs]) [2]. Supporting structures, particularly the crural diaphragm, fail to bolster the LES when hiatal herniation (HH) occurs [3]. Gastric volume is increased by large meals, increased gastric secretion (typified by gastrinomas in Zollinger-Ellison syndrome [ZES]), delayed gastric emptying, or duodenogastric reflux. Intragastric pressure is increased in various settings that may produce both tonic increases in pressure or more abrupt increases. These factors may interact; for example, during cough LES support increases for protection, unless a hiatal hernia is present [3].

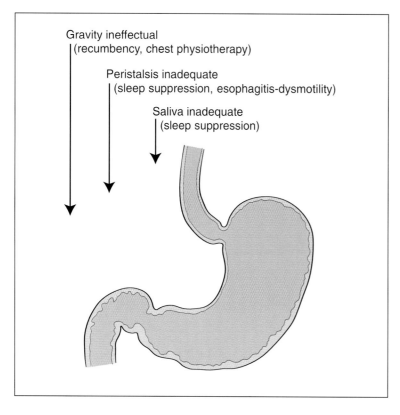

FIGURE 4-2.

Clearance of reflux episodes (duration). Physiologic reflux episodes are rapidly cleared by gravitational forces (in the upright position), propulsive peristaltic forces, and salivary washdown and neutralization of residual acid [4]. These protective factors are hindered during sleep [5], when recumbency, decreased salivation, and infrequent swallowing naturally occur. In healthy children this has little effect because physiologic transient lower esophageal sphincter relaxations are rare during sleep [5]. Peristaltic clearance may be impaired by weak or disorganized waves, as well as by infrequent swallowing; that this sort of impairment may be caused by esophagitis is considered the basis of vicious cycles of esophagitis and esophageal dysmotility [6-9].

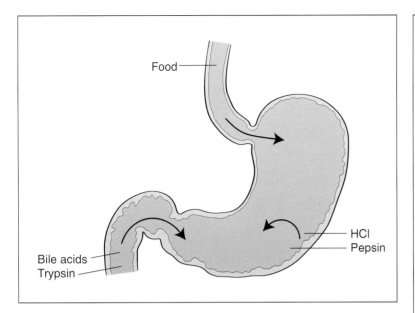

FIGURE 4-3.

Harmful components of refluxate. Although gastric hydrochloric acid (HCl) is the most prominent noxious component of refluxate and the basis of many diagnostic and therapeutic strategies, gastric pepsin, bile acids, and pancreatic trypsin also play a role [10–14]. The central role of HCl is heightened by its role in converting pepsinogen to pepsin. Nutrients, either acidic (promoting esophagitis) or not (promoting malnutrition or respiratory disease depending on where they go when refluxed), are also potentially harmful components of the refluxate.

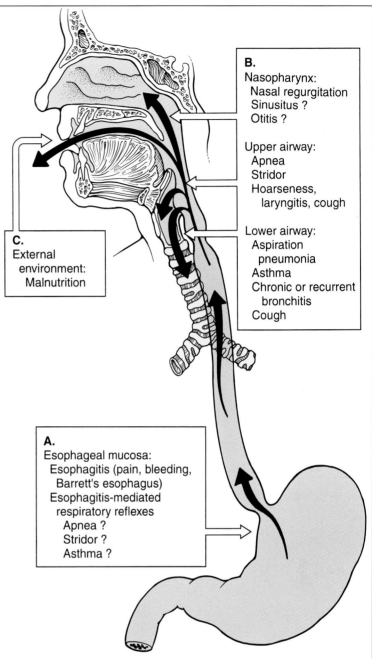

B.
Nasopharynx:
  Nasal regurgitation
  Sinusitus ?
  Otitis ?

Upper airway:
  Apnea
  Stridor
  Hoarseness,
    laryngitis, cough

Lower airway:
  Aspiration
    pneumonia
  Asthma
  Chronic or recurrent
    bronchitis
  Cough

C.
External
environment:
Malnutrition

A.
Esophageal mucosa:
  Esophagitis (pain, bleeding,
    Barrett's esophagus)
  Esophagitis-mediated
    respiratory reflexes
    Apnea ?
    Stridor ?
    Asthma ?

FIGURE 4-4.

A–C, Harmful destinations of the refluxate. Perhaps because of immature protective reflexes or other factors, the destination of the refluxate plays a larger role in young children than in adults with gastroesophageal reflux disease. The classic destination of refluxate—the esophagus—is responsible for esophagitis and its diverse esophageal sequelae (*eg*, pain, bleeding, stricture, Barrett's esophagus, and malignancy). An esophageal destination may also provoke respiratory symptoms through reflex mechanisms. Other hazardous targets of the refluxate are the lower and upper airways, including the nasopharynx. Finally, the external environment is indirectly a harmful destination because of implied caloric loss.

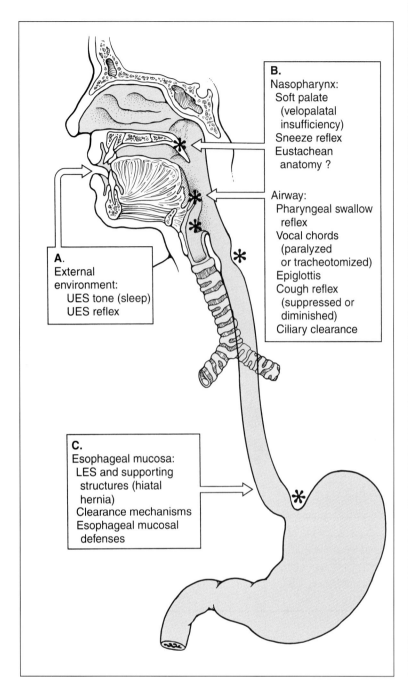

FIGURE 4-5.

A–C, Protection of vulnerable targets of the refluxate. Although the lower esophageal sphincter (LES*) and its supporting structures represent the primary first-line defense against harmful effects of reflux, these are reinforced by the clearance mechanisms previously discussed and by esophageal mucosal defenses against injury [15]. Protection against reflux-related tissue damage proximal to the esophagus is provided first by the upper esophageal sphincter (UES*)—and its reflexively augmented tone during gastroesophageal reflux—and then by the structures that protect the airway during either swallowing or reflux—the epiglottis*, vocal cords*, and soft palate* [16–21]. The swallow reflex, which occurs when the pharynx is stimulated, is an elaborate mechanism that removes refluxate from a dangerous location at the crossroads of the airway and the gastrointestinal tract. The cough and sneeze reflexes clear the lower airway and nasal passages when matter does enter the respiratory tract. In parentheses are some factors that may impair these protections, such as sleep state, velopalatal insufficiency, cough suppression, and tracheotomy.

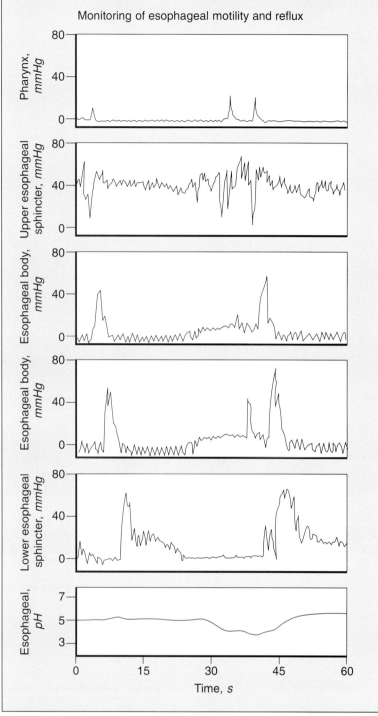

FIGURE 4-6.

Example of a transient lower esophageal sphincter relaxation (TLESR) causing a reflux episode. The top five channels are manometric tracings from the pharynx, the upper esophageal sphincter (UES), the esophageal body (two ports), and the lower esophageal sphincter (LES) (a Dent sleeve) of a child. The bottom channel is a distal esophageal pH probe. Abolition of LES pressure in the form of TLESR occurs about 20 seconds into the tracing, about 15 seconds after the initial swallow complex. The ensuing reflux episode is documented both by a pH drop in the bottom channel and by a pressure rise (a "common cavity" phenomenon) in the esophageal body.

An initial pharynx-protecting reflex increase in UES pressure is followed by two primary peristaltic sequences, which result in clearance of both bulk (pressure) and acid from the esophageal body. (*Adapted from* Orenstein [27] from data provided by Drs. J. Dent and G. P. Davidson, Adelaide, Australia.)

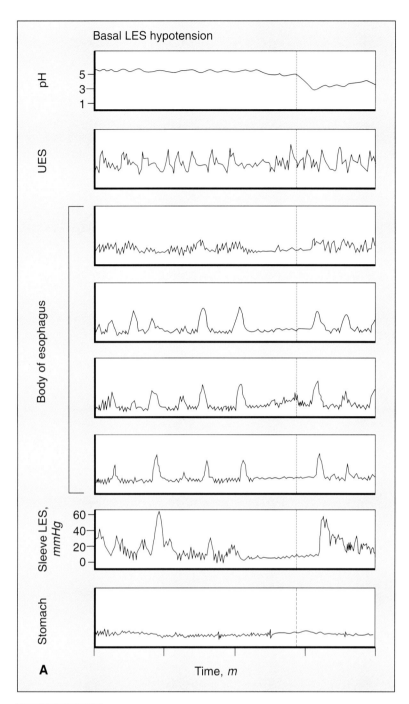

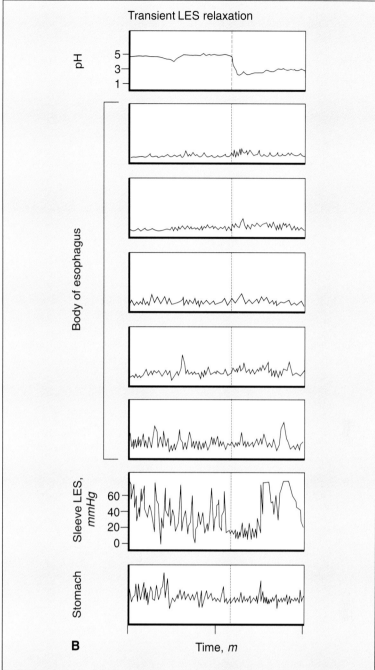

FIGURE 4-7.

Examples of reflux episodes provoked by basal lower esophageal sphincter (LES) hypotonia (**A**), a transient LES relaxation (TLESR) (**B**), and increased abdominal pressure (**C**) in children. The top channel is distal esophageal pH, and the next seven manometric channels document pressures in the upper esophageal sphincter (UES), the esophageal body (four channels), the LES (a Dent sleeve), and the stomach [22]. The reflux episodes defined in the top channel are provoked by the three different mechanisms, as

(*continued on next page*)

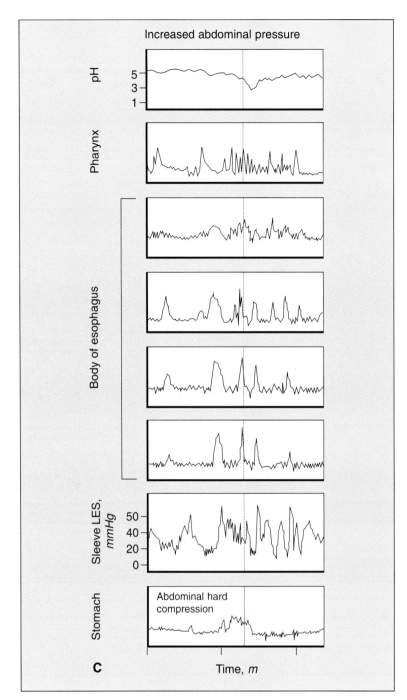

Increased abdominal pressure

pH

Pharynx

Body of esophagus

Sleeve LES, *mmHg*

Stomach

Abdominal hard compression

C

Time, *m*

FIGURE 4-7. (*CONTINUED*)

shown in the LES sleeve and the gastric channels. Temporary lowering of LES pressure is important, however, for each of the three examples: in the first, a somewhat prolonged TLESR is ongoing at the time the acid refluxes; in the third, it appears that the reflux episode does not occur until a swallow-associated LESR is superimposed on an ongoing increase in gastric pressure. (*Adapted from* Werlin *et al.* [22].)

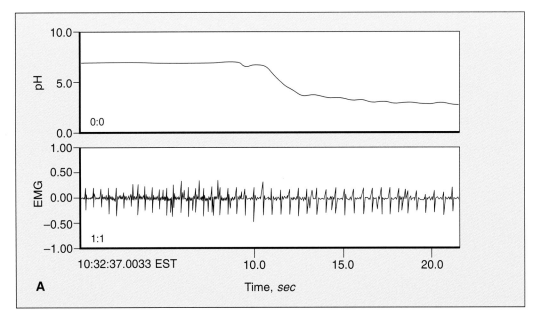

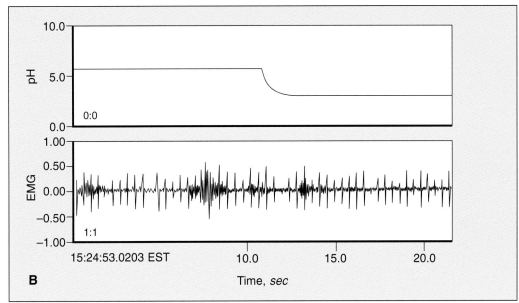

FIGURE 4-8.

The role of abdominal muscle contraction in determining whether refluxate will be regurgitated by an infant. Top channel, distal esophageal pH. Bottom channel, rectus abdominis surface electromyographic (EMG) tracing with superimposed electrocardiographic artifact. **A**, Reflux that is not accompanied by regurgitation is more likely to show no rectus abdominis contraction, in contrast with reflux with regurgitation (**B**). (*Adapted from* Orenstein *et al.* [23].)

Neuromuscular mediators

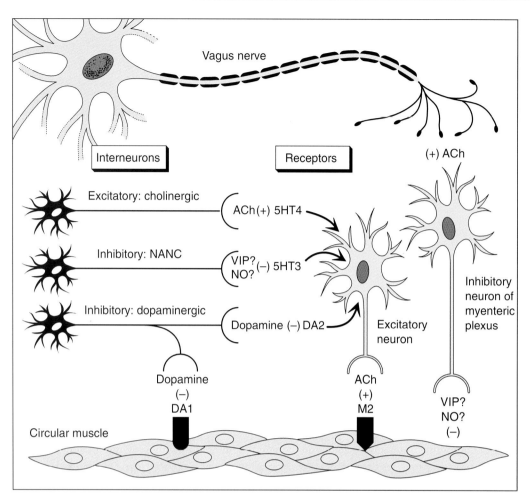

FIGURE 4-9

Neuromuscular mediators and the lower esophageal sphincter (LES). The tonic contraction of the LES circular muscle is modulated by complex neural input, which is still incompletely understood. Excitatory input on the muscle's M2 receptors is mediated by acetylcholine (ACh). These excitatory neurons are controlled in turn by excitatory input from cholinergic interneurons in the myenteric plexus that stimulate 5HT4 receptors and by inhibitory input from dopaminergic interneurons on DA2 receptors and from nonadrenergic, noncholinergic interneurons producing nitric oxide (NO) or vasoactive inhibitory peptide (VIP) that affect 5HT3 receptors. Direct inhibitory input on the circular muscle is also provided by dopaminergic interneurons acting on DA1 receptors and by inhibitory neurons producing NO or VIP when stimulated by ACh output from the vagus nerve [24]. Prokinetic agents block dopaminergic inhibition of the LES (metoclopramide) or enhance cholinergic stimulation of the LES (cisapride and bethanechol). DA—dopamine; HT—hydroxytryptamine; M—muscarinic; NANC—nonadrenergic, noncholinergic; VIP—vasoactive inhibitory peptide; (+)—excitatory; (–)—inhibitory.

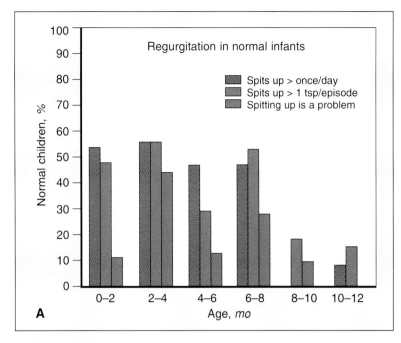

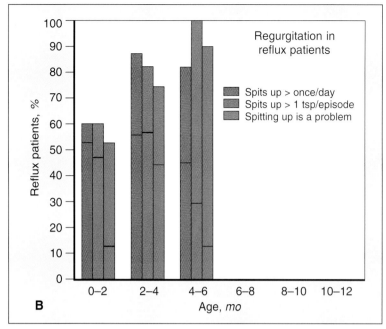

FIGURE 4-10.

Regurgitation in normal infants and in those presenting with gastro-esophageal reflux disease (GERD). Regurgitation is the most evident manifestation of GERD in young children but also commonly occurs in normal infants. A, Quantification and characterization of regurgitation by age in normal infants as they mature through the first year of life was assessed by a standardized questionnaire in 100 children being seen for well-child care in an outpatient clinic [25]. B, The same questionnaire was administered to 69 children upon presentation with GERD [25]; only the first 6 months are represented because of the rarity of presentation of infants with reflux disease after 6 months of age. The horizontal lines reproduce the normal values from *panel A*, for comparison. Salient findings in normal infants are the presence of daily regurgitation greater than 1 teaspoonful in nearly half of them under 8 months of age, with an abrupt decrease thereafter, and the peak at 2 to 4 months of age of regurgitation regarded as a problem in nearly 50% of normal babies. Similar proportions of babies with GERD and normal babies have daily regurgitation of more than 1 teaspoonful in the first 2 months of age, but parents of the GERD infants are more apt to define it as a problem. In addition, there is an abrupt increase in the proportion of infants regurgitating daily more than 1 teaspoonful after 2 months of age in those presenting with GERD [26].

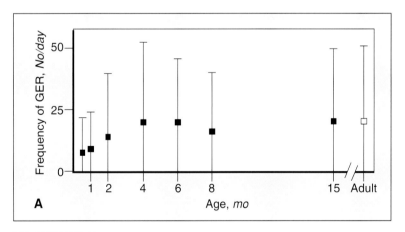

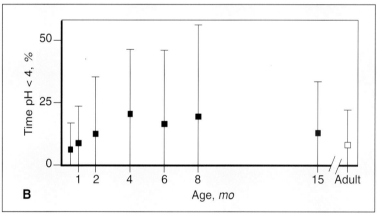

FIGURE 4-11.

A–B, Reflux quantification in normal infants and adults by pH probe. Studies in 285 normal infants and in 15 normal adults provide information on the frequency and duration of acid reflux episodes in normal children and adults taking a normal diet [28,29]. These data suggest that values for normal adults and infants are more similar than often assumed, although the buffering capacity of the usual infant milk formula diet must be considered in interpreting these values. Data are mean ±2SD. GER—gastroesophageal reflux. (*From* Orenstein [27]; with permission; *Data from* Vandenplas *et al.* [28] and Johnson *et al.* [29].)

TABLE 4-1. FLUOROSCOPIC REFLUX

	NUMBER OF REFLUX EPISODES IN 5 MINUTES	
AGE	NORMAL CHILDREN	CHILDREN WITH REFLUX DISEASE
0–1.5 months	<4	3.7 ± 0.3
1.5–6 months	<3	3.2 ± 0.3
6–12 months	<3	2.2 ± 0.4
1–1.5 years	<2	1.7 ± 0.1
1.5–6 years	<2	0.8 ± 0.1
6–12 years	<1	0.8 ± 0.1
12–18 years	<1	2.1 ± 0.2

TABLE 4-1.

Reflux quantification during barium fluoroscopy in normal children and those with reflux disease. Fluoroscopically-detected reflux rates of up to 4 episodes per 5 minutes in infants and less than 1 episode per 5 minutes in adults [30] contrast with the previous graph showing a pH probe reflux frequency in normal infants of less than 50 (ie, mean + 2 SD) episodes per 24-hour period (ie, < 2 episodes per hour) in the last illustration. The postprandial observation for the barium study, however, and the ability to detect nonacidic reflux, are the most likely reasons for the greater frequency of reflux episodes detected during fluoroscopy. (*Data from* Cleveland *et al.* [30].)

■ PRESENTING SYMPTOMS

Regurgitation and failure to thrive

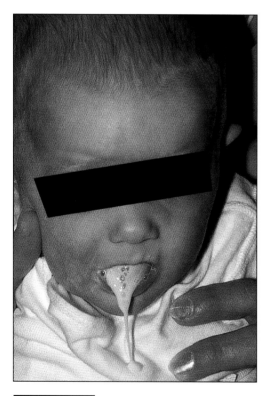

FIGURE 4-12.

Regurgitation is the most prominent presenting symptom of reflux disease in young children. This is in contrast with older children and adults, for whom "heartburn" is the most common symptom.

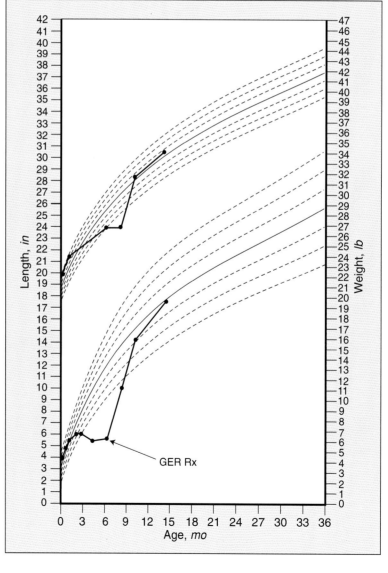

FIGURE 4-13.

Failure to thrive and poor weight gain, eventually affecting height percentiles, are the result of regurgitant reflux. The child whose data are shown gained weight well for the first 2 months and then had regurgitation causing caloric losses and no weight gain for the next 4 months. At that point (GER Rx), aggressive management of the child's reflux permitted catch-up weight gain, returning her to her previous percentiles during the next 4 to 6 months. Typically, her plateau of height gain lagged behind the weight plateau, both as her gastroesophageal reflux disease was developing and as it was treated. GER—gastroesophageal reflux.

Stimulation of central vomiting center:
Drugs; toxins
Metabolic disease
Diabetic ketoacidosis, diabetes insipidus, lactic acidosis, adrenal insufficiency
Phenylketonuria, maple-syrup-urine disease, methylmalonic acidemia
Hereditary fructose intolerance, galactosemia, tyrosinemia
Hyperammonemia, Reye's syndrome, fatty acid oxidation disorders
Uremia, renal tubular acidosis

Stimulation of supramedullary receptors:
Improper feeding and psychobehavioral problems
Overfeeding, air feeding, baby bouncing
Psychogenic, volitional
Vestibular disease, "motion sickness"
Increased intracranial pressure
Subdural effusion or hematoma
Hydrocephalus
Cerebral edema or tumor
Meningoencephalitis, Reye's syndrome

Stimulation of peripheral receptors:
Pharyngeal: gag reflex sinusitis post-nasal drip
Esophageal (nonreflux)
Obstruction—stricture, ring, stenosis, foreign body
Dysmotility—esophageal body dysmotility, achalasia
Gastric
Obstruction—pyloric stenosis, web, foreign body, bezoar
Dysmotility—impaired gastric emptying
Peptic ulcer disease
Intestinal
Infection, enterotoxin, appendicitis
Allergy—cow's milk, soy, eosinophilic gastroenteritis
Obstruction
Web, stenosis, superior mesenteric artery syndrome
Volvulus, Intussusception
Adhesions
Meconium ileus, meconium plug, Hirschsprung's disease
Hepatobiliary: hepatitis, cholecystitis
Pancreatic: pancreatitis
Urinary: urinary infection, pyelonephritis
Generalized: sepsis, peritonitis

TABLE 4-2.

Differential diagnosis of regurgitation and vomiting. Although regurgitant reflux is often recognized clinically, caution must be exercised to avoid missing other causes for the vomiting. (*Adapted from* Orenstein [26].)

Esophagitis symptoms

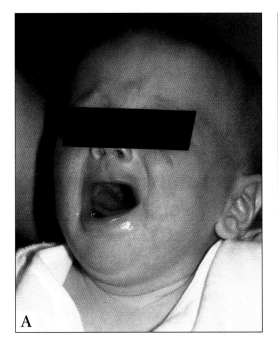

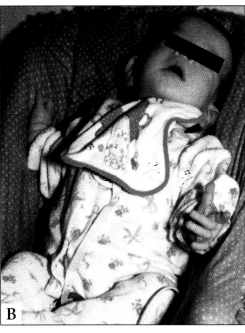

FIGURE 4-14.

Symptoms of infantile reflux esophagitis. **A,** "Crying and irritability," commonly believed to be a sensitive indicator of esophagitis in infants, occur in most, but not all, such infants with esophagitis, but also in many infants without esophagitis. **B,** "Arching" (torso hyperextension) occurs in infants with esophagitis in a proportion similar to that of those with crying and irritability, but is far more specifically diagnostic for esophagitis than crying.

(*continued on next page*)

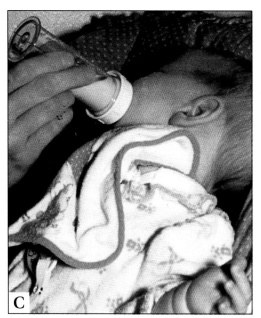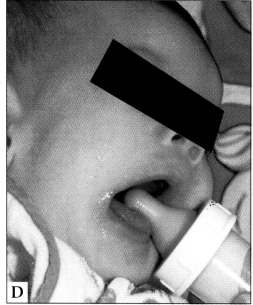

FIGURE 4-14. (CONTINUED)

C, "Refusing feedings even when hungry" occurs in slightly less than half of infants with esophagitis but occurs so infrequently in infants without esophagitis that it is fairly specific. D, "Gagging and choking on feedings" also occurs somewhat more frequently in infants with esophagitis than those without, although not significantly so [26].

TABLE 4-3. SYMPTOMS OF INFANTILE REFLUX ESOPHAGITIS

	ARCHING	REFUSAL OF FEEDINGS	CHOKING OR GAGGING	REGURGITATION	FUSSINESS
Esophagitis* (n=20)	55	40	55	80	55
Normals* (n=20)	20	15	30	70	55
P <	.05	.10	Not significant	Not significant	Not significant
Sensitivity	.55	.40	.55	.80	55
Specificity	.80	.85	.70	.30	.45

*Data represent infants positive for the symptom, %.

TABLE 4-3.

Questionnaire data on symptoms of infantile reflux esophagitis. Of symptomatic infants evaluated for histologic esophagitis, 20 had completely normal esophageal biopsies and 20 had definite esophagitis. Questionnaire data [25] on these 20 normal infants and 20 infants with esophagitis were contrasted by χ^2 test to determine the utility of various symptoms for predicting esophagitis [31]. Sensitivity and specificity of the symptoms were calculated. Although regurgitation is sensitive for esophagitis, it is nonspecific because of the number of regurgitating infants who do not have esophagitis. In contrast, arching, refusal of feedings even when hungry, and choking or gagging on feedings were not very sensitive but were more specific indicators of esophagitis. Fussiness and irritability, although often considered an important symptom of esophagitis in infants, were not very sensitive or specific. (*From* Orenstein *et al.* [31]; with permission.)

TABLE 4-4. DIFFERENTIAL DIAGNOSIS OF IRRITABILITY AND PAIN FROM ESOPHAGITIS

Infants: Nonspecific irritability
   "Colic"
   Parent-infant dysfunction
   Nutrient intolerance
   Otitis
   Urinary tract infection
   Miscellaneous other causes

Older children: Chest or epigastric pain or dysphagia
   Cardiac pain
   Pulmonary, mediastinal, chest wall pain
     (eg, costrochondritis)
   Nonesophagitis upper gastrointestinal inflammation
     Peptic ulcer disease
     Pancreatitis
     Hepatitis, cholangitis, cholecystitis, cholelithiasis
   Nonesophagitis dysphagia
   Functional, malingering

TABLE 4-4.

Differential diagnosis of irritability and pain. In infants, irritability has a wide diversity of causes, including esophagitis. In older children, who can describe chest pain, epigastric pain, or dysphagia, the differential diagnosis is narrower but remains important. (*Adapted from* Orenstein [25].)

TABLE 4-5. SYMPTOMS AND COMPLICATIONS OF ESOPHAGITIS

"Heartburn," odynophagia

Hematemesis, hemoccult-positive stools, anemia

Stricture

Barrett's metaplastic epithelium
    (especially intestinal)

Adenocarcinoma

TABLE 4-5.

Symptoms and complications of esophagitis. Esophagitis may be manifest in older children by complaints of heartburn or odynophagia. Hematemesis or subtler manifestations of chronic erosive esophagitis, such as anemia or hemoccult positive stools, occurs occasionally. Chronic severe reflux damage may result in esophageal strictures (*see* Fig. 4-31); occasionally these children will have no complaints referable to esophagitis until their esophageal lumen is obstructed. Chronic mucosal damage by refluxate may also result in intestinal or gastric metaplasia of the epithelium—Barrett's esophagus. These epithelial changes may coexist with reflux strictures or be independent of them. Recent data suggest that only the intestinal metaplasia (with goblet cells and brush border) has malignant potential; esophageal gastric metaplasia must be distinguished from hiatal herniation and "inlet patch" in any case. Barrett's metaplasia warrants aggressive management, and although very rarely in children, Barrett's metaplasia *has* progressed to adenocarcinoma.

Respiratory symptoms

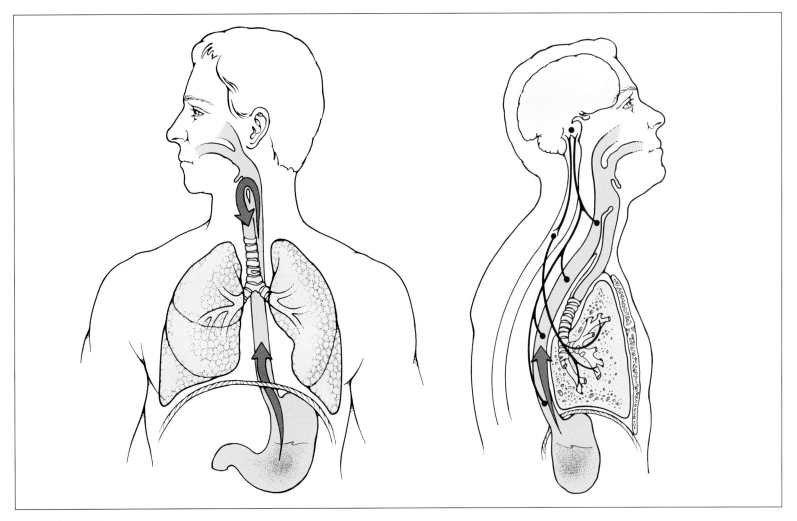

FIGURE 4-15.

Dualistic view of the pathophysiology of reflux-mediated respiratory disease: aspiration versus esophagorespiratory reflexes. Initially, the link between reflux and the respiratory diseases it seemed to provoke was presumed to be aspiration; subsequently vagal reflexes with esophageal afferents and pulmonary efferents were identified. (*Adapted from* Barish *et al.* [32].)

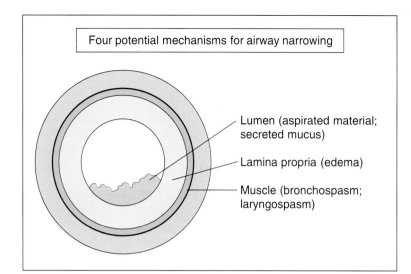

Four potential mechanisms for airway narrowing

Lumen (aspirated material; secreted mucus)

Lamina propria (edema)

Muscle (bronchospasm; laryngospasm)

FIGURE 4-16.

Four potential mechanisms for airway narrowing. This diagram illustrates possible sites for narrowing of the lower airway (producing asthma, cough, or pneumonia) or the upper airway (producing stridor or apnea) [33]. Aspirated or secreted material, edema, or muscular spasm may each be a locus of airway obstruction. (*Adapted from* Putnam *et al.* [33].)

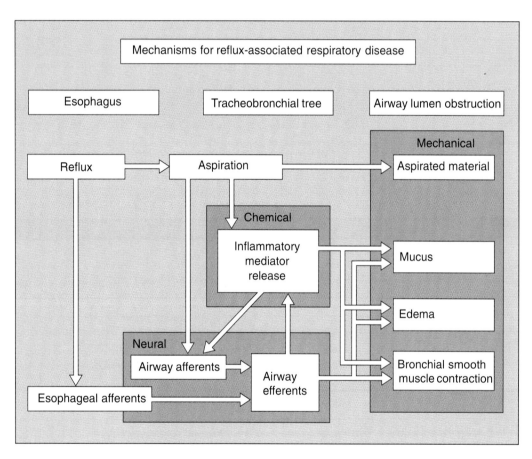

Mechanisms for reflux-associated respiratory disease

Esophagus

Tracheobronchial tree

Airway lumen obstruction

Reflux

Aspiration

Mechanical

Aspirated material

Chemical

Inflammatory mediator release

Mucus

Edema

Neural

Airway afferents

Airway efferents

Bronchial smooth muscle contraction

Esophageal afferents

FIGURE 4-17.

A more complex schematic of the pathophysiology of reflux-mediated respiratory disease. This diagram illustrates a more complex view of the interactions between reflux and respiratory disease [33]. The right panel "airway lumen obstruction," has the same four loci of obstruction discussed in Fig. 4-16. On the left, reflux is shown to stimulate esophageal afferents or to cause obstruction of the tracheobronchial tree directly by aspiration. Now, however, more has been described of the likely neural and chemical mediators between the esophageal afferents and the lumen obstruction by mucus, edema, or muscle spasm, and similarly between the aspirated material and lumen obstruction; these interactions are illustrated. (*Adapted from* Putnam *et al.* [33]; with permission.)

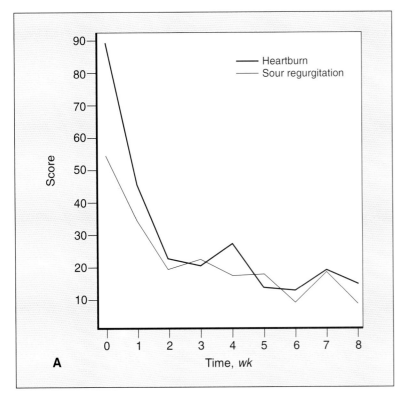

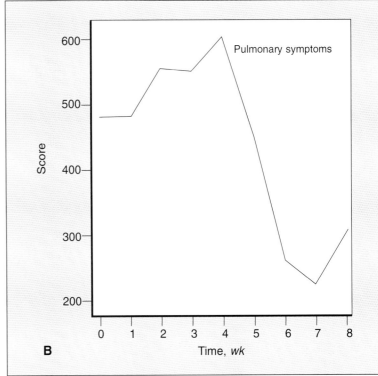

FIGURE 4-18.

Reflux-mediated bronchospasm (asthma). Reflux has been implicated as contributing to asthma in a subset of children. It should be considered particularly in those who do not have a prominent atopic component, who have symptoms of reflux (*eg*, heartburn), who have a prominent nocturnal component, or who have inadequate response to standard asthma treatment. Steroid-dependent asthmatic patients, in particular, have much to gain from the clinician's considering reflux as a potential contributor. Studies have suggested that esophagitis may be a prerequisite and that reflux-associated bronchospasm may require particularly aggressive therapy of the reflux. In adults a course of antireflux therapy induces a more rapid response of the esophagitis symptoms (**A**) than the respiratory symptoms (**B**). Respiratory symptoms lasted 5 or 6 weeks before any improvement was detected and continued to improve for at least several weeks after that. (*Adapted from* Harper *et al.* [34].)

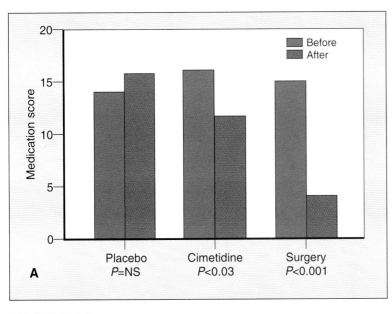

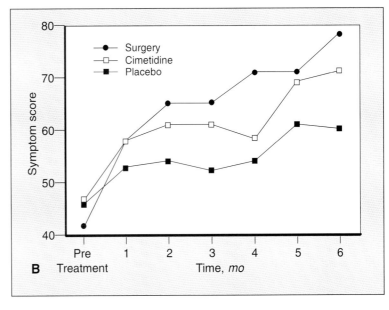

FIGURE 4-19.

Medical and surgical therapy for reflux-associated asthma. Another study in adults demonstrates better improvement in asthma after fundoplication than after pharmacotherapy (**A** and **B**) and that improvement after both sorts of therapy continued to increase up to at least 6 months (**B**) [34]. Higher scores are *less* symptomic. These data provide the impetus for aggressive and prolonged therapy of reflux in asthmatic children: a course of 6 months of cisapride plus omeprazole prior to reassessment could be justified. NS—not significant. (*Adapted from* Larrain *et al.* [35].)

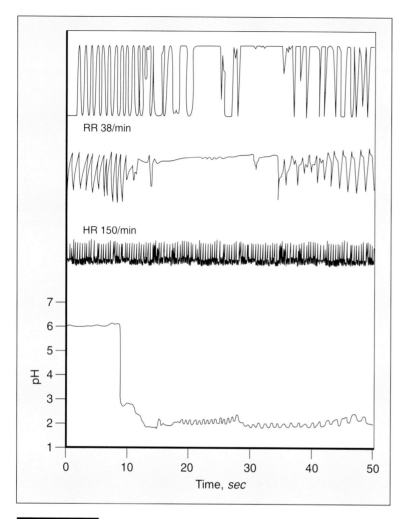

DIAGNOSIS	N	%
Known cause		
Digestive	1107	47
Gastroesophageal reflux	770	20
Infection	152	
Aspiration	105	
Malformations	75	
Dumping syndrome	5	
Neurologic	683	29
Vasovagal syndrome	376	
Epilepsy	150	
Infection	150	
Subdural hematoma	5	
Malformation	2	
Respiratory	353	15
Infection	275	
Airway abnormality	74	
Alveolar hypoventilation	4	
Cardiovascular	82	3.5
Infection	35	
Cardiomyopathy	18	
Arrhythmia	18	
Congenital malformation	11	
Metabolic and Endocrine	59	2.5
Hypoglycemia	23	
Hypocalcemia	12	
Food intolerance	10	
Reye's syndrome	6	
Hypothyroidism	2	
Nonesterified fatty acid metabolism deficiency	2	
Leigh's syndrome	1	
Carnitine	1	
Menke's syndrome	1	
Fructosemia	1	
Miscellaneous	71	3
Accidents	39	
Sepsis	11	
Munchausen's syndrome	8	
Nutritional error	7	
Drug effect	6	
Total	2355	62
Unknown cause		
Apparently minor incident	874	23
Apparently severe incident (idiopathic ALTE)	570	15
Total	1444	38

FIGURE 4-20.

Reflux-mediated apnea. In infants, obstructive apnea, characterized by cessation of air flow (second channel from top—nasal thermistor) during persisting chest wall movement (first channel—impedance pneumotachogram) has been shown by many types of studies to be provoked by spontaneous gastroesophageal reflux (fourth channel–distal esophageal pH probe) [36]. It is as yet uncertain whether the refluxate must be acidic to provoke the response, and whether the afferents are laryngeal or can be esophageal, and whether esophagitis must be present for esophageal afferents to provoke the laryngospasm. (*Adapted from* Herbst *et al.* [36].)

TABLE 4-6.

Differential diagnosis of infantile apnea or an acute life-threatening event (ALTE). Because the diagnosis of apnea caused by reflux is usually presumptive, care must be taken to keep the broad differential diagnosis in mind. This table gives the relative frequencies of etiologies in 3799 infants who were carefully and systematically evaluated. (*Modified from* Kahn *et al.* [37].)

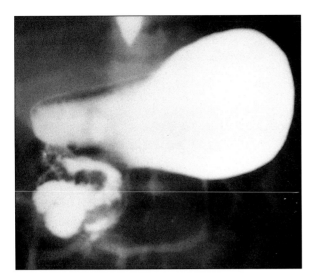

FIGURE 4-32.

Differential diagnosis of infantile vomiting—malrotation. The reflux episode in Fig. 4-27 occurred in this baby with malrotation shortly before her death from volvulus. The differential diagnosis of infantile vomiting (*see* Table 4-2) includes potentially lethal metabolic and anatomic disorders that must be distinguished from simple gastroesophageal reflux. This differentiation is made more difficult by the projectile character of reflux in some infants.

Scintigraphy

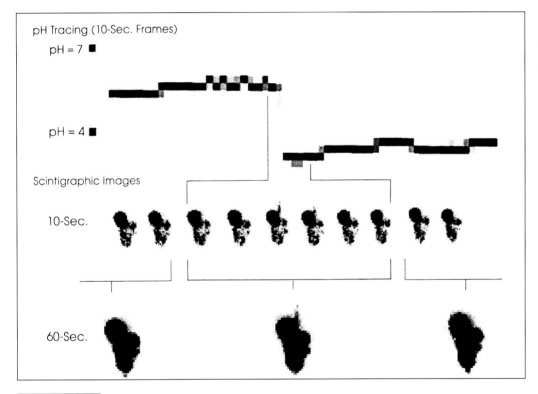

FIGURE 4-33.

Relationships between scintigraphic and pH probe studies. The central image at the bottom of the figure is a posterior view of a child's gastrointestinal tract during a scintigraphic study after a feeding of technetium 99m-labeled apple juice (half-life ~6hr) [56]. It shows labeled refluxate in the esophagus, which is absent from the images just before (to the left) and just after (to the right). These images, obtained by continuous gamma camera monitoring during three contiguous 60-second periods, can be compared with those above, which represent the 10-second segments making up the 60-second periods. These briefer images show that the bulk of the refluxate was in the esophagus only during the central 20 seconds of the 60 seconds represented by the bottom central image. A simultaneous distal esophageal pH probe study was also transmitted into the gamma camera's computer and is displayed by the coarse points (each representing 10 seconds) in the top channel. The distal esophageal pH is initially above 5, corresponding to the first two images in the row directly below, and to the

first single image in the bottom row. Halfway across the figure, the pH abruptly drops to below 4, representing acidic reflux entering the distal esophagus. The six central bracketed 10-second images just below correspond to the six points surrounding this moment of reflux. Although the scintigraphically-imaged volume of refluxate and the pH-probe– imaged acidity of refluxate began simultaneously in this example, it can be seen that the volume of the reflux is cleared within 20 seconds, whereas the residual acid has not been cleared to above pH 4 even by the far right of the figure, several minutes later. Other authors have also compared simultaneous pH probe and scintigraphic representations of gastroesophageal reflux in children [57,58]. Such scintigraphic studies are capable of imaging the gastrointestinal tract for hours while the technetium remains detectable, generating time-activity curves of "condensed dynamic images" [59] of the esophagus and stomach; however, the logistic issue of controlling for patient movement in these prolonged computerized analyses makes simple images more practical for children. Techniques differ greatly among institutions; one should beware of "diagnosing reflux" on the basis of an image or two disclosing reflux episodes—they are not specific for reflux disease. Scintigraphy can also document delayed gastric emptying (consider the type of food given and the source of the normal values used) [60–64] and aspiration (although it is insensitive, like most methods) [65–68]. (*Adapted from* Orenstein *et al.* [56]; with permission.)

Endoscopy

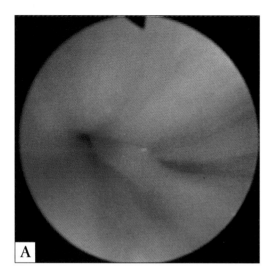

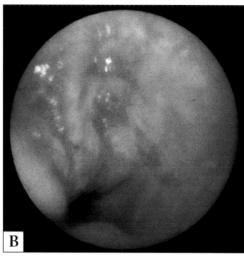

FIGURE 4-34.

Endoscopic view of normal esophageal mucosa and erosive esophagitis in two children. **A,** The smooth pink mucosa of the normal esophagus contrasts with **B,** The eroded, bleeding mucosa of the esophagus with severe esophagitis. Histologic esophagitis may be present even in endoscopically normal-appearing mucosa, and subtle changes including erythema, formerly considered to represent mild endoscopic esophagitis, have been found to be nonspecific, at least in children [69]. Histologic samples should be taken during endoscopic evaluation to increase the sensitivity and specificity of the findings. (*From* Orenstein [55]; with permission.)

Histology

TABLE 4-8. HISTOLOGIC MARKERS FOR ESOPHAGITIS

MARKER	NORMAL (N=6)	ESOPHAGITIS (N=27)
Basal cell thickness	< 25%	39 ± 7%
Papillary height	< 53%	53 ± 10%
Epithelial eosinophils	0%	> 0 in 7/27
Epithelial neutrophils	0%	> 0 in 4/27

TABLE 4-8.

Normal values for histologic assessment of reflux esophagitis. Contrasting values for several parameters in infants with reflux esophagitis with those in normal infants who died suddenly in accidents gives normal ranges comparable with those determined in normal adults. (*Data from* Black *et al.* [71].)

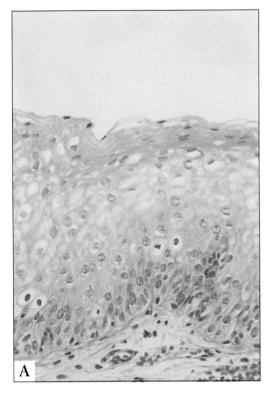

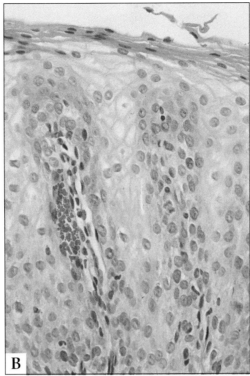

FIGURE 4-35.

Examples of normal esophageal histology and esophagitis as defined by morphometric changes in two infants. **A,** Normal esophageal epithelium from a 2-month-old boy evaluated because of bronchospasm; the basal layer is less than 20% of the total epithelial height and the papilla are clearly less than 50% of the height. **B,** An esophageal biopsy from a 5-month-old boy with vomiting, cough, and failure to thrive, in which the papillae are about 90% of the total epithelial height and the basal layer is about as tall as the papillae. (Original magnification × 200.)

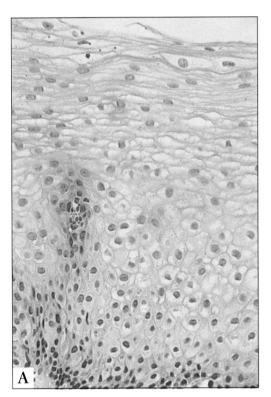

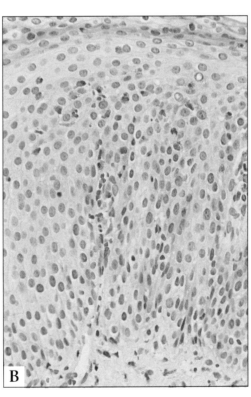

FIGURE 4-36.

Examples of normal esophageal histology and esophagitis marked by inflammatory infiltrates in two older infants. **A,** Normal epithelium from a 14-month-old with apnea and choking during feedings. **B,** Marked esophagitis with basal layer and papillae extending nearly to the lumenal margin and with prominent infiltration by eosinophils, from a 10-month-old girl with emesis, failure to thrive, and refusal to eat. (Original magnification × 200.) (*From* Orenstein [55]; with permission.)

Symptom-based algorithms for use of diagnostic techniques in infants

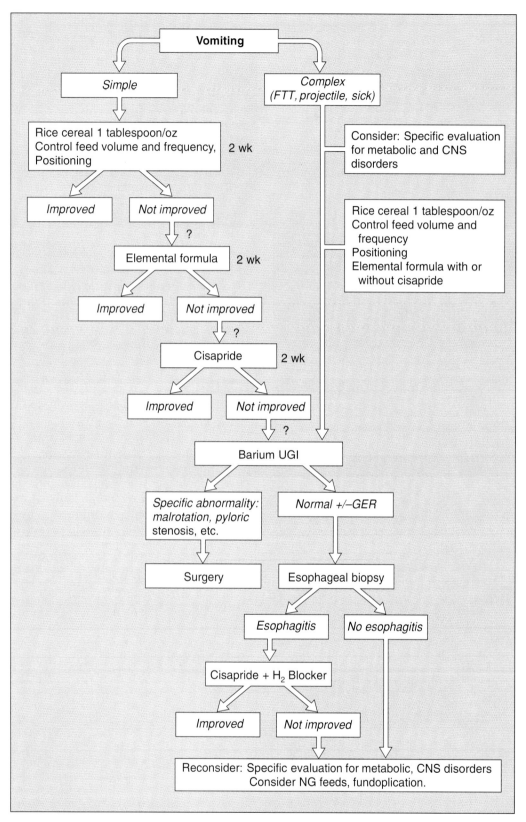

FIGURE 4-37.

Diagnosis of reflux disease in the vomiting infant. This algorhithm illustrates one possible way to approach the infant whose vomiting suggests gastroesophageal reflux (GER) as the cause. Vomiting without weight loss, irritability, or projectile quality is termed *simple vomiting* (*ie*, regurgitation—it is not "vomiting" as strictly defined), and can be approached with trials of empiric therapy, initially comprised of "conservative" antireflux therapy, then adding an elemental formula (Pregestimil [Mead Johnson] or Alimentum [Ross]) for 2 weeks to address the issue of formula protein intolerance or allergy. A therapeutic trial of cisapride before investigations may be useful, even in an infant who is otherwise well and thriving. Infants who fail to improve after this degree of empiric therapy and infants who present with "complex" vomiting should be evaluated radiographically to exclude structural abnormalities that may require surgical therapy. In complex vomiting, while awaiting the radiographic results, evaluation for metabolic or neurologic disease, as well as empiric use of elemental formula and "conservative" antireflux therapy should be considered. If the results of the barium study do not show any abnormality other than reflux, I use esophageal histology to determine whether to add acid suppression to the prokinetic agent. The absence of esophagitis or the failure to respond to optimal pharmacotherapy suggests the need to reconsider other primary etiologies. CNS—central nervous system; FTT—failure to thrive; NG—nasogastric tube; UGI—upper gastrointestinal radiography.

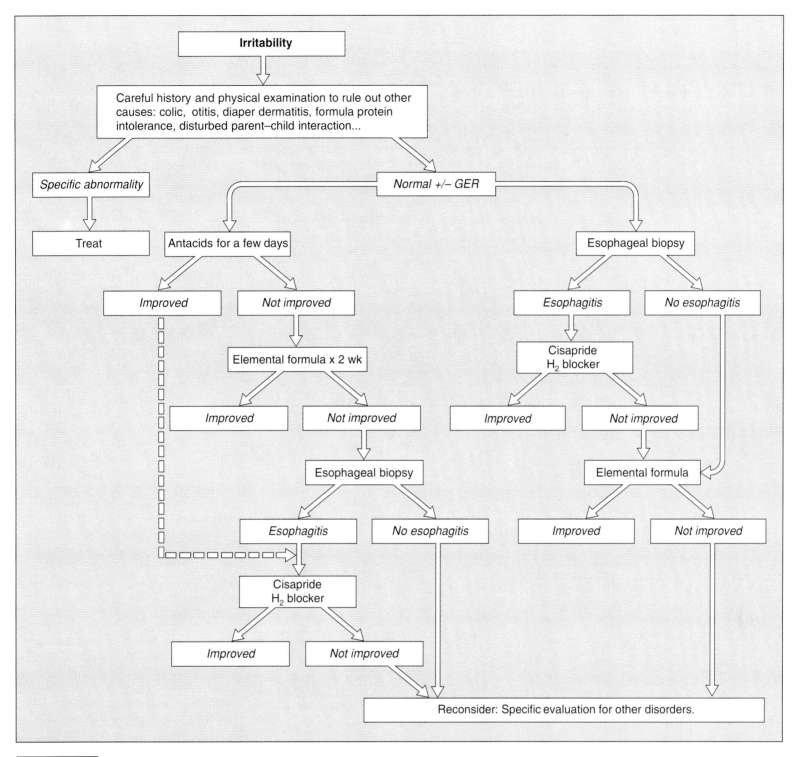

FIGURE 4-38.

Diagnosis of reflux disease in the irritable infant. The irritable infant is often described as having "colic," but many are also suspected of having esophagitis. The clinician should beware of early closure on the diagnosis of esophagitis. If esophagitis is still suspected after careful history and physical examination, there are two different strategies. The first uses a simple blind esophageal suction biopsy to confirm or deny esophagitis and to dictate its therapy with acid suppression and prokinetic therapy; the second strategy uses brief empiric therapy with antacids to suggest whether more prolonged empiric therapy with acid suppression and a prokinetic agent are warranted. Trials of elemental formula to treat formula protein intolerance or allergy remain prominent in both schematics; I have seen a fair number of infants with symptoms strongly suggesting that reflux esophagitis responds to this therapy.

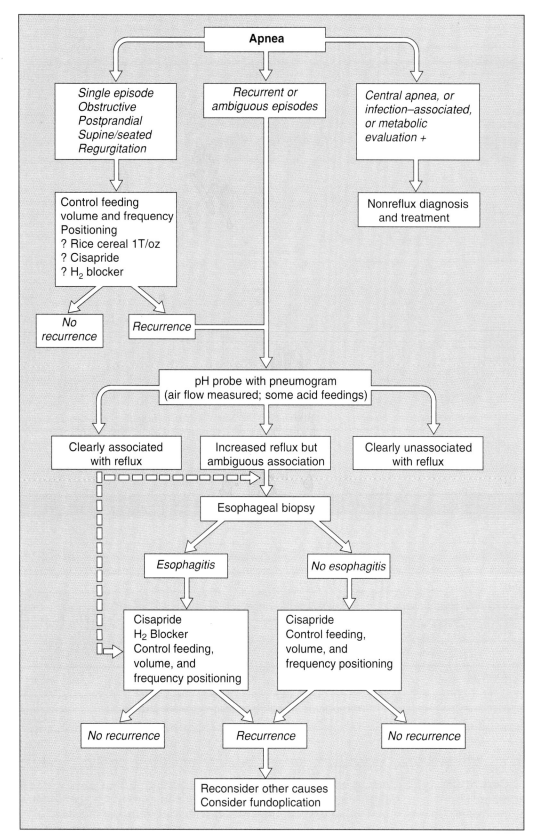

FIGURE 4-39.

Diagnosis of reflux disease in the infant with apnea. Apnea is a difficult symptom to evaluate: the history is often garbled by the frantic parent; events of it are rare and recurrences unpredictable, and the differential diagnosis is broad (*see* Fig. 4-21). The diagnosis of the cause of single episodes often rests largely on the history. Single episodes that appear obstructive (*ie*, respiratory efforts seem to continue; the baby may be stiff and struggling to breathe), occur within the hour after feeding, and that occur in positions provocative for reflux (supine or seated) are often reflux-related, particularly when regurgitation through the mouth or nose accompanies the episode. If the historical evidence for reflux is great, conservative therapy and (possibly) pharmacotherapy could be instituted without formal evaluation for reflux disease. In contrast, apnea that appears clearly "central" (*ie*, the baby seems initially limp and "forgetting to breathe"), or apnea in a baby who appears ill from possible infectious or metabolic disease, requires that the nonreflux etiology be evaluated and treated. The most difficult apneas are the recurrent or ambiguous episodes; their etiology may be clarified by the use of a pH probe linked to a pneumocardiogram (which must include a measure of air flow such as a nasal thermistor or end tidal CO_2) during a 24-hour study in which at least some acid feedings (*eg*, apple juice) are used to permit detection of postprandial reflux. If such study clarifies that reflux episodes precede apnea, conservative therapy and use of a prokinetic agent are warranted and acid suppression probably is as well, although one might demand that esophagitis be documented before adding acid suppression to therapy. Episodes of presumed reflux–associated apnea recurring on maximal medical therapy mandate reconsideration of other causes as well as consideration of fundoplication. Parents of all babies who have had an apnea should receive instruction in infant cardiopulmonary resuscitation; the benefit of monitoring in these babies is controversial.

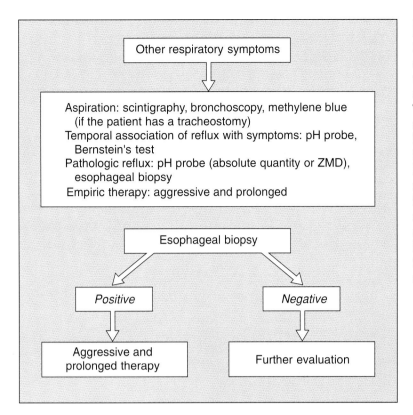

Figure 4-40.

Diagnosis of reflux disease in the infant with other respiratory symptoms. This collection of symptoms does not readily lend itself to depiction in a flow diagram. The presentations are too diverse, and the diagnostic tests too varied, to present a simple approach. Thus, this diagram simply indicates the utilities of the various tests: scintigraphy, bronchoscopy, or methylene blue in the feedings of a baby with a tracheostomy are all used to diagnose aspiration. In the absence of immune deficiency or a history of ingestion, histologic esophagitis almost always indicates reflux disease and mandates therapy. Thus, esophageal histology comprises a useful initial test, particularly because many of the reflexive airway responses to gastroesophageal reflux may require a background of esophagitis to permit their occurrence. That therapy of reflux must be aggressive and prolonged when reflux is responsible for respiratory disease must also be kept in mind (*see* Figs. 4-18 and 4-19, and Table 4-7). ZMD—mean duration of reflux during sleep.

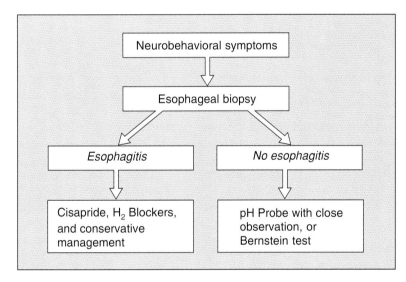

Figure 4-41.

Diagnosis of reflux disease in the infant with neurobehavioral symptoms. Again, and for similar reasons, evaluating esophageal histology provides a useful starting point. If esophagitis is not present and the symptoms are frequent, a pH probe with close observation for the symptom may be useful; alternatively, a modified Bernstein test may provide the same information more efficiently.

TABLE 4-9. COST-EFFECTIVENESS CONSIDERATIONS IN THE DESIGN OF DIAGNOSTIC STRATEGIES (CHARGES AT CHILDREN'S HOSPITAL OF PITTSBURGH; SUBJECTIVE ESTIMATES OF RISKS AND EFFECTIVENESS)

DIAGNOSTIC TOOL	COST			EFFECTIVENESS (+ TO ++++)			
	$ (5 KG PATIENT)	TIME STAFF/PATIENT	RISK, DISCOMFORT	SENSITIVITY	SPECIFICITY	POSITIVE PV	NEGATIVE PV
Empiric therapy							
Positioning and milk thickening × 2 mo	<15	min/hr*	0	++	++		
Cimetidine × 2 mo	25	min/hr*	1	++	++		
Cisapride × 2 mo	100	min/hr*	1	++	++		
Imaging							
Fluoroscopy (UGI)	550	hr/hrs	1.5	++	+++		
Scintigraphy	1000	hr/hrs	1.2	+	++		
Histology							
Endoscopy and biopsy	2200-3300	hr/hrs	3	0.25 of Bx	+++		0.3 of Bx
Blind suction biopsy	1300†	mins/min	1.5	+++	+++		
Detection of acid							
pH probe	1400	hrs/day	2	++++	++		
Specialized							
pH probe and pneumogram	2200	hrs/day	2	++	+++		
Modified Bernstein's test	400	hr/hrs	1	+	+++		
Methylene blue NG feeds	10	min/hr	0	+	++++		

*Thickening of formula and avoidance of prone or seated position for 2 months. Time to diagnosis is much longer than the time to do the test: days to weeks if positive diagnosis; indefinite if negative.
†Paid lower, if at all, currently.

TABLE 4-9.

Cost-effectiveness considerations in the design of diagnostic strategies with estimates of the costs and efficacies of various diagnostic tools. Costs include staff and patient time as well as risks of morbidity and discomfort on a noneconomic basis. Effectiveness is estimated in terms of sensitivity and specificity for the diagnosis of gastro-esophageal reflux disease; specific data regarding sensitivity and negative predictive value are available only for endoscopic biopsy compared with suction biopsy. The roles of empiric therapy and suction biopsy may be greater in the future than they have been thus far; in contrast, there may in the future be less use for pH probes and for endoscopic evaluation of infantile esophagitis. PV—predicted value; Bx—biopsy; NG—nasogastric; UGI—upper gastrointestinal.

TABLE 4-10. THERAPY FOR GASTROESOPHAGEAL REFLUX DISEASE

I. Conservative

    A. Position—prone, or completely upright (avoid supine, seated)

    B. Thicken infant feedings—1 T of dry rice cereal/oz of formula
        (= 30 cal/oz, if original formula is 20 cal/oz)

    C. Fast before bed

    D. Avoid large meals, obesity, tight clothing

    E. Avoid foods and medications which lower LES tone, delay
        gastric emptying, or increase gastric acidity

        1. Fatty foods, citrus, tomato, carbonated beverages, coffee,
           alcohol, smoke exposure

        2. Anticholinergics, adrenergics, xanthines (theophylline,
           caffeine), calcium channel blockers, prostaglandins

II. Pharmacologic*

    A. Prokinetic

        1. Metoclopramide (0.1 mg/kg/dose qid: 0–30 min AC, HS)
           {restlessness, drowsiness, dystonic reactions—antidote:
           diphenhydramine}
           {{gastrointestinal obstruction, perforation, hemorrhage;
           pheochromocytoma; extrapyramidal risk}}

        2. Bethanechol (0.1–0.3 mg/kg/dose tid or qid: 30–60 min AC, HS)
           {cholinergic—hypotension, flushing, headache,
           bronchospasm, salivation, abdominal cramping}
           {{urinary or gastrointestinal obstruction, perforation, hemorrhage,
           recent surgery, peritonitis; hypotension; bradycardia;
           epilepsy; asthma; hyperthyroidism; peptic ulcer}}

        3. Domperidone (0.2–0.3–?0.6 mg/kg/dose tid or qid: AC, HS)
           {drug not available in United States}

        4. Cisapride (0.2–0.3 mg/kg/dose tid-qid: 0–30 min AC, HS)
           {diarrhea; cardiac arrhythmias}
           {{concurrent treatment with erythromycin, fluconozole, and
           related antibiotics may provoke fatal arrhythmias}}

B. Anti-acid

    1. Cimetidine (5–10 mg/kg/dose qid: AC, HS)
       {headache, confusion, pancytopenia, gynecomastia,
       cholestasis}

    2. Ranitidine (2–5 mg/kg/dose bid–tid)
       {similar to cimetidine, less gynecomastia, more hepatitis}

    3. Famotidine, nizatidine (incompletely defined for children;
       adult 40 mg HS, 300 mg HS, respectively)

    4. Omeprazole (adult 20 mg qam; pediatric 0.6 mg/kg/dose qam)

    5. Antacids (0.5–1.0 mL/kg/dose, 3–8x a day: 1–2 hr PC, HS)
       {diarrhea, constipation, hypophosphatemia, hypercalcemia}

C. Barrier or miscellaneous mechanism

    1. Sucralfate slurry (1 g in 5–15 mL solution, qid: PC, HS)—
       protects against bile salts, trypsin, acid
       {constipation, gastric concretions, potential binding of other
       medications}

    2. Alginic acid–antacid (2 g 3–8x a day: PC)

III. Surgical

    A. Fundoplication (complete vs loose wrap; ± gastrostomy,
       ± pyloroplasty)

    B. Gastrojejunostomy feedings

---

*Usual initial course is 8 weeks.
() = common doses; {} = partial list of side effects; {{}} = partial list of contraindications.

TABLE 4-10.

Therapy for pediatric gastroesophageal reflux disease (GERD). Traditionally, therapeutic measures for GERD are divided into three categories: "conservative measures," pharmacotherapy, and surgical therapy. Specifics of these types of treatment are included in the table. AC—before meals; HS—before bed; LES—lower esophageal sphincter; PC—after meals; qam—each morning. (*Adapted from* Orenstein [26].)

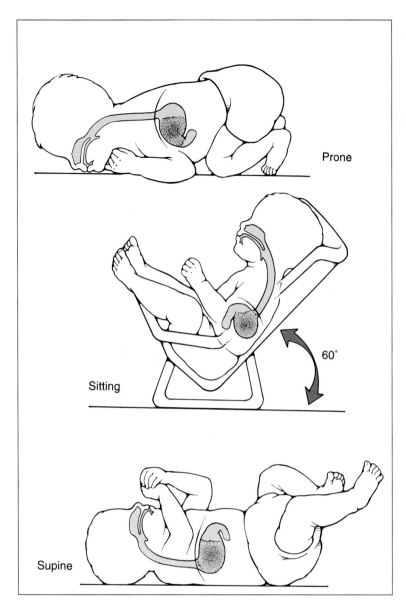

Prone

Sitting

60°

Supine

FIGURE 4-42.

Effects of positioning for infantile gastroesophageal reflux. This figure illustrates the effects of seated, prone, and supine positions on the air-to-fluid interface in the infant's stomach and provides a rationale for avoiding both supine and seated positions in infantile gastroesophageal reflux disease [72]. The effects diagrammed have also been demonstrated fluoroscopically [73,74]. (*Adapted from* Ramenofsky *et al.* [72].)

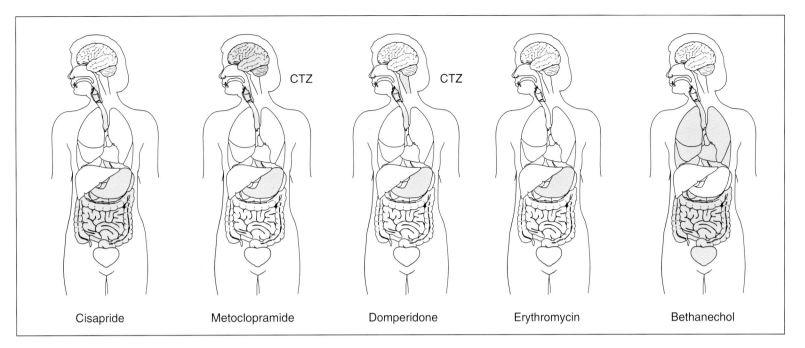

| Cisapride | Metoclopramide | Domperidone | Erythromycin | Bethanechol |

FIGURE 4-43.

Sites of action of five prokinetic agents. Four of these five agents have been used to treat gastroesophageal reflux disease in children; erythromycin's limited locus of action makes it unsuitable in comparison. Metoclopramide's central nervous system effects induce most of its side effects and make it a less favorable drug than cisapride, which is probably the optimal prokinetic at present. (*Adapted from* Hyman [74a]; with permission.)

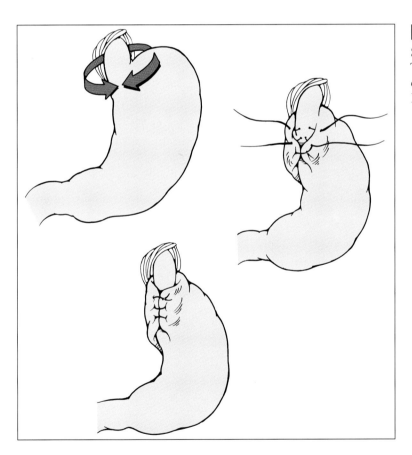

FIGURE 4-44.

Surgical therapy for gastroesophageal reflux disease: fundoplication. This diagram shows formation of a Nissen fundoplication, the most effective antireflux procedure [75]. (*see* Volume 3 on Stomach and Duodenum for more detail). (*Adapted from* Schatzlein *et al.* [75].)

TABLE 4-11. COST-EFFECTIVENESS CONSIDERATIONS IN THE DESIGN OF THERAPEUTIC STRATEGIES

Treatment	Cost			Effectiveness	
	$ (5 kg pt)	Time to start Rx	Risks	% Cure	Time to cure
Conservative Therapy					
Positioning and milk thickening × 2 mo	15	day	+	+	4–6 mo
Antacids × 2 mo	40	day	+	++	4–6 mo
Pharmacotherapy					
Cimetidine × 2 mo	25	day	++	+++	4–6 mo
Ranitidine × 2 mo	100	day	++	+++	4–6 mo
Cisapride × 2 mo	100	day	+	+++	4–6 mo
Metoclopramide × 2 mo	6	day	+++	++-	4–6 mo
Bethanechol × 2 mo	125	day	++	++-	4–6 mo
Surgical Therapy					
Fundoplication	10,000	week	++++	++++	week(s)
Miscellaneous Therapy					
Nasogastric drip feeds × 2 mo	?100	days	+++	?	?
Nasojejunal (elemental) feeds × 2 mo	1300 +350	week	+++	?	?

TABLE 4-11.

Cost-effectiveness considerations in the design of therapeutic strategies. Estimates of the costs and efficacies of various therapies for gastroesophageal reflux disease are shown. "Conservative" therapy is used for all patients with reflux disease and can be instituted even for infants with physiologic reflux if the parents desire. Pharmacotherapy is effective for nearly all children with reflux disease. The most useful prokinetic and acid suppressors for most patients are cisapride plus a histamine–H$_2$ receptor antagonist.

The low cost and dosing frequency, similar to that of prokinetic agents (four times daily), lead me to favor generic cimetidine as the antisecretory agent. Omeprazole is not included in the table because it is impractical for infants, although it has been used in older children with intractable symptoms or respiratory disease mandating aggressive therapy [76]. Tube feedings or surgery are reserved for the occasional patient whose disease remains intractable [77].

REFERENCES

1. Mittal R: The spincter mechanism at the lower end of the esophagus: An overview. *Dysphagia* 1993, 8:347–350.
2. Dent J, Davidson GP, Barnes BE, *et al.*: The mechanism of gastroesophagheal reflux in children. *Aust Paediatr J* 1981, 17:125.
3. Sloan S, Rademaker AW, Kahrilas PJ: Determinants of gastroesophageal junction incompetence: Hiatal hernia, lower esophageal sphincter, or both. *Ann Intern Med* 1992, 117:977–982.
4. Helm JF, Dodds WJ, Pelc LR, *et al.*: Effect of esophageal emptying and saliva on clearance of acid from the esophagus. *N Engl J Med* 1984, 310:284–288.
5. Sondheimer JM: Clearance of spontaneous gastroesophageal reflux in awake and sleeping infants. *Gastroenterology* 1989, 97:821–826.
6. Gill RC, Bowes KL, Murphy PD, Kingma YJ: Esophageal motor abnormalities in gastroesophageal reflux and the effects of fundoplication. *Gastroenterology* 1986, 91:364–369.
7. Kahrilas P, Dodds W, Hogan W, *et al.*: Esophageal peristaltic dysfunction in peptic esophagitis. *Gastroenterology* 1986, 91:897–904.
8. Triadafilopoulos G, Castillo T: Nonpropulsive esophageal contractions and gastroesophageal reflux. *Am J Gastroenterol* 1991, 86:153–159.
9. Mahony M, Migliavacca M, Spitz L, Milla P: Motor disorders of the oesophagus in gastro-oesophageal reflux. *Arch Dis Child* 1988, 63:1333–1338.
10. Tovar J, Wang W, Eizaguirre I: Simultaneous gastroesophageal pH monitoring and the diagnosis of alkaline reflux. *J Pediatr Surg* 1993, 28:1386–1392.
11. Stein H, Feussner H, Kauer W, *et al.*: Alkaline gastroesophageal reflux: Assessment by ambulatory esophageal aspiration and pH monitoring. *Am J Surg* 1994, 167:163–168.
12. Stein HJ, Barlow AP, DeMeester TR, Hinder RA: Complications of gastroesophageal reflux disease: Role of the lower esophageal sphincter, esophageal acid and acid/alkaline exposure, and duodenogastric reflux. *Ann Surg* 1992, 216:35–43.
13. Vandenplas Y, Loeb H: Alkaline gastroesophageal reflux in infancy. *J Pediatr Gastroenterol Nutr* 1991, 12:448–452.

14. Malthaner R, Newman K, Parry R, *et al.*: Alkaline gastroesophageal reflux in infants and children. *J Pediatr Surg* 1991, 26:986–991.

15. Orlando R: Esophageal epithelial defenses against acid injury. *Am J Gastroenterol* 1994, 89:S48–S52.

16. Kahrilas P, Dodds W, Dent J, *et al.*: Effect of sleep, spontaneous gastroesophageal reflux, and a meal on upper esophageal sphincter pressure in normal human volunteers. *Gastroenterology* 1987, 92:466–471.

17. Lang I, Shaker R: An update on the physiology of the components of the upper esophageal sphincter. *Dysphagia* 1994, 9:229–232.

18. Shaker R, Ren J, Kern M, *et al.*: Mechanisms of airway protection and upper esophageal sphincter opening during belching. *Am J Physiol* 1992, 262:G621–G628.

19. Sondheimer JM: Upper esophageal sphincter and pharyngoesophageal motor function in infants with and without gastroesophageal reflux. *Gastroenterology* 1983, 85:301–305.

20. Staiano A, Cucchiara S, De VB, *et al.*: Disorders of upper esophageal sphincter motility in children. *J Pediatr Gastroenterol Nutr* 1987, 6:892–898.

21. Winship D: Upper esophageal sphincter: Does it care about reflux? *Gastroenterology* 1983, 85:470–472.

22. Werlin SL, Dodds WJ, Hogan WJ, Arndorfer RC: Mechanisms of gastroesophageal reflux in children. *J Pediatr* 1980, 97:244–249.

23. Orenstein S, Dent J, Deneault L, *et al.*: Regurgitant reflux vs. non-regurgitant reflux, is preceded by rectus abdominis contraction in infants. *Neurogastroenterol Mot* 1994, 6:271–277.

24. Orenstein S: Gastroesophageal reflux. In *Pediatric Gastrointestinal Motility, Clinical Spectra of Chronic Enteric Neuromuscular Disorders.* Edited by Hyman P, DiLorenzo C. New York: Academy Professional Information Services, Inc.; 1994; 55–88.

25. Orenstein SR, Shalaby TM, Cohn JF: Gastroesophageal reflux symptoms in 100 normals: Diagnostic validity of the Infant Gastrointestinal Reflux Questionnaire [abstract]. *J Pediatr Gastroenterol Nutr* 1995, 21:333.

26. Orenstein SR, Cohn JF, Shalaby TM, Kartan R: Reliability and validity of an infant gastroesophageal reflux questionnaire. *Clin Pediatr* 1993, 32:472–484.

27. Orenstein SR: Gastroesophageal reflux. *Curr Probl Pediatr* 1991, 193–241.

28. Vandenplas Y, Sacre-Smits L: Continuous 24-hour esophageal pH monitoring in 285 asymptomatic infants 0–15 months old. *J Pediatr Gastroenterol Nutr* 1987, 6:220–224.

29. Johnson L, DeMeester T: Twenty-four-hour pH monitoring of the distal esophagus: A quantitative measure of gastroesophageal reflux. *Am J Gastroenterol* 1974, 62:325–332.

30. Cleveland RH, Kushner DC, Schwartz AN: Gastroesophageal reflux in children: Results of a standardized fluoroscopic approach. *Am J Roentgenol* 1983, 141:53–56.

31. Orenstein S, Putnam P, Shalaby T, *et al.*: Symptoms of infantile reflux esophagitis, using validated techniques for symptoms and histopathology. *Gastroenterology* 1994, 106:A153.

32. Barish CF, Wu WC, Castell DO: Respiratory complications of gastroesophageal reflux. *Arch Intern Med* 1985, 145:1882–1888.

33. Putnam PE, Ricker DH, Orenstein SR: Gastroesophageal reflux. In *Respiratory Control Disorders in Infants and Children.* Edited by Beckerman R, Brouilette R, Hunt C. Baltimore: Williams & Wilkins; 1992: 322–341.

34. Harper P, Bergner A, Kaye M: Antireflux treatment for asthma: Improvement in patients with associated gastroesophageal reflux. *Arch Intern Med* 1987, 147:56–60.

35. Larrain A, Carrasco E, Galleguillos F, *et al*: Medical and surgical treatment of non-allergic asthma associated with gastroesophageal reflux. *Chest* 1991, 99:1330–1336.

36. Herbst JJ, Minton SD, Book LS: Gastroesophageal reflux causing respiratory distress and apnea in newborn infants. *J Pediatr* 1979, 95:763–768.

37. Kahn A, Rebuffat E, Franco P, *et al.*: Apparent life-threatening events and apnea of infancy. In *Respiratory Control Disorders in Infants and Children.* Edited by Beckerman R, Brouilette R, Hunt C. Baltimore: Williams & Wilkins; 1992:178–189.

38. Orenstein SR, Orenstein DM, Whitington PF: Gastroesophageal reflux causing stridor. *Chest* 1983, 84:301–302.

39. Pellegrini C, DeMeester T, Johnson L, Skinner D: Gastroesophageal reflux and pulmonary aspiration: Incidence, functional abnormality, and results of surgical therapy. *Surgery* 1979, 86:110–119.

40. Puntis J, Smith H, Buick R, Booth I: Effect of dystonic movements on oesophageal peristalsis in Sandifer's syndrome. *Arch Dis Child* 1989, 64:1311–1313.

41. Friesen CA, Hayes R, Hodge C, Roberts CC: Comparison of methods of assessing 24-hour intraesophageal pH recordings in children. *J Pediatr Gastroenterol Nutr* 1992, 14:252–255.

42. Hampton FJ, MacFadyen UM, Mayberry JF: Variations in results of simultaneous ambulatory pH monitoring. *Dig Dis Sci* 1992, 37:506–512.

43. Wiener G, Morgan T, Copper J, *et al.*: Ambulatory 24-hour esophageal pH monitoring: Reproducibility and variability of pH parameters. *Dig Dis Sci* 1988, 33:1127–1133.

44. Sondheimer JM: Continuous monitoring of distal esophageal pH: A diagnostic test for gastroesophageal reflux in infants. *J Pediatr* 1980, 96:804–807.

45. Euler AR, Byrne WJ: Twenty-four-hour esophageal intraluminal pH probe testing: A comparative analysis. *Gastroenterology* 1981, 80:957–961.

46. Eizaguirre I, Tovar JA: Predicting preoperatively the outcome of respiratory symptoms of gastroesophageal reflux. *J Pediatr Surg* 1992, 27:848–851.

47. Halpern LM, Jolley SG, Tunnell WP, *et al.*: The mean duration of gastroesophageal reflux during sleep as an indicator of respiratory symptoms from gastroesophageal reflux in children. *J Pediatr Surg* 1991, 26:686–690.

48. Vandenplas Y, Franckx GA, Pipeleers MM, *et al.*: Area under pH 4: Advantages of a new parameter in the interpretation of esophageal pH monitoring data in infants. *J Pediatr Gastroenterol Nutr* 1989, 9:34–39.

49. Tovar J, Izquierdo M, Eizaguirre I: The area under pH curve: A single-figure parameter representative of esophageal acid exposure. *J Pediatr Surg* 1991, 26:163–167.

50. Jolley S, Johnson D, Herbst J, *et al.*: An assessment of gastroesophageal reflux in children by extended monitoring of the distal esophagus. *Surgery* 1978, 84:16–22.

51. Strobel CT, Byrne WJ, Ament ME, Euler AR: Correlation of esophageal lengths in children with height: Application to the Tuttle test without prior esophageal manometry. *J Pediatr* 1979, 94:81–84.

52. Putnam PE, Orenstein SR: Determining esophageal length from crown-rump length. *J Pediatr Gastroenterol Nutr* 1991, 13:354–359.

53. Jolley SG, Tunell WP, Carson JA, *et al.*: The accuracy of abbreviated esophageal pH monitoring in children. *J Pediatr Surg* 1984, 19:848–854.

54. Putnam PE, Orenstein SR: Crown-rump length and pH probe length [Author's Reply]. *J Pediatr Gastroenterol Nutr* 1992, 15:222–223.

55. Orenstein SR: Gastroesophageal reflux. *Pediatr Rev* 1992, 13:178.

56. Orenstein SR, Klein HA, Rosenthal MS: Scintigraphic images for quantifying pediatric gastroesophaeal reflux: A study of simultaneous scinitigraphy and pH probe using multiplexed data and acid feedings. *J Nucl Med* 1993, 34:1228–1234.

57. Vandenplas Y, Derde M, Piepsz A: Evaluation of reflux episodes during simultaneous esophageal pH monitoring and gastroesophageal reflux scintigraphy in children. *J Pediatr Gastroenterol Nutr* 1992, 14:256–260.

58. Tolia V, Kuhns L, Kauffman RE: Comparison of simultaneous esophageal pH monitoring and scintigraphy in infants with gastroesophageal reflux. *Am J Gastroenterol* 1993, 88:661–664.

59. Klein H: Esophageal and other condensed dynamic images. *Clin Nucl Med* 1985, 10:530–531.

60. DiLorenzo C, Piepsz A, Ham H, Cadranel S: Gastric emptying with gastro-oesophageal reflux. *Arch Dis Child* 1987, 62:449–453.

61. Hillemeier AC, Lange R, McCallum R, *et al.*: Delayed gastric emptying in infants with gastroesophageal reflux. *J Pediatr* 1981, 98:190–193.

62. Tolia V, Lin C-H, Kuhns L: Gastric emptying using three different formulas in infants with gastroesophageal reflux. *J Pediatr Gastroenterol Nutr* 1992, 15:297–301.

63. Jolley SG, Leonard JC, Tunell WP: Gastric emptying in children with gastroesophageal reflux. I. An estimate of effective gastric emptying. *J Pediatr Surg* 1987, 22:923–926.

64. Andres JM, Mathias JR, Clech MH, Davis RH: Gastric emptying in infants with gastroesophageal reflux. Measurement with a technetium-99m-labeled semisolid meal. *Dig Dis Sci* 1988, 33:393–399.

65. Arasu TS, Franken EA, Wyllie R, *et al.*: The gastroesophageal (GE) scintiscan in detection of GE reflux and pulmonary aspiration in children. *Ann Radiol* 1980, 23:187–192.

66. Fawcett HD, Hayden CK, Adams JC, Swischuk LE: How useful is gastroesophageal reflux scintigraphy in suspected childhood aspiration? *Pediatr Radiol* 1988, 18:311–313.

67. McVeagh P, Howman-Giles R, Kemp A: Pulmonary aspiration studied by radionuclide milk scanning and barium swallow roentgenography. *Am J Dis Child* 1987, 141:917–921.

68. Miller JH: How useful is gastroesophageal reflux scinitigraphy in suspected childhood aspiration? *Pediatr Radiol* 1988, 19:70.

69. Biller J, Winter H, Grand R: Is endoscopy of benefit in the diagnosis of esophagitis in children? *Pediatr Res* 1982, 157A.

70. Blackstone MO: *Endoscopic Interpretation: Normal and Pathologic Appearances of the Gastrointestinal Tract.* New York: Raven Press; 1984; 11–21.

71. Black DD, Haggitt RC, Orenstein SR, Whitington PF: Esophagitis in infants: morphometric histologic diagnosis and correlation with measures of gastroesophageal reflux. *Gastroenterology* 1990, 98:1408–1414.

72. Ramenofsky ML, Leape LL: Continuous upper esophageal pH monitoring in infants and children with gastroesophaeal reflux, pneumonia, and apneic spells. *J Pediatr Surg* 1981, 16:374–378.

73. Orenstein SR, Whitington PF, Orenstein DM: The infant seat as treatment for gastroesophageal reflux. *N Engl J Med* 1983, 309:760–763.

74. Orenstein SR, Whitington PF: Positioning for prevention of infant gastroesophageal reflux. *J Pediatr* 1983, 103:534–537.

74a. Hyman PE: Gastroesophageal Reflux: One reason why baby won't eat. *J Pediatr* 1994, 125(suppl):S103–S109.

75. Schatzlein M, Ballantine T, Thirunavukkarasu S, *et al.*: Gastroesophageal reflux in infants and children. *Arch Surg* 1979, 114:505–510.

76. Gunasekaran T, Hassall E: Efficacy and safety of omeprazole for severe gastroesophageal reflux in children. *J Pediatr* 1993, 123:148–154.

77. Albanese C, Towbin R, Ulman I, *et al.*: Percutaneous gastrojejun-ostomy versus Nissen fundoplication for enteral feeding of the neurologically impaired child with gastroesophageal reflux. *J Pediatr* 1993, 123:371–375.

Peptic Ulcer Disease and Helicobacter pylori–Related Gastroduodenal Disease in Pediatrics

Chapter

5

VASUNDHARA TOLIA

The term *acid-peptic disorders* encompasses a variety of lesions of the gastroduodenal mucosa as seen during endoscopy or on histology. The endoscopic lesions include hemorrhages, erosions, ulcers, or inflammatory conditions limited to the mucosa without surface erosions. These nonulcerating lesions may cause identical symptoms as ulcers and are therefore discussed in the same context [1].

Peptic ulcer disease is diagnosed in the pediatric population when there is an index of suspicion and routine use of endoscopy. An ulcer is the result of an imbalance between aggressive and defensive factors in the gastroduodenal mucosa [2]. Part of that imbalance is related to infection with *Helicobacter pylori* [3,4].

Peptic ulcers are described by their location (gastric or duodenal) or etiology (primary versus secondary). Primary peptic ulcers are not associated with systemic disease, whereas secondary peptic ulcers are associated with some precipitating factors. These factors include underlying systemic disease, head trauma, sepsis, burns, and intake of ulcerogenic medications [5]. Secondary ulcers usually present acutely and are not associated with a positive family history of peptic ulcer or recurrence, except those associated with intake of nonsteroidal anti-inflammatory agents (NSAIDs). The majority of primary duodenal and gastric antral ulcers are associated with *H. pylori* infection [4].

Although secondary ulcers are more common in younger children, primary ulcers have been reported even in neonates [5]. Infants present with symptoms such as vomiting, feeding difficulty, unexplained crying, anemia, or with a complication such as bleeding, perforation, or obstruction. Abdominal pain and nausea are typical symptoms in older children and adolescents [6].

Gastritis is defined as an inflammatory process involving the gastric mucosa on visual inspection or under the microscope.

There is poor correlation between the histologic abnormalities and endoscopic observations in the assessment of gastritis. An endoscopically normal-appearing mucosa may be inflamed under the microscope, and a diffusely red mucosa on endoscopy may reveal very few abnormalities on histology. Therefore, any discussion of gastritis and duodenitis is incomplete without inclusion of both endoscopic and histologic findings [7,8].

H. pylori plays a major role in the pathogenesis of peptic ulcer disease, although the exact mechanism is not clear [9]. Strain variability and host resistance probably contribute to the different outcomes of infection in different individuals [10]. *H. pylori* infection may also increase the risk of developing gastric adenocarcinoma and lymphoma [11]. Furthermore, *H. pylori* infection may cause nonulcer dyspepsia in adults and children [12–14].

The symptoms of nonulcerating *H. pylori* infection can include abdominal pain, nausea, vomiting, and halitosis [15]. A wide range of differential diagnoses, including infectious, structural, inflammatory, and functional causes affecting other gastrointestinal and nongastrointestinal intraabdominal organs, should be considered.

Endoscopy is the most reliable tool for diagnosing acid-peptic diseases [16]. Single- or double-contrast barium studies are not as reliable, with a high incidence of false positive results caused by overreading of soft findings of pylorospasm and thickened folds [17,18]. Moreover, besides ulcers, other lesions such as mucosal hemorrhages, erosions, nodularity, and duodenitis are identified with endoscopy. Biopsies from different areas of esophagus, stomach, and duodenum for histologic and other evaluations, such as culture, are often useful in the absence of visual abnormalities [19].

H. pylori infection can be diagnosed by endoscopic biopsy (histology, urease test, or culture), serologic testing, or urea breath test [20]. Eradication of *H. pylori* decreases the recurrence rate of peptic ulcer disease [21,22].

Surgery is necessary for perforation. For gastrointestinal bleeding, initial management should include fluid resuscitation followed by more individualized treatment based on the condition of the patient and presence of associated disease [22]. Diagnosis of the cause of bleeding can be accomplished by endoscopy after stabilizing the patient with special attention for assessing stigmata of recent hemorrhage and consideration of using therapeutic maneuvers such as heater probe, variceal injection, and banding as necessary for ongoing bleeding. For patients at risk for stress ulcers, a protocol for suppressing gastric acidity can be employed [23].

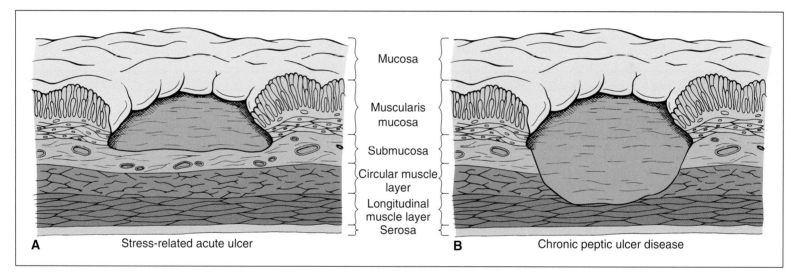

FIGURE 5-1.

There are three categories of gastroduodenal mucosal damage. The first leads to a denudation of the superficial layers of mucosa, which is discernible through a scanning microscope as exposure of lamina propria occurs following exposure to some foods and medications. These superficial "wear and tear" lesions are repaired by cell migration without cell division. These lesions are generally visible only under the microscope.

This diagram illustrates the next two stages of damage to the mucosa. **A,** In acute ulcer or erosion, the damage is limited only to the lamina propria and this lesion can be typically seen in the acid producing areas of the body and fundus [24]. **B,** The third stage of injury penetrates through the muscularis mucosa and results in a localized but deep defect in the epithelium known as chronic ulcer. (*Adapted from* Brown [25].)

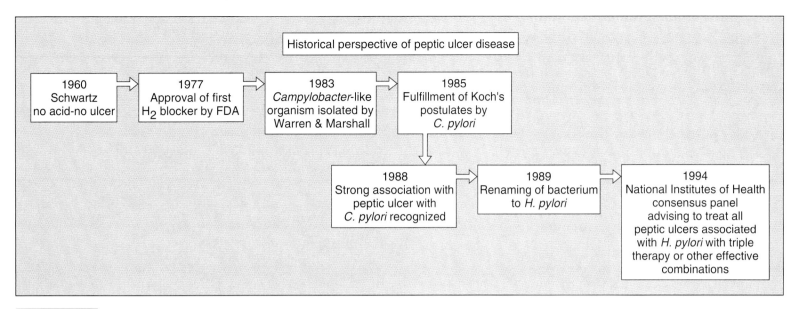

FIGURE 5-2.

Peptic ulcer disease was traditionally considered to be secondary to hyperacidity, and Schwartz's dictum of "no acid-no ulcer" needs to be modified to "no *Helicobacter pylori*-no gastritis-no ulcer, atrophy or cancer" [26]. The history of pathophysiological insights toward understanding peptic ulcer disease are depicted in this diagram. *H. pylori* is the most important factor in the pathogenesis of peptic ulcer disease.

TABLE 5-1. POTENTIAL MECHANISMS IN THE PATHOGENESIS OF PEPTIC ULCERS

PROTECTIVE FACTORS	AGGRESSIVE FACTORS
Cytoprotection	*H. pylori* infection
	Bile and pancreatic reflux
Mucus bicarbonate layer	Excess acid and pepsin
Prostaglandins	Stress
Epithelial resistance	Medications
Preservation of vascular flow	Alcohol
Epithelial cell renewal	Smoking
	Unknown

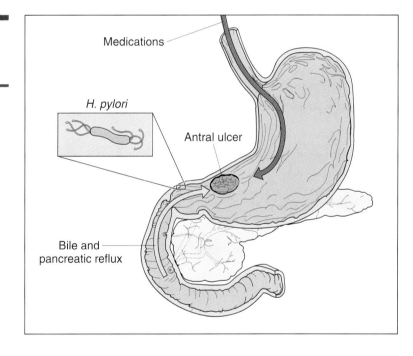

TABLE 5-1 AND FIGURE 5-3.

Improved understanding of the gastric physiology and mechanisms of injury suggest that the pathogenesis of ulcers is multifactorial. A delicate balance of the aggressive and protective factors shown in this table maintain the homeostasis of the gastroduodenal region. The defense mechanisms contribute towards maintaining integrity of the mucosa by cytoprotection [6].

Gastric ulcers can be caused by medications that directly injure the mucosa and inhibit prostaglandin synthesis. Duodenogastric reflux of bile and pancreatic juices may irritate the gastric mucosa.

Infection with *Helicobacter pylori* is coexistent in 70% to 80% of patients with gastric ulcers and more than 90% of patients with duodenal ulcers [4]. However, excessive acid and pepsin secretion may contribute towards the occurrence of duodenal ulcer in the absence of *H. pylori*. Prostaglandins have a multifactorial defense role by inhibiting gastric secretion, increasing bicarbonate secretion, preventing deep tissue injury, stimulating healing of damaged epithelium, and maintaining adequate circulation [27].

TABLE 5-2. PRESENTING SYMPTOMS OF PEPTIC ULCERS AT DIFFERENT AGES

SYMPTOMS	NEWBORN	1 MONTH TO 6 YEARS	> 6 YEARS
Vomiting	+	+	±
Feeding problems	+	+	-
Irritability	+	+	-
Abdominal pain	-	±	+
Gastrointestinal bleeding	+	+	+
Association of pain with meals	-	-	+

TABLE 5-2.

The presenting symptoms of primary peptic ulcer vary with the age of the child [2,3,5]. In the neonates, the most common symptoms of peptic disease include vomiting, feeding difficulty, irritability, failure to thrive, gastrointestinal bleeding, pyloric outlet obstruction, and perforation. In infants and young children, between a month to 6 years of age, vomiting, unexplained crying, feeding problems, and occult or overt bleeding are the major symptoms. When abdominal pain occurs in infants who cannot speak, their behavior may change. Intractable fussiness, food refusal, and failure to thrive may be caused by abdominal pain. In older children and adolescents, the symptoms are similar to those in adults. Epigastric or periumbilical pain with nocturnal awakening, a temporal association to meals, nausea, vomiting, and heartburn can occur with different degrees of severity.

Tomomasa and coworkers [28] analyzed 13 ulcer-related symptoms and signs in children 6 to 15 years of age; they concluded that a combination of epigastric pain associated with meals, positive family history of peptic ulcer, vomiting, and bleeding were most suggestive of ulcers in children. Stress or secondary ulcers present with catastrophic events like massive hemorrhage or perforation.

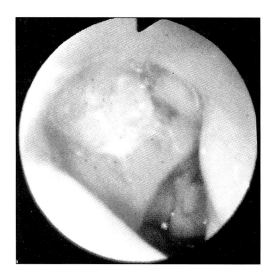

FIGURE 5-4.

Diagnosis of peptic disease. Studies comparing radiologic and endoscopic techniques in children have shown that radiology identifies 50% to 90% of duodenal ulcers demonstrated by endoscopy [29]. In addition, there is a high risk of false-positive and false-negative radiologic diagnoses in children. Although the double-contrast barium studies are superior to single-contrast studies in demonstrating mucosal lesions, these tests are uncomfortable to patients, and overinterpretation of nonspecific findings, such as pylorospasm and thickened folds, may lead to erroneous diagnoses.

Endoscopy is safe and accurate in the hands of an experienced gastroenterologist. It offers the advantage of obtaining targeted mucosal biopsies from different areas for histology and other special tests. Endoscopic visualization cannot reliably detect mucosal disease; therefore, biopsies are an integral part of the endoscopic exam [19]. This figure shows a duodenal ulcer with sharp edges in the duodenal bulb.

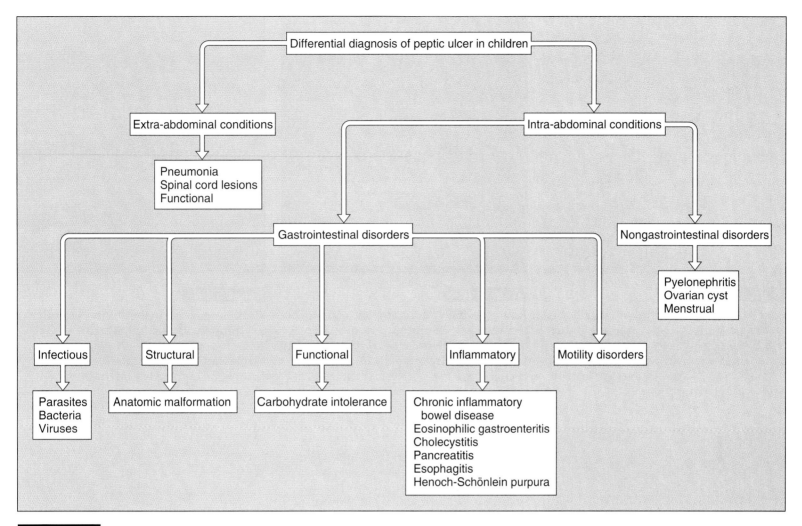

FIGURE 5-5.

Many conditions mimic some or all of the symptoms of peptic disease. These can be broadly classified into extra-abdominal and intra-abdominal disorders. The intra-abdominal category can be further subdivided into gastrointestinal and nongastrointestinal diseases. Special consideration needs to be given to differentiating the very common functional recurrent abdominal pain of childhood from peptic disease. Long duration of symptoms is not a reliable distinguishing factor. In a study of 100 children with ulcers, the mean interval between the onset of symptoms and diagnosis was 1.8 years. A delay of 4.8 years for diagnosis has been reported for symptoms beginning of early childhood [30].

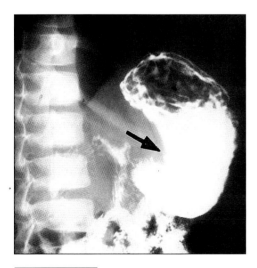

FIGURE 5-6.

Barium study of the upper gastrointestinal tract demonstrating an ulcer niche (*arrow*) on the lesser curvature of the stomach indicating a gastric ulcer. Rest of the stomach and duodenal bulb are normal in appearance.

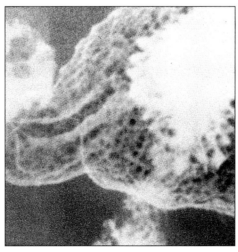

FIGURE 5-7.

Nodularity of the gastric antrum seen on an air-contrast barium study. This has been typically described in association with *Helicobacter pylori* gastritis.

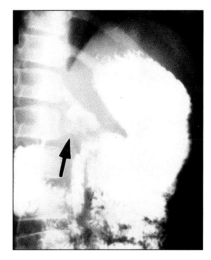

FIGURE 5-8.

Deformed duodenal bulb (*arrow*) on barium study. In such a finding, it is not possible to decide if an active crater is present without performing an upper endoscopy. An active giant ulcer could be present in the bulb, so that it may have been permanently deformed due to scarring.

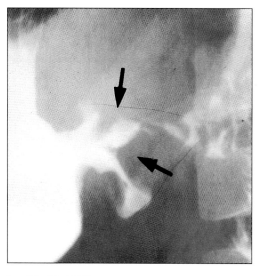

FIGURE 5-9.

Typical clover-leaf deformity of the duodenal bulb signifying an acute ulcer in a deformed bulb. *Arrows* point to the retraction of the upper and lower margins of the duodenum toward the ulcer. Normally the bulb is triangular and appears smooth.

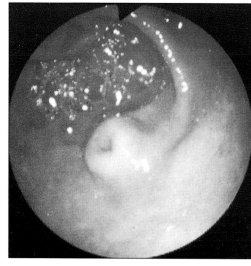

FIGURE 5-10.

Pancreatic rest in the prepyloric region. This elevation is a submucosal ectopic pancreas in gastric antrum with typical apical dimple. It should not be confused with an ulcer. Such a lesion is generally an incidental finding and does not cause symptoms.

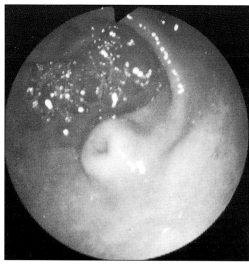

FIGURE 5-11.

Multiple erosions in the antrum secondary to aspirin. Note the confluence of several neighboring erosions with erythematous, hemorrhagic borders of the lesions. Such lesions can eventually lead to chronic ulcers.

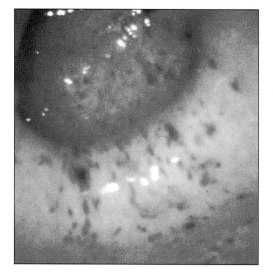

FIGURE 5-12.

Hemorrhagic gastritis in the antrum. Fresh and older submucosal hemorrhages (discrete and confluent) are seen. Brownish discoloration is seen, suggesting old hemorrhages because recent lesions are bright red.

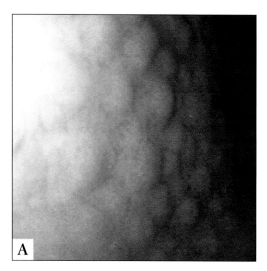

A

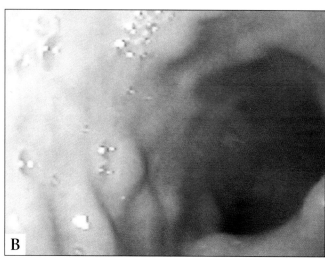

B

FIGURE 5-13.

A–B, Antrum nodularity as described in *Helicobacter pylori* infection. The spectrum of gross endoscopic findings in patients with *H. pylori* gastritis can vary from completely normal to nodularity, nonspecific gastritis, and ulcers [31]. The nodules become more prominent following an antral biopsy, as the oozing blood outlines the nodules similar to the appearance in an intravital stain.

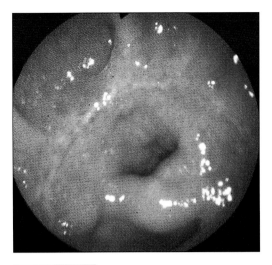

FIGURE 5-14.

Pseudodiverticulum in a scarred and deformed duodenal bulb secondary to a previously healed ulcer. The lumen is in the center and the diverticulum is between the 9 o'clock and 12 o'clock positions. On barium study, it could resemble the radiograph seen in Figure 5-8.

TABLE 5-3. COMPLICATIONS OF PEPTIC ULCER

Hemorrhage	Penetration
Perforation	Partial obstruction

TABLE 5-3.

Major complications of peptic ulcer are hemorrhage, perforation, and gastric outlet obstruction. Hemorrhage presents as hematemesis or melena, although occult bleeding is more frequent than overt bleeding. Massive hemorrhage occurs with stress ulcers. Perforation of the ulcer causes a surgical emergency and is more common in neonates and younger children with acute ulcers secondary to stress. Posteriorly located duodenal ulcer may burrow into the pancreas, causing deep pain secondary to penetration of the ulcer. Gastric outlet obstruction is an uncommon complication because of inflammation and edema within the pyloric channel. Pyloric channel ulcer may heal with fibrosis, resulting in partial obstruction [6]. Crohn's disease of the gastroduodenal area should be considered in the differential diagnosis of such a complication.

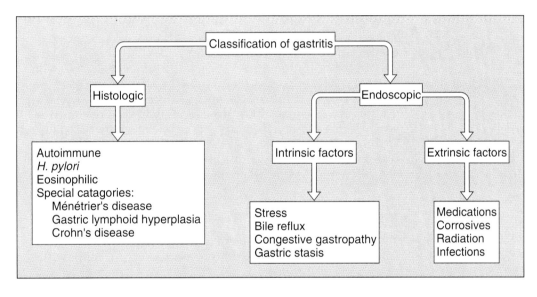

FIGURE 5-15.

Classification of gastritis. The diagnosis of gastritis can be made only by histology, as endoscopic appearances of the gastric mucosa are often misleading. In the classification on gastritis, major categories are "true" or histologic gastritis and endoscopic gastritis. Histologic gastritis involves a dynamic and often progressive lesion [32]. The findings on histology are dependent on the stage of the disease process (ie, types of inflammatory cells and the degree of damage to the glandular structures.) Autoimmune or Type A gastritis secondary to genetic and autoimmune basis is rare in children. Type B or antral gastritis most commonly caused by *Helicobacter pylori* infection is seen in 11% to 32% of children undergoing endoscopy [2,3,31].

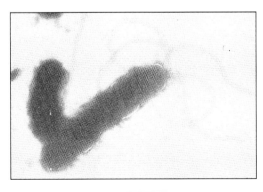

TABLE 5-4. BIOLOGY OF *H. PYLORI*

Gram-negative, spiral-shaped bacillus

Flagellated, motile

Located in the gastric mucosa

FIGURE 5-16 AND TABLE 5-4.

Helicobacter pylori is a gram-negative, spiral-shaped bacillus with flagella at one end. It lives in the interface between the surface of the gastric epithelial cells and the overlying mucous gel layer, around the junction between epithelial cells. *H. pylori* produces urease, which increases the juxta-mucosal pH. This may account for its ability to survive in the hostile acidic environment of the stomach. Other features that enable it to colonize the stomach include its motility and its ability to adhere to the mucosa. However, how it escapes the bactericidal effects of gastric acid, colonizes the gastric mucosa, and damages the underlying epithelial cells is not well understood [33].

TABLE 5-5. EPIDEMIOLOGY OF *H. PYLORI*

Worldwide distribution

No gender predisposition

Higher prevalence in:

    Developing countries

    Older age

    Blacks

    White hispanics

    Lower socioeconomic status

    Institutionalized people

    Gastroenterologists and nurses

TABLE 5-5.

The only known reservoir of *Helicobacter pylori* is humans. The prevalence of infection in healthy people increases with age; 50% of people over 60 years of age are infected. The prevalence is higher in blacks than in whites and is inversely related to socioeconomic status. Clusters of infections in families, custodial institutions, and nursing homes suggest that *H. pylori* is spread by close personal contact. It is not known if transmission is primarily fecal-oral or oral-oral. The organism has been detected by the polymerase chain reaction in feces, dental plaque, and saliva [34–36].

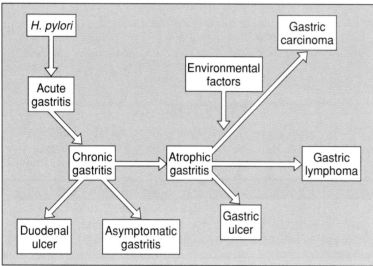

FIGURE 5-17.

Pathogenesis and possible outcomes of *Helicobacter pylori*–induced injury. Although *H. pylori* infection produces inflammation, only a minority of those infected develop peptic ulcers. In fact, a majority of hosts are asymptomatic despite an inflammatory response composed of polymorphs, monocytes, lymphocytes, and plasma cells within the lamina propria, and damage to the mucosal epithelial glands of the antrum and fundus. *H. pylori* infections may persist for decades, even for life.

    DNA hybridization studies suggest that strains associated with duodenal ulcer are distinct from those causing superficial chronic gastritis [10]. In some people, intense inflammation may ensue as a result of inadequate down-regulation of the immune response, whereas in a subset of patients with peptic ulcer disease, abnormalities in gastrin physiology may result in G-cell hyperfunction and abnormalities in gastric acid secretion [37]. (*Adapted from* Blaser and Soll [38]; with permission.)

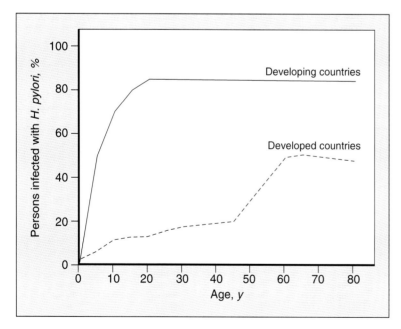

FIGURE 5-18.

In developing countries, rates of acquisition of *Helicobacter pylori* infection are higher than in other countries; 50% of children are infected by the time they are 10 years old. This pattern suggests a chronic source of infection. Possibly, infection between parents and children only occurs occasionally, but the presence of incontinent ambulant children amplifies the infectivity in a family group [39]. Large family size and lower socioeconomic status predispose to a higher prevalence of *H. pylori* in adulthood. In developed countries, only a small percentage of children are infected with *H. pylori*; 50% of individuals between 50 and 60 years of age are infected. This pattern of infection in developed countries suggest a cohort effect rather than increased exposure or increase in infection with age [40]. (*Adapted from* Marshall [4].)

TABLE 5-6. PRESENTING SYMPTOMS IN 104 CHILDREN WITH *H. PYLORI* GASTRITIS

SYMPTOM	PERCENTAGE
Abdominal pain	60
Vomiting	31
Hematemesis	20
Failure to thrive (< 5th percentile weight/age)	13
Melena	6
Chest pain	6
Diarrhea	4
Dysphagia	3

TABLE 5-6.

The spectrum of *Helicobacter pylori* infection in children is diverse and not always associated with ulcer [41–43]. Udall *et al.* [15] retrospectively reviewed data in 104 *H. pylori*–positive children between 1 and 17 years of age over a 7-year period. Although more than one symptom was present in many children, the frequency and approximate distribution of major symptoms are shown in this table. Although not a part of this series, protein-losing enteropathy has also been reported from *H. pylori* infection [44].

DIAGNOSING *HELICOBACTER PYLORI* INFECTION

TABLE 5-7. DIAGNOSTIC TESTS FOR *H. PYLORI*

TEST	SENSITIVITY	SPECIFICITY	COST*	FOLLOW-UP USE?
Invasive tests (each requires endoscopy)				
Histology	93–99	95–99[†]	$$$	Yes
Culture	77–92	100[†]	$$$	Yes
Biopsy urease test	89–98	93–98	$	Yes
Noninvasive tests				
^{13}C-urea breath test	90–100	98–100	$$	Yes
^{14}C-urea breath test	90–97	89–100	$$	Yes
Serology	88–99	86–95	$	Not for short-term use

*Excluding cost of endoscopy if required.
[†]Estimated.

TABLE 5-7.

Diagnosing *Helicobacter pylori* infection. Tests to detect *H. pylori* infection are shown in this table [45]. These tests can be classified as invasive (requiring endoscopy) or noninvasive. Although they are all sensitive and specific, they have advantages and disadvantages. Usually, documentation of an organism by culture confirms the infection; however, *H. pylori* culture is a tedious and difficult task because of the fastidious nature of the organism. Culture of *H. pylori* should be performed if the antibiotic sensitivity of the organism is required. It would be indicated if the patient has antibiotic allergies or had failed previous therapies or in countries where *H. pylori* has a high level of background antibiotic resistance [40]. (*Adapted from* Graham [45]; with permission.)

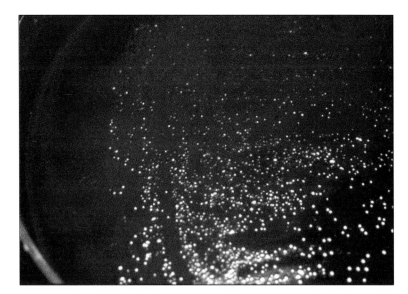

FIGURE 5-19.

Helicobacter pylori colonies grown on brain-heart infusion agar. (*From* Graham [45]; with permission.)

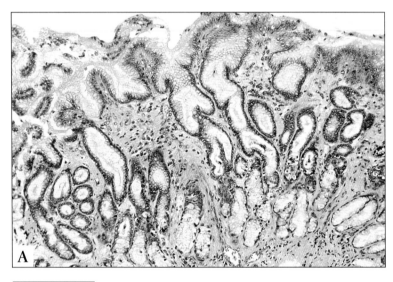

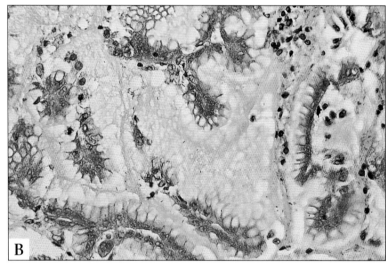

FIGURE 5-20.

Histology of *Helicobacter pylori*. Histology of the biopsy is very sensitive (93%–99%) and specific (95%–99%), especially if biopsies are obtained from different areas of the stomach to avoid the possibility of a false-negative study in case the infection was patchy [45,46]. Generally, routine hematoxylin and eosin staining is adequate (**A**); Giemsa or silver stains facilitate identification of the organism as (**B**). Histologic assessment is also helpful in diagnosing the severity of inflammation and in excluding unsuspected lesions, such as mucosa-associated lymphoma-type lesions [46].

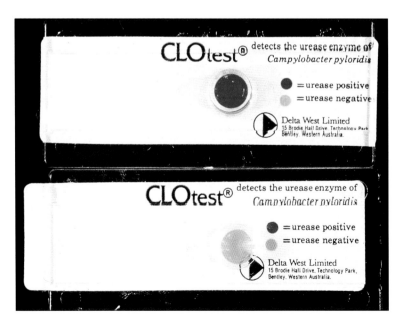

FIGURE 5-21.

The rapid urease test. The rapid urease test involves inoculation of the biopsy specimens into a liquid or gel medium containing urea and phenol red, which turns pink if the pH rises above 6.0. Such a change occurs when urea in the gel is metabolized to ammonia by the urease of the organism. One such test, called CLO test (Delta West Limited, Bentley, Western Australia), is shown in this figure. Its low cost and dependability make it the most quick and desirable endoscopic method of diagnosis [47]. The rapid urease test is 89% to 98% sensitive and 93% to 98% specific.

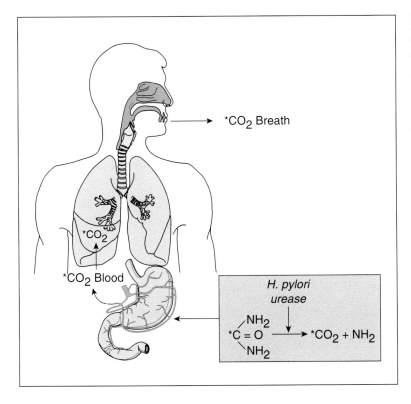

FIGURE 5-22.

The noninvasive serologic and breath tests do not require endoscopy. The enzyme-linked immunosorbent assay is simple, inexpensive, and commercially available. Usually immunoglobulin G antibody is elevated in persons with *Helicobacter pylori* infection. Because *H. pylori* is a chronic infection that does not resolve spontaneously, elevated immunoglobulin G indicates active infection unless the patient is known to have been treated in the preceding 2 years. Although the antibody titers fall after *H. pylori* eradication, the rate of decline is uncertain [48,49].

The principle of labeled urea ^{13}C or ^{14}C breath test. Breath tests using ^{13}C or ^{14}C label are highly specific and very sensitive measures of the presence of *H. pylori* urease [52]. They indicate cure of *H. pylori* 4 weeks after antibiotic therapy, at a time when serologic antibody tests still give a positive result. False-negative tests occur if patients take Pepto-bismol (Proctor & Gamble, Cincinnati, OH) or antibiotics a few days before the test. ^{13}C is nonradioactive but expensive. On the other hand, ^{14}C exposes the patient to a small radiation dose, but is simple to perform. Data in the pediatric population with breath tests are limited [51].

In practice, endoscopy is still necessary to diagnose the actual pathology, *ie*, the location of ulcer, inflammation, or both, along with at least two biopsies from the gastric antrum for CLO test (Delta West Limited, Bentley, Western Australia). When ^{13}C tests are available, they will be the ideal, noninvasive method to assess the response to treatment.

Asterisks indicate radioactivity.

TREATMENT OF ACID-PEPTIC DISEASES

TABLE 5-8. MECHANISMS OF ACTION OF COMMONLY USED MEDICATIONS FOR PEPTIC ULCERS

Enhancing mucosal resistance	Acid control	*H. pylori* eradication
Sucralfate	Neutralization—antacids	Antibiotics
Prostaglandin	Supression	
Bismuth preparations	Anticholinergics	
	H_2-receptor blockers	
	Proton pump inhibitors	

TABLE 5-8.

Avoidance of known precipitating factors, such as ulcerogenic medications, ethanol, and stress ulcer prophylaxis, should be advocated if appropriate. No specific dietary restrictions are necessary except avoidance of alcohol, caffeine, smoking, and foods that provoke symptoms in that particular patient. Management of peptic ulcer and related nonulcerating inflammatory conditions is dependent on the *Helicobacter pylori* status of the individual. Although antacids, H_2 receptor antagonists, synthetic prostaglandins, and other cytoprotective agents are effective in ulcer healing, they do not alter *H. pylori* colonization. Many

studies in adults have demonstrated that resolution of clinical symptoms and endoscopic healing of ulcers occur more rapidly if antibiotic therapy is used in addition to standard anti-ulcer regimen [53]. Furthermore, recurrence of ulcers has also been dramatically reduced by eradication of *H. pylori* [21]. Thus, standard anti-ulcer therapy, anti-*Helicobacter* therapy, or a combination of both may need to be used, depending on the individual patient [2,3,6]. Although this table describes all available anti-ulcer agents, H_2 blockers are most frequently used because of their convenience, dosing ease, and safety profile.

TABLE 5-9. TREATMENT REGIMENS FOR *HELICOBACTER PYLORI* INFECTION

Therapy	Drug 1	Drug 2	Drug 3	Notes*	Success rate, %
Triple	Tetracycline HCl 500 mg qid	Metronidazole 250 mg tid	Bismuth subsalicylate† 2 tablets qid	With meals for 14 days plus an antisecretory drug	>90
Triple	Tetracycline HCl 500 mg qid	Clarithromycin 500 mg tid	Bismuth subsalicylate 2 tablets qid	With meals for 14 days plus an antisecretory drug	>90
Triple	Amoxicillin 500 mg qid	Clarithromycin 500 mg tid	Bismuth subsalicylate 2 tablets qid	With meals for 14 days plus an antisecretory drug	>90
Triple	Amoxicillin 500 mg qid	Metronidazole 250 mg tid	Bismuth subsalicylate 2 tablets qid	With meals for 14 days plus an antisecretory drug	>80
Double	Clarithromycin 250 mg bid	Metronidazole 500 mg bid	Omeprazole 20 mg bid	For 7–14 days	>90
Double	Amoxicillin 750 mg tid	Clarithromycin 500 mg tid		With meals for 14 days plus an antisecretory drug	>90
Double	Amoxicillin 750 mg tid	Metronidazole 500 mg tid		With meals for 14 days plus an antisecretory drug	>85
Double	Clarithromycin 500 mg tid	Omeprazole 40 mg qam		With meals for 14 days	65–75
Double	Amoxicillin 750 mg tid	Omeprazole 40 mg tid		With meals for 14 days	>90
Double‡	Amoxicillin 1 g tid	Omeprazole 20 mg bid		With meals for 14 days	35–60

*Generally, one should continue an antisecretory drug for 6 weeks to ensure ulcer healing.
†Bismuth subsalicylate is the only bismuth compound available in the US; bismuth subcitrate can be substituted.
‡This outcome is based on my impression and estimates based on review of the available data as well as on the results of clinical trials. This particular combination at these or lower dosages is not recommended.

TABLE 5-9.

The most frequently recommended regimens for *Helicobacter pylori* treatment [45]. In resistant cases, alternative therapeutic regimens may need to be used. It is possible that preantibiotic treatment with omeprazole may induce the organism to take on the spherical shape. These coccoid forms of the bacteria appear to be less sensitive to antimicrobials than the flagellated form. Preliminary experience in children suggests that triple therapy is superior to double therapy [54]. Concomitant antisecretory therapy for 6 weeks may accelerate ulcer healing and provide symptom relief. bid—twice a day; qam—every morning; qid—four times a day; tid—three times a day. (*Adapted from* Graham [45].)

STRESS ULCERS

TABLE 5-10. CAUSES OF SECONDARY OR STRESS ULCERS

In newborn	Infants and children
Shock	Shock
Sepsis	Burns
Dehydration	Head injury
Traumatic delivery	Postoperative status
Severe respiratory distress	Sepsis
Hypoglycemia	Any other serious illness
Cardiac condition	

TABLE 5-10.

Causes of stress ulcers. In infants, stress ulceration is associated with antecedent or concurrent shock, sepsis, respiratory or cardiac insufficiency, traumatic delivery, hypoglycemia, and severe dehydration. In older children, trauma, head injury, shock, severe burns, sepsis, postsurgical state, or any other life-threatening illness can cause stress ulcer [6].

TABLE 5-11. STRESS ULCER

POSSIBLE MECHANISM OF OCCURRENCE
Catastrophic illness
↓
Ischemia, hypotension
↓
Gastric hypoperfusion
↓
Back diffusion of H+ ions
↓
Disruption of mucosal integrity
↓
Acute ulcer

PRESENTATION
Perforation
Massive hemorrhage

TABLE 5-11.

In stress ulcer, microcirculation in the gastric mucosa is decreased, leading to mucosal ischemia, which leads to hemorrhage or perforation [55].

Perforation is a common mode of presentation in neonates, although it can occur at any age. Sudden deterioration in the clinical condition of the patient with abdominal rigidity, guarding, and rebound tenderness suggest perforation. Free intra-abdominal air seen on radiograph confirms perforation, and emergent surgical intervention is usually necessary [2,4,6]. Massive bleeding presents with hematemesis, melena, both, or circulatory collapse. Vigorous cardiovascular resuscitation, provision of adequate venous access to sustain intravascular volume with blood, and colloids are the mainstay of treatment during such emergencies. Although in the majority of patients bleeding ceases spontaneously within 24 to 48 hours, it is important to establish the actual source of bleeding to target specific treatment. This can generally be established by endoscopy once the patient has been stabilized. During endoscopy, it is important to establish the cause of bleeding to assess for stigmata of recent hemorrhage to predict possible rebleeding and to provide therapy if active bleeding is ongoing. Therapeutic endoscopy using sclerotherapy is routine; however, heater probe and lasers are still in the preliminary stages in the pediatric population and available only in a few centers.

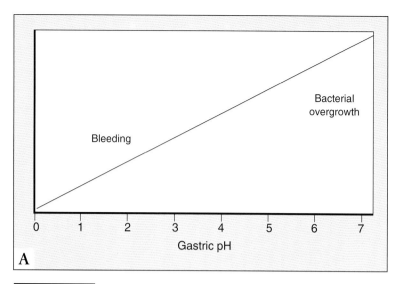

FIGURE 5-23.

A, Gastric complications in the critically ill child. Many pediatric intensive care units routinely administer antacids or histamine receptor antagonists to achieve a gastric pH of 4 or higher to decrease the incidence of stress-related erosions and ulcers [56]. Sucralfate is as effective as antacids or H_2-receptor blockers for prevention of stress ulcers but cannot be used in renal insufficiency

[57]. Alkalinization of gastric pH with antacids or antisecretory medications can allow bacterial overgrowth and subsequent airway colonization leading to nosocomial pneumonia. In a randomized pediatric study comparing four different treatments, nosocomial pneumonia was not a significant complication [58]. **B,** This figure shows multiple healing erosions in the body of the stomach.

UPPER GASTROINTESTINAL BLEEDING

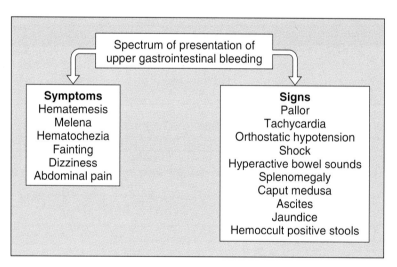

FIGURE 5-24.

Upper gastrointestinal bleeding. Upper gastrointestinal bleeding originates from a source proximal to the ligament of Treitz [59] and can present as hematemesis, melena, or hematochezia. Hematemesis denotes vomiting of either bright red blood or coffee-ground like material. Melena describes the passage of dark black stools, whereas hematochezia is the passage of bright red or maroon blood. The latter is usually associated with lower gastrointestinal bleeding; however, massive upper gastrointestinal bleeding may present as hematochezia.

TABLE 5-12. ASSESSMENT AND STABILIZATION OF PATIENTS WITH GASTROINTESTINAL BLEEDING

Establish intravenous access: for mild shock—one intravenous catheter; for moderate or severe shock—two intravenous catheters

Rapidly infuse saline, lactated Ringer's solution, or Plasmanate (Miles, Inc, Elkhart, IN) (10 mL/kg/10 minute until vital signs are normal)

Aspirate gastric contents to determine the need for lavage

Monitor vital signs, urine output, skin perfusion, and orthostatic changes in pulse and blood pressure for early recognition of shock

Transfuse with packed red blood cells to return oxygen-carrying capacity to normal

Strict intake and output records

TABLE 5-12.

Assessment and stabilization of patients with gastrointestinal bleeding. Emergent assessment with correction of the hemodynamic status is the most important aspect of management of such patients. Placement of nasogastric tube is a must to assess if the bleeding is ongoing. However, a negative nasogastric aspirate does not completely exclude the possibility of a source of bleeding distal to the pylorus. Gastric lavage with saline at room temperature can also be performed through the nasogastric tube. This table outlines a management plan [60].

TABLE 5-13. EVALUATION OF PATIENTS WITH GASTROINTESTINAL BLEEDING

HISTORY	Past bleeding Retching Abdominal pain Medications Quality and quantity of blood loss

PHYSICAL EXAMINATION	Pulse
	Blood pressure (lying and sitting)
	Evaluate for
	  ascites,
	  hepatosplenomegaly, and
	  caput medusa
	Stool color and hemoccult

LABORATORY	Type and cross match CBC, platelet count, and reticulocyte count PT, PTT, ALT, AST, BUN, guaiac, or hematest suspected blood

TABLE 5-13.

Evaluation of patients with gastrointestinal bleeding. Following resuscitation, a history and complete examination helps to delineate possible diagnoses. The key factors in differential diagnoses of upper gastrointestinal bleeding are the patient age, severity of bleeding, history of previous abdominal pain, bleeding, or any systemic illness, and signs of liver disease on examination, such as splenomegaly, spider angiomata, jaundice, edema, or ascites. There may be a history of ingestion of medications, such as aspirin, iron, nonsteroidal anti-inflammatory agents, and caustic substances, or a sharp foreign body. Vomiting and retching prior to the onset of bleeding suggest a Mallory-Weiss tear. A schema to elicit specific points in history and to determine on physical and laboratory examination is illustrated in this table [22,60]. ALT—alanine aminotransferase; AST—aspartate aminotransferase; BUN—blood urea nitrogen; CBC—complete blood count; PT—prothrombin time; PTT—partial thromboplastin time.

TABLE 5-14. DIFFERENTIAL DIAGNOSIS OF UPPER GASTROINTESTINAL BLEEDING

AGE GROUP	COMMON CAUSES	LESS COMMON CAUSES
Neonates (0–30 days)	Swallowed maternal blood Gastritis Duodenitis Peptic ulcer	Coagulopathy Vascular malformations Gastric/esophageal duplication Leiomyoma
Infants (30 days–1 year)	Gastritis and gastric ulcer Esophagitis Duodenitis	Esophageal varices Foreign body Aortoesophageal fistula
Children (1–12 years)	Esophagitis Esophageal varices Gastris and gastric ulcer Duodenal ulcer Mallory-Weiss tear Nasopharyngeal bleeding	Leiomyoma Salicylates Vascular malformation Hematocelia
Adolescents (12 years–adult)	Duodenal ulcer Esophagitis Esophageal varices Gastritis Mallory-Weiss tear	Thrombocytopenia Dieulafoy's lesion Hemobilia

TABLE 5-14.

Differential diagnosis of upper gastrointestinal bleeding. The etiology of upper gastrointestinal bleeding can vary according to the age of the patient. The differential diagnosis at different ages is outlined in this table. Both common and rare etiologies are included. Diseases associated with coagulopathy or thrombocytopenia can lead to bleeding secondary to any interruption of mucosal integrity.

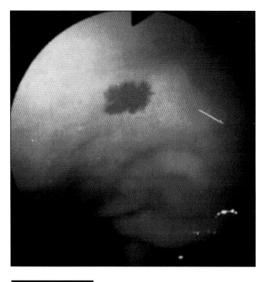

FIGURE 5-25.

Gastric angiodysplasia on endoscopy.

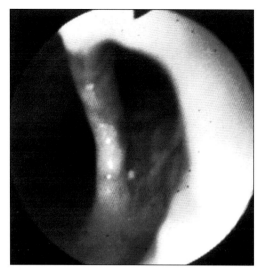

FIGURE 5-26.

Endoscopic view of the opening of esophageal duplication. Esophageal lumen is seen on the right.

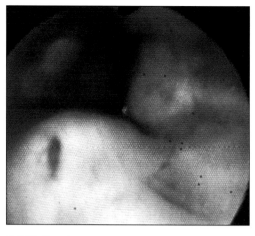

FIGURE 5-27.

Endoscopic view of an esophageal varix immediately after sclerosant injection. Note the blanched mucosa around the intravariceal injection site.

TABLE 5-15. SUGGESTED TESTS IN EVALUATING UPPER GASTROINTESTINAL BLEEDING

Esophagogastroduodenoscopy	Barium studies
99^{m}Tc Erythrocyte Scan	Enteroscopy
Arteriography	

TABLE 5-15.

Suggested tests in evaluating upper gastrointestinal bleeding. Following resuscitation, stabilization, physical examination, and availability of laboratory test results, one can proceed with an upper endoscopy. The largest possible scope that can be used safely should be used. Moreover, during endoscopy, it is sometimes possible to apply therapeutic interventions such as sclerotherapy or banding for varices and heater probe or injection for ulcers. Generally, endoscopy should be performed within 12 to 24 hours of presentation, because superficial mucosal lesions may heal and the diagnosis of gastritis may be missed. Rarely, emergent endoscopy may be needed if massive bleeding continues unabated, to target therapy (generally impossible in the presence of copious amount of blood), or to determine the need for surgery. However, if the endoscopy fails to reveal a bleeding site and bleeding is ongoing, then a 99^{m}Tc-labeled erythrocyte scan may localize the bleeding source. The erythrocyte scan is less invasive than angiography (which can be used later if the lesion is still not identified and bleeding continues). Angiography also allows therapeutic interventions such as selective infusion of vasopressin or embolization of bleeding vessel [63]. Barium does not allow these other studies to be performed by precluding adequate visualization, so contrast radiograph studies should be considered only if all other tests are nondiagnostic. Rarely, enteroscopy to evaluate jejunum and ileum may be necessary.

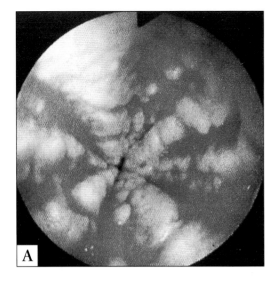

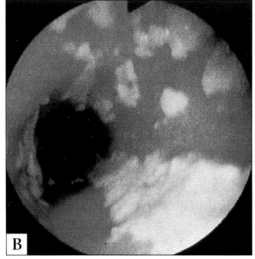

FIGURE 5-28.

A, Severe candida esophagitis with erosions and exudates, causing upper gastrointestinal bleeding. B, Close-up of esophagus showing satellite lesions with exudates of raw areas following attempts at suctioning the exudates.

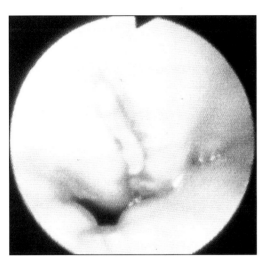

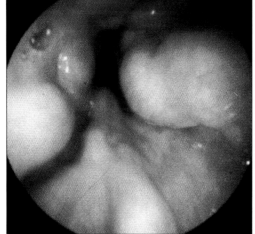

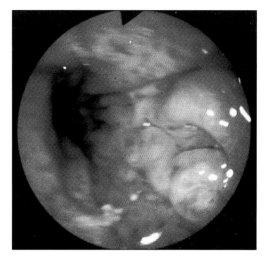

FIGURE 5-29.

Mallory-Weiss tear seen as a healing vertical deep erosion at gastroesophageal junction.

FIGURE 5-30.

Esophageal varices seen as beaded tortuous prominences along distal esophagus.

FIGURE 5-31.

Congestive gastropathy as seen in portal hypertension.

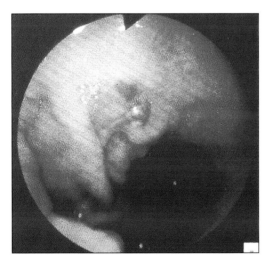

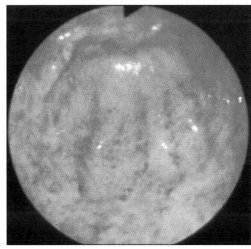

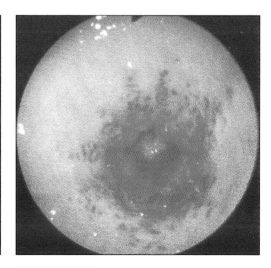

FIGURE 5-32.

Dieulafoy's lesion [64]. Dieulafoy's lesion is a distinctive vascular abnormality found almost exclusively in the proximal stomach. It can cause acute or recurrent massive upper gastrointestinal bleeding resulting from rupture of a small submucosal artery into the gastric lumen.

FIGURE 5-33.

Hemorrhagic gastritis in antrum.

FIGURE 5-34.

Antral telangiectasia.

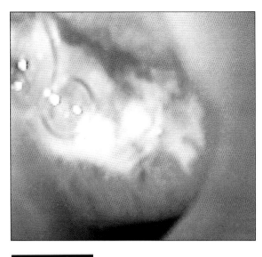

FIGURE 5-35.

Ulcer associated with *Helicobacter pylori,* causing bleeding.

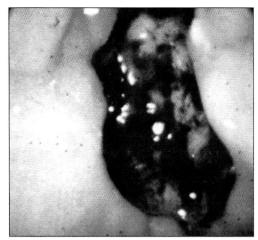

FIGURE 5-36.

Duodenal ulcer with black slough adhering to the ulcer base.

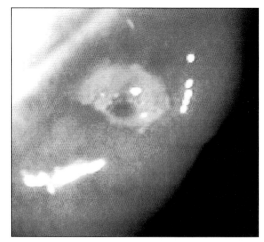

FIGURE 5-37.

Bleeding gastric ulcer with protruding vessel.

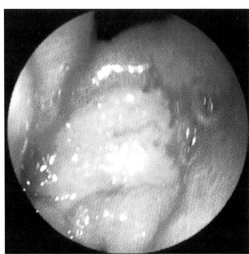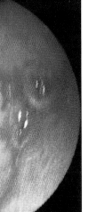

FIGURE 5-38.

Duodenal ulcer with oozing blood.

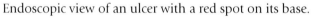

TABLE 5-16. STIGMATA OF RECENT HEMORRHAGE

Presence of red spot	Active oozing
Presence of slough	Arterial spurting

TABLE 5-16.

Stigmata of recent hemorrhage. The terms *visible vessel* and *sentinel clot* both refer to a protruding red or white mount, 2 to 3 mm in diameter, situated in the base of a peptic ulcer that has recently bled [65]. Rebleeding is an important and potentially preventable factor contributing to the mortality of patients with peptic ulcer bleeding. The endoscopic criteria of recent hemorrhage may be helpful to predict which ulcers will rebleed and require therapeutic intervention.

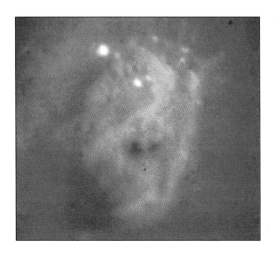

FIGURE 5-39.

Endoscopic view of an ulcer with a red spot on its base.

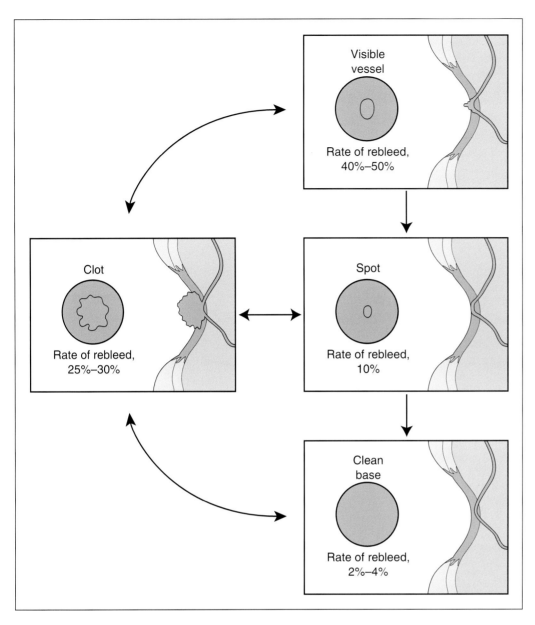

FIGURE 5-40.

The absence of stigmata of recent hemorrhage in a peptic ulcer base reliably predicts negligible risk of further bleeding. The visible vessel probably implies some increased risk of major rebleeding, but by itself is not a sufficiently reliable indicator to select patients for invasive therapy. The combination of endoscopic stigmata and clinical features of major hemorrhage should be used to provide a more reliable prediction of rebleeding. An adherent clot covering an ulcer should not be disturbed unless the criteria for therapeutic intervention have been fulfilled and the endoscopist is prepared to treat arterial hemorrhage. While healing, stigmata of recent hemorrhage evolve through a sequence of phases, a visible vessel may or may not appear as an adherent clot and then as a red or black flat spot before disappearing [67].

TABLE 5-17. RISK FACTORS CONTRIBUTING TO MORBIDITY AND MORTALITY IN PATIENTS WITH GASTROINTESTINAL BLEEDING

Very young age

Associated illness

Coagulopathy

Immunosuppression

Magnitude of bleeding (hemodymanic consequences, transfusion requirement)

Inaccurate diagnosis

Bleeding during hospitalization

Rebleeding

Endoscopic features (*eg*, arterial spurting, visible spurting, variceal source)

TABLE 5-17.

Risk factors contributing to morbidity and mortality in patients with upper gastrointestinal bleeding. In approximately 85% of patients with acute gastrointestinal bleeding, the bleeding stops spontaneously. Therapeutic interventions need to be focused on only the remaining 15% of patients. This high-risk group requires early identification so that appropriate therapy can be given. Although no large studies have been conducted in children to determine the outcome of upper gastrointestinal bleeding, these risk factors have been adapted from adult studies including age, vital signs, comorbid conditions, and stigmata of recent hemorrhage as seen endoscopy [22,56].

TABLE 5-18. RECENT ADVANCES IN THE THERAPY OF GASTROINTESTINAL BLEEDING

Specialized management teams

Pharmacotherapy

    Vasopression and nitroglycerine

    Somatostatin and octreotide

    β-blockers

Endoscopic therapy

    Laser

    Bipolar electrocautery

    Heater probe

    Injection therapy for ulcers

    Variceal sclerosis and band ligation

    Cyanoacrylate injection of gastric varices

Angiographic therapy

    Arterial embolization

    Transjugular intrahepatic protosystemic shunts

Stress ulcer prophylaxis

Mucosal cytoprotective therapy in users of nonsteroidal anti-inflammatory drugs

Early hospital discharge in absence of high-risk prognositc factors

TABLE 5-18.

Recent advances in the therapy of gastrointestinal bleeding. The ideal management of high-risk bleeders includes a multidisciplinary team combining the medical and surgical aspects of care. Such an organized approach with well-defined management policies and early intensive medical and surgical intervention may reduce the morbidity and mortality associated with acute upper gastrointestinal bleeding.

REFERENCES

1. Weber A: Primary gastroduodenal diseases: Gastritis and gastroduodenal peptic ulcers. In *Pediatric Clinical Gastroenterology.* Eds Roy, Silvermann, Alagille, 4th edition, Mosby & Co.; 1995:182–195.

2. George DE, Glassman M: Peptic ulcer disease in children. *Gastrointest Endosc Clin North Am* 1994, 4:23–37.

3. Sherman P: Peptic ulcer disease in children: Diagnosis, treatment, and the implication of Helicobacter pylori. *Gastroenterol Clin North Am* 1994, 23:4:707–725.

4. Marshall BJ: Helicobacter pylori. *Am J Gastroenterol* 1994, 89:S116–S128.

5. Tolia V, Dubois RS: Peptic ulcer disease in children and adolescents: a ten-year experience. *Clin Pediatr* 1983, 2:665–669.

6. Gryboski JD, Moyer MS: Peptic ulcer in children. In *Pediatric Gastrointestinal Disease.* Eds Wyllie, Hyams. WB Saunders; 1993:447–467.

7. McCallum RW, Singh D, Wollman J: Endoscopic and histologic correlations of the duodenal bulb. *Arch Pathol Lab Med* 1979, 103:169–172.

8. Sircus W: Duodenitis: A clinical endoscopic and histo-pathologic study. *Q J Med* 1985, 56:593–600.

9. Nomura A, Stemmermann GN, Chyou PH, Perez-Perez GI, Blaser MJ: Helicobacter pylori infection and the risk for duodenal and gastric ulceration. *Ann Int Med* 1994, 120:977–981.

10. Yoshimura HH, Evans DG, Graham DY: DNA-DNA hybridization demonstrates apparent genetic differences between Helicobacter pylori from patients with duodenal ulcer and asymptomatic gastritis. *Dig Dis Sci* 1993, 38:1128–1131.

11. Van Dam J, Scully RE, Shapiro RB, Graeme Cook F: Case records of the Massachusetts General Hospital. *N Engl J Med* 1995, 332:1153–1159.

12. Talley NJ: A critique of therapeutic trials in Helicobacter pylori positive functional dyspepsia. *Gastroenterology* 1994, 106:1174–1183.

13. Tolia V: Helicobacter pylori in pediatric non-ulcer dyspepsia: Pathogen or commensal? *Am J Gastroenterol* 1995, 90:865–868.

14. McCarthur C, Saunders N, Feldman W: Helicobacter pylori, gastroduodenal disease and recurrent abdominal pain in children. *JAMA* 1995, 273:729–734.

15. Udall J, Khoshoo V, Paipilla-Mooroy S, Correa-Gracian H, Brown RF, Schmidt-Sommerfield E, Adam-Noel R, Mannick EE, Tang SC, Craver RD: Helicobacter pylori infection in children: Associated features. *Pediatr Research* 1995, 37:4,part 2:132A.

16. Miller V, Doig CM: Upper gastrointestinal tract endoscopy. *Arch Dis Child* 1984, 57:1100–1102.

17. Dooley CP, Larsen AW, Stace NH, *et al.*: Double contrast barium meal and upper gastrointestinal endoscopy: A comparative study. *Ann Int Med* 1984, 101:538–545.

18. Levine MS, Rubesin SE, Herlinger H, *et al.*: Double contrast upper gastrointestinal examination: Technique and interpretation. *Radiology* 1988, 168:593–602.

19. Carpenter HA, Talley NJ: Gastroscopy is incomplete without biopsy: Clinical relevance in distinguishing gastropathy from gastritis. *Gastroenterology* 1995, 108:917–926.

20. Loffeld RJLF, Stobberingh E, Arends JW: A review of diagnostic techniques for Helicobacter pylori infection. *Dig Dis Sci* 1993, 11:173–180.

21. Graham DY, Law GM, Klein PD, *et al.*: Effect of treatment of Helicobacter pylori infection on the long-term recurrence of gastric or duodenal ulcer. *Ann Intern Med* 1992, 116:705–708.

22. Treem WR: Gastrointestinal bleeding in children. *Gastrointest Endosc Clin North Am* 1994, 4:75–97.

23. Peterson W: Prevention of upper gastrointestinal bleeding. *N Engl J Med* 1994, 330:6:428–429.

24. Caruse I, Bianchi Parro G: Gastroscopic evaluation of anti-inflammatory agents. *Br Med J* 1980, 280:75–78.

25. Brown KE, Peura DA: Stress-related mycosal damage: Which ICU patients are at greatest risk? *J Critical Illness* 1991, 6:1215–1224.

26. Thomson ABR: Helicobacter pylori and gastroduodenal pathology. *Canadian J Gastroenterol* 1993 7(4):353–358.

27. Rachmilewitz D, Ligumsky M, Filch A, *et al.*: Role of endogenous gastric prostanoids in the pathogenesis and therapy of duodenal therapy. *Gastroenterol* 1986, 90:963–969.

28. Tomomasa T, Hsu JY, Shigeta M, *et al.*: Statistical analysis of symptoms and signs in pediatric patients with peptic ulcers. *J Pediatr Gastroenterol Nutr* 1986, 5:711–715.

29. Drumm B, Rhoads JM, Stringer DA, *et al.*: Peptic ulcer disease in children: Etiology, clinical findings and clinical course. *Pediatrics* 1988, 982:410–414.

30. Murphy MS, Eastham EJ, Jimenez M, *et al.*: Duodenal ulceration: Review of 100 cases. *Arch Dis Child* 1987, 62:544–558.

31. Czinn SJ: Helicobacter pylori gastroduodenal disease in infants and children. In *Pediatric Gastrointestinal Disease*. Eds Wylllie, Hyams. WB Saunders, 1993; 429–434.

32. Anand BS, Graham DY: Gastritis and duodenitis. In *Management of Gastrointestinal Diseases*. Eds Winawer SJ. New York: Gower Medical Publishing; 1992, Chapter 4.

33. Falk GW: Current status of Helicobacter pylori in peptic ulcer disease. *Cleve Clin J Med* 1995, 62:95–104.

34. Graham D, Malaty H, Evans D, Evans DJ, Klein P: Epidemiology of Helicobacter pylori in an asymptomatic population in the United States: Effect of age, race, and socieconomic status. *Gastroenterology* 1991, 100:1495–1501.

35. Malaty H, Graham D: Importance of childhood socioeconomic status on the current prevalence of Helicobacter pylori infection. *Gut* 1994, 35:742–745.

36. Whitaker CJ, Dubiel AJ, Gaplin OP: Social and geographical risk factors in Helicobacter pylori infection. *Epidemiol Infect* 1993, 111:63–70.

37. Blaser MJ: Hypotheses on the pathogenesis and natural history of Helicobacter pylori-induced inflammation. *Gastroenterology* 1992, 102:720–727.

38. Blaser MJ, Soll AH: *Helicobacter pylori: Pathophysiology and Epidemiology*. Edited by Graham DY. Deerfield, IL: Discovery International; 1995. 12–18.

39. Vincent P, Gottrand F, Pernes P, *et al.*: High prevalence of Helicobacter pylori infection in co-habiting children: Epidemiology of a cluster with special emaphsis on molecular typing. *Gut* 1994, 35:313–316.

40. Mendall M, Goggin PM, Molineaux N, *et al.*: Childhood living conditions and Helicobacter pylori seropositivity in adult life. *Lancet* 1992, 339:896–897,

41. Glassman MS: Helicobacter pylori-associated diseases in children. A clinical summary. *Clin Pediatr* 1992, 31:481–487.

42. Tolia V, Chang CH, Brennan S, Newell D, Thirimoorthi MC: Occurrence and diagnosis of Campylobacter pylori infection in children. *Int Pediatr* 1990, 5:37–41.

43. Heldenberg D, Wagner Y, Heldengerg E, *et al.*: The role of Helicobacter pylori in children with recurrent abdominal pain. *Am J Gastroenterol* 1995, 90:906–909.

44. Hill ID, Sinclair-Smith C, Lastovica AJ, Bowie MD, Emms M: Transient protein-losing enteropathy associated with acute gastritis and Campylobacter pylori. *Arch Dis Child* 1987, 62:1215–1219.

45. Graham DY: *Helicobacter pylori Diagnosis and Treatment*. Deerfield, IL: Discovery International, 1995; 2–8.

46. Berthel JS, Everett ED: Diagnosis of Campylobacter pylori infections: The "gold standard" and the alternatives. *Rev Infect Dis* 1990, 12:S107–S114.

47. Marshall BJ, Warren JR, Francis GI, Langston SR, Goodwin CS, Blincow ED: Rapid urease test in the management of Campylobacter pylori disease-associated gastritis. *Am J Gastroenterol* 1987, 182:200–210.

48. Thomas JE, Whatmore AM, Barer MR, *et al.*: Serodiagnosis of Helicobacter pylori infection in childhood. *J Clin Microbiol* 1990, 28:2641–2646.

49. Glassman MS, Dallal S, Berezin SH, *et al.*: Helicobacter pylori-related gastroduodenal disease in children. Diagnosis utility of enzyme-linked immunosorbent assay. *Dig Dis Sci* 1990, 35:993–997.

50. Atherton JC, Spiller RC: The urea breath test for Helicobacter pylori. *Gut* 1994, 35:723–725.

51. Vandenplas Y, Blecker L, Devroker T, *et al.*: Contribution of ^{13}C breath test to the detection of Helicobacter pylori gastritis in children. *Pediatrics* 1992, 19:608–611.

52. Graham DY, Go MF: Helicobacter pylori: Current status. *Gastroenterology* 1993, 105:279–282.

53. Sung JJY, Chung SCS, Ling TKW, *et al.*: Antibacterial treatment of gastric ulcers associated with Helicobacter pylori. *N Engl J Med* 1995, 332:139–142.

54. Dohil R, Israel DM, Hassall E: Omeprazole and amoxicillin for H. pylori-associated duodenal ulcer disease in children. *Gastrointest Endosc* 1995, 41:4:A:158–335.

55. Weber A: Secondary peptic ulcerations and gastritis. In *Pediatric Clinical Gastroenterology*, 4th ed. Eds Roy, Silverman, Alagille. Mosby & Co., 1995:195–205.

56. Cochran EB, Phelps SJ, Tolley EA, Stidham GL: Prevalence of and risk factors for upper gastrointestinal tract bleeding in critically ill pediatric patients. *Crit Care Med* 1992, 20:1519–1523.

57. Driks MR, Craven DE, Celli BR: Nosocomial pneumonia in intubated patients given sucralfate as compared with antacids or histamine-type 2 blockers. The role of gastric colonization. *N Engl J Med* 1987, 317:1376–1381.

58. Lieh-Lai MW, Hassan N, Meert KL, Theodorou A, Tolia V, Sarnaik AP: Stress gastrointestinal hemorrhage and nosocomial pneumonia in mechanically-ventilated children receiving stress ulcer prophylaxis. *Pediatr Res* 1993, 33:36A.

59. Weber A: Gastrointestinal bleeding. In *Pediatric Clinical Gastroenterology*, 4th ed. Eds Roy, Silverman, Alagille. Mosby & Co., 1995; 205–215.

60. Olson AD, Hillemeier CA: Gastrointestinal hemorrhage. In *Pediatric Gastrointestinal Disease*. Eds Wyllie, Hyams. Saunders; 1993; 250–270.

61. Misiewicz JJ, Bartram CI, Cotton PB, *et al.*: *Atlas of Clinical Gastroenterology*. London: Gower Medical Publishing; 1990.

62. Bozymski EM, London JE: Miscellaneous diseases of the esophagus. In *Atlas of Gastroenterology*. Edited by Yamada Y, Alpers D, Owyang C, *et al.* Philadelphia: JB Lippincott; 1991:148–155.

63. Gostout CJ: Acute gastrointestinal bleeding - a common problem revisited. *Mayo Clin Proc* 1988, 63:596–604.

64. Reilly H III, Al-Kawas F: Dieulafoy's lesion diagnosis and management. *Dig Dis Sci* 1991, 36:1702–1707.

65. Johnson JH: The sentinel clot/visible vessel revisited. *Gastrointest Endosc* 1986, 32:238–289.

66. Swain CP, Storey DW, Brown SG, *et al.*: Nature of the bleeding vessel in recurrently bleeding gastric ulcers. *Gastroenterol* 1986, 90:595–608.

67. Yang CC, Shin JS, Lix XZ, Hsu PI, Chen KW, Lin CY: The natural history (fading time) of stigmata of recent hemorrhage in peptic ulcer disease. *Gastrointest Endosc* 1994, 40:562–566.

Chapter 6

Diarrheal Disease in Infants and Children

JON A. VANDERHOOF

Diarrhea is a common complaint among pediatric patients. The differential diagnosis of diarrhea in children is extensive and varies considerably based on the patient's age. Diarrhea is most commonly defined either as an increase in stool frequency or as a loosened consistency of the stool. Because the number of stools may vary considerably, consistency is perhaps the more important factor. A normal infant passes 5 to 10 g per kilogram of stool per day; volume in excess of that is generally considered as diarrhea. By 3 years of age, stool loss in excess of 200 g per day defines diarrhea in both children and adults.

The pathophysiology of diarrhea in children is the same as that seen in adults. Osmotic diarrhea, secretory diarrhea, inflammatory diarrhea, and occasionally, motility disturbances can all produce loosening of the stools. Often, especially in inflammatory disorders, more than a single mechanism is involved.

In children, diarrhea is considered to be acute if its duration is shorter than 2 weeks. Most acute diarrhea has an infectious origin. Viral pathogens typically injure the small intestine, producing watery stools primarily through osmotic and secretory mechanisms. Bacterial pathogens primarily involve the colon; an inflammatory mechanism, as well as secretory or osmotic components, is usually important. Consequently, bacterial pathogens typically produce bloody, mucoserous stools with associated crampy abdominal pain; viral pathogens most commonly present with watery stools and vomiting.

The differential diagnosis of chronic diarrhea varies more with age than acute diarrhea. In small infants, common causes of chronic diarrhea include milk protein enterocolitis, which may develop into intractable or protracted diarrhea of infancy, as well as infectious pathogens such as *Giardia lamblia*. Less common disorders include microvillous inclusion disease, autoimmune enteropathy, Hirschsprung's disease, and several congenital disorders related to transport and malabsorptive factors. In toddlers 1 to 2 years old, chronic nonspecific diarrhea, otherwise known as irritable colon of infancy or toddler diarrhea, is the most common cause. Infectious pathogens such as Giardia play a role. Inflammatory bowel disease, primarily ulcerative colitis, may be seen in this age group. Small bowel disorders, including celiac disease, frequently present around this time. In school-age children, inflammatory bowel disease becomes a more important cause of chronic diarrhea. Loose stools and abdominal pain are a common presentation of primary acquired lactase deficiency common after 5 years of age. Finally, chronic constipation with overflow, *ie*, encopresis, is often misinterpreted as diarrhea in children of this age.

Endoscopy for endoscopic biopsy of both the small and large intestine is often helpful in making a definitive diagnosis in infants and children of all ages with chronic diarrhea. Except in the toddler with intermittent loose runny stools, chronic diarrhea is usually a manifestation of organic disease and merits diagnostic evaluation. The images shown in this chapter are obtained from children of various ages; they include photographs, pathologic and biopsy specimens, and endoscopic pictures obtained from infants and children with several diarrheal diseases. The figures selected are designed to help the clinician formulate a differential diagnosis and interpret the results of diagnostic studies.

■ SMALL-BOWEL DISORDERS

Celiac disease

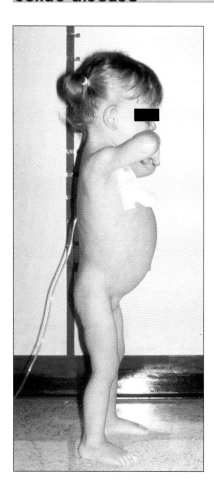

FIGURE 6-1.

Child with celiac disease. Note the protuberant abdomen and the marked muscle wasting and evidence of malnutrition. Children with celiac disease may exhibit no unusual findings on physical examination and rarely are as severely affected as this girl. This photograph was selected to demonstrate the physical findings. This child responded very well to a strict gluten-free diet that she must follow for the rest of her life.

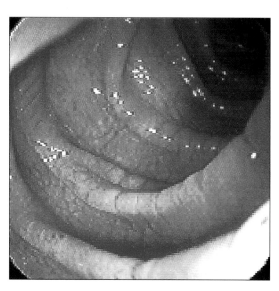

FIGURE 6-2.

Endoscopic image from the proximal small intestine of a patient with celiac sprue. Note the "scalloped" appearance of the small bowel. Although this image strongly suggests celiac disease, the findings are nonspecific. Confirmation by biopsy as well as clinical response to a gluten-free diet are necessary to confirm the diagnosis. (*Courtesy of* Stuart S. Kaufman, MD, Creighton University, Omaha, NE.)

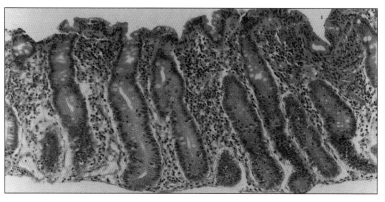

FIGURE 6-3.

Biopsy specimen obtained from a patient with celiac disease. This is the classic flat lesion of celiac sprue. No villi are visible because the epithelium is totally flat. An intense inflammatory infiltrate is present in the lamina propria, primarily mononuclear cells. A marked increase in mitotic epithelial cell activity is present in the crypts, another hallmark of celiac disease. The surface epithelium has lost its polarity, with the normal basal orientation of the nuclei disturbed. Although these findings are common in celiac disease, they are also nonspecific and may occur, in extreme cases, from a variety of small intestinal disorders. (*Courtesy of* Robert Kruger, MD, Children's Hospital, Omaha, NE.)

Jejunal biopsy

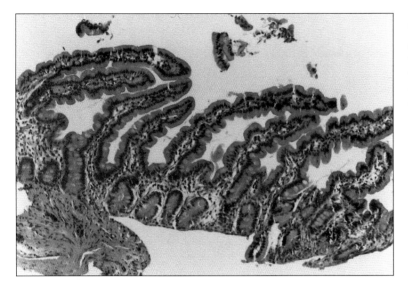

FIGURE 6-4.

Jejunal biopsy specimen from a normal infant for comparison with celiac disease. The villi are roughly four to five times as tall as the crypts are deep, known as a 4-to-1 villus-to-crypt ratio. The epithelial cells have nice polarity with basally oriented nuclei. A normal complement of plasma cells and lymphocytes is present in the lamina propria. Eosinophils are present only in small numbers and neutrophils are absent. The average crypt contains two or fewer mitotic epithelial cells. (*Courtesy of* Robert Kruger, MD, Children's Hospital, Omaha, NE.)

Milk protein–induced enteritis

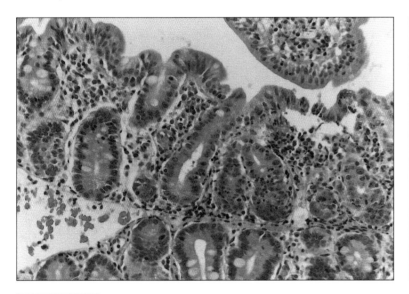

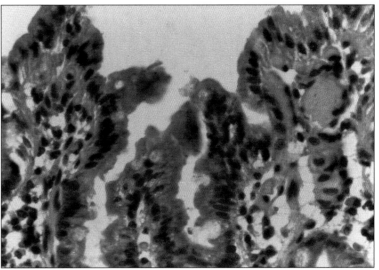

FIGURE 6-5.

Jejunal biopsy specimen of an infant with a milk protein–induced enteritis. Milk-protein intolerance may produce various histologic abnormalities in the small intestine. These may vary from a totally flat biopsy similar to that seen in celiac disease to essentially normal findings. Because the lesion is patchy, several biopsies must be obtained; a wide variety of lesions are typically seen in the same patient at the same time. Small intestinal involvement is characterized by partial villus destruction with modest degrees of crypt cell hyperplasia. The lamina propria is infiltrated with a mixture of lymphocytes, plasma cells, eosinophils, and occasionally neutrophils. (*Courtesy of* Robert Kruger, MD, Children's Hospital, Omaha, NE.)

FIGURE 6-6.

Magnified jejunal biopsy specimen obtained from an infant with milk protein–induced enteritis. The epithelium loses its distinct polarity. Nuclei are no longer basally oriented in all of the epithelial cells. Mononuclear cells can be seen migrating through the surface epithelium. (*Courtesy of* Robert Kruger, MD, Children's Hospital, Omaha, NE.)

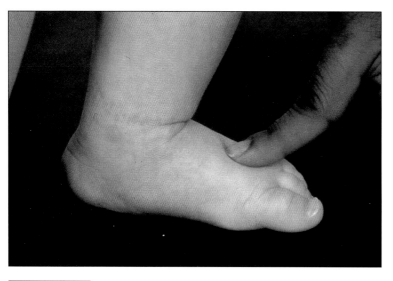

FIGURE 6-7.

Edema in an infant with protein-losing enteropathy resulting from cow milk–protein intolerance. During the first 3 months of life, cow milk–protein intolerance typically presents with irritability, diarrhea, and blood in the stool. During the second 6 months of life, however, small bowel disease may predominate. In this clinical setting, hypoproteinemia, iron deficiency anemia, and edema may characterize the findings. The infant in this figure, who has cow milk–protein intolerance, has marked edema produced by hypoproteinemia secondary to gastrointestinal protein loss.

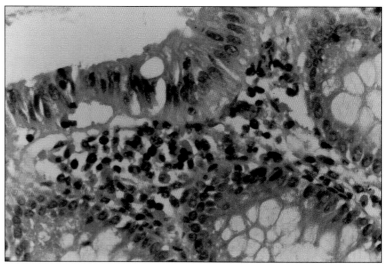

FIGURE 6-8.

Rectal biopsy specimen obtained from an infant with milk protein–induced colitis. The predominant feature is an increase in the number of eosinophils present in the lamina propria. At least six eosinophils per high powered field are required to be diagnostic. The changes are patchy, and at least three biopsies should be obtained to make the diagnosis adequately. Neutrophils, as well as increased plasma cells and lymphocytes, may also be present in the lamina propria. Because these changes are nonspecific, the diagnosis must be made in terms of the overall clinical presentation. (*Courtesy of* Robert Kruger, MD, Children's Hospital, Omaha, NE.)

Small intestine biopsy

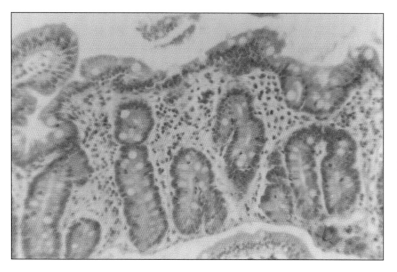

FIGURE 6-9.

Typical biopsy specimen from the small intestine of a patient with intractable diarrhea of infancy. This disorder is characterized by mild to moderate injury to the small intestinal epithelium. Because the lesion is patchy, biopsies may be normal in some areas and totally flat in others. The lesion is highly variable and is a poor predictor of outcome or duration of therapy. The inflammatory response is usually not as intense as is seen in celiac disease nor is the proliferation of mitotic epithelial cells in the crypts as pronounced as in celiac disease. (*Courtesy of* Robert Kruger, MD, Children's Hospital, Omaha, NE.)

Giardiasis

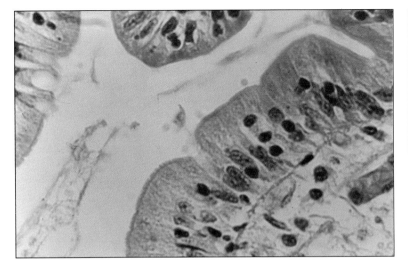

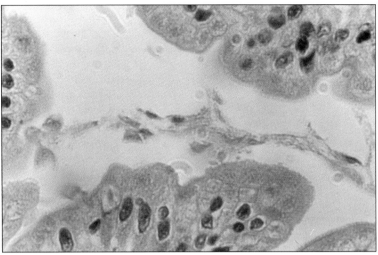

FIGURE 6-10.

Giardiasis in biopsy specimen of small intestine. The inflammatory response and degree of villus injury are variable in this disease. Diagnosis can, however, be made by demonstrating the presence of crescent-shaped organisms adhering or in close proximity to the mucosal surface. Often, the karyosomes in the organisms appear as eyes looking back at the clinician through the microscope if the organisms are optimally oriented. Although biopsies of the small intestine have traditionally provided the most accurate means of diagnosing giardiasis, assessment of the presence of *Giardia* antigen in the stool is now also a commonly accepted method.

FIGURE 6-11.

Another view of a small-bowel biopsy specimen from a patient with giardiasis. Again, the crescent-shaped organisms are present in close proximity to the mucosal surface.

Abetalipoproteinemia

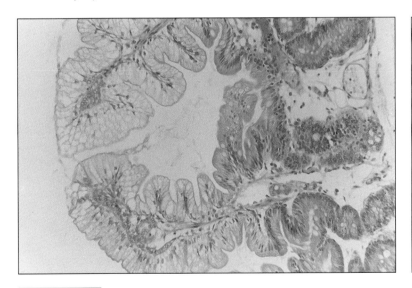

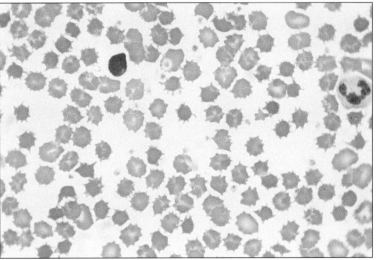

FIGURE 6-12.

Biopsy specimen of small intestine from a patient with abetalipo-proteinemia. These patients are incapable of producing chylomicrons. As a consequence, such patients cannot transport fat out of the mucosal epithelial cells. Fat accumulates in the cells, giving them an appearance resembling pale-colored balloons, even during fasting, as is seen in this biopsy specimen. Steatorrhea, acanthocytosis, and failure to thrive commonly occur. (*Courtesy of* David R. Mack, MD, University of Nebraska, Omaha, NE.)

FIGURE 6-13.

Acanthocytosis in abetalipoproteinemia. In addition to the biopsy findings in the small intestine, patients with abetalipoproteinemia often have characteristic peripheral blood smears demonstrating acanthocytes. This figure demonstrates these spiny-appearing erythrocytes characteristic of abetalipoproteinemia.

Chylomicron inclusion disease

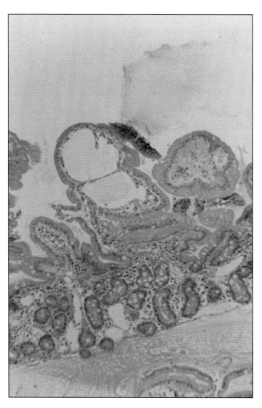

FIGURE 6-14.

Electron microscopic biopsy specimen obtained from a patient with chylomicron inclusion disease. This disorder, also known as *congenital microvillus atrophy*, presents in infants with symptoms of severe diarrhea and malabsorption. Patients generally require lifelong parenteral nutrition. Intestinal transplantation has recently been employed in the treatment of this disorder. In both the small bowel and colon, intestinal epithelial cells demonstrate cytoplasmic vacuoles containing microvillus structures as seen in this specimen. Electron microscopic examination is required for diagnosis of this rare disorder. (*Courtesy of* E. Cutz, MD, Toronto, Ontario, Canada.)

Intestinal lymphangiectasia

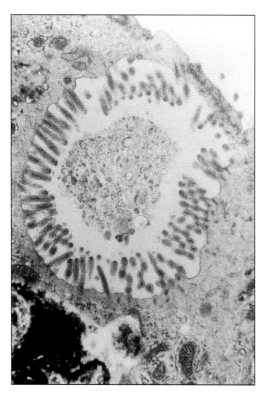

FIGURE 6-15.

A biopsy specimen from proximal small intestine of a patient with intestinal lymphangiectasia. Note the dilated lacteal causing gross dilatation of the villus in the center of the figure. These patients have fat malabsorption and lymphocytopenia in their peripheral blood because of the loss of lymphocytes in the gut. Dilated lacteals in the villus rupture, causing loss of fat, protein, and lymphocytes into the gut lumen. The disorder is commonly treated using enteral feeding formulas containing medium-chain triglycerides that can be absorbed without transportation through lymphatics; however, high carbohydrate, low-fat formulas, such as found in some elemental diets, may be even more effective in the treatment of this disorder.

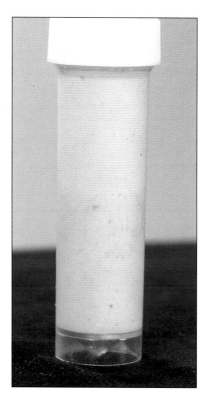

FIGURE 6-16.

Stool sample from a patient with intestinal lymphangiectasia. Marked steatorrhea may occur in this disorder. This stool sample contains large amounts of lipid.

Steatorrhea

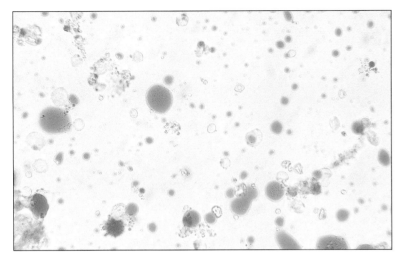

FIGURE 6-17.

Steatorrhea by fecal Sudan stain. This photomicrograph stool sample demonstrates the presence of large amounts of fat by Sudan stain. This test is qualitative and should only be used as a screening tool for gross steatorrhea, but in this particular patient it reveals the presence of a large amount of fat in the stool.

Pathogen-related disorders

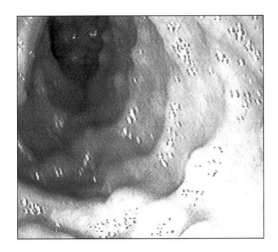

FIGURE 6-18.

Endoscopic image of the jejunum of a patient with an unusual lymphoproliferative disease. Lymphoid proliferation in the small intestine is uncommon. It is often stimulated by a viral process. It is seen most frequently in immunosuppressed patients, especially in patients following transplantation of the small intestine or in those with immunodeficiency disorders. The Epstein-Barr virus is perhaps the most common cause. In the nonimmunosuppressed patient the disorder may be benign, whereby it may regress spontaneously or respond to corticosteroid therapy.

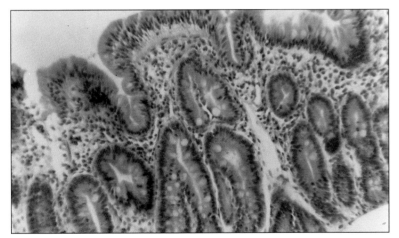

FIGURE 6-19.

Small-bowel biopsy specimen from a patient with rotavirus enteritis. Most viruses result in injury to the proximal small intestine. The lesion is not unlike many other small-bowel disorders with partial flattening of the villi, increase in inflammatory cells, and loss of polarity of the surface epithelium. The lesion is often quite patchy and variable, as are many other small intestinal lesions. Combined secretory and osmotic diarrhea occurs in these patients, in whom the disorder is typically transient.

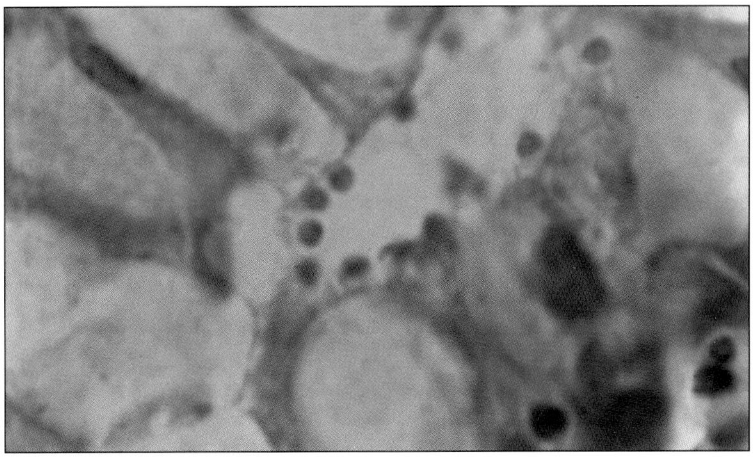

FIGURE 6-20.

Magnified biopsy specimen from the small intestine of an infant with cryptosporidium. These small, round organisms are frequently found adhering to the epithelium. They are associated with the self-limited infectious enterocolitis in immunocompetent patients, but in immunodeficient patients, the disorder may result in severe diarrhea and malabsorption and is often fatal. Treatment is generally not rewarding. Although the organism is commonly thought to reside predominantly in the small intestine, it may also cause colitis. (*Courtesy of* Robert Kruger, MD, Children's Hospital, Omaha, NE.)

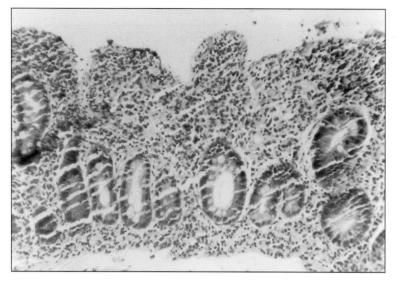

FIGURE 6-21.

Biopsy specimen of proximal small intestine of a child with auto-immune enteropathy. This disorder is characterized by severe diarrhea and malabsorption beginning during the first 6 months of life. The disorder may improve after treatment with corticosteroids with or without cyclosporine, but healing is often incomplete. Children typically require long-term home parenteral nutrition. Severe malabsorption prevents the reinstitution of adequate enteral feedings. Hyperglycemia from pancreatic endocrine involvement is also common. The microscopic lesion is characterized by an intense mixed inflammatory-cell infiltrate. Marked polymorphonuclear infiltration is typical. Loss of the surface epithelium and small intestinal crypt abscesses may be seen.

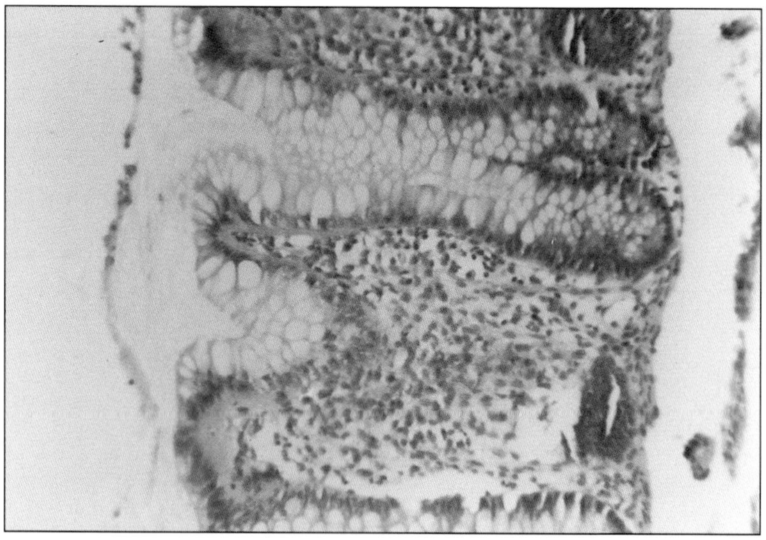

FIGURE 6-22.

Rectal biopsy specimen in a patient with autoimmune enteropathy. Inflammation extends throughout the gastrointestinal tract and into the colon in some patients. In this patient, a mixed inflammatory cell infiltrate is present in the lamina propria with some overlying purulent matter. Colonic inflammation is not always present and is usually not as severe as small intestinal inflammation. (*Courtesy of* Robert Kruger, MD, Children's Hospital, Omaha, NE.)

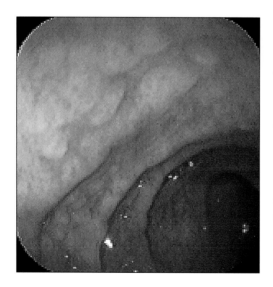

FIGURE 6-23.

Endoscopic image of the duodenum of a patient with autoimmune enteropathy. This is the same patient whose biopsy specimens were shown in Figures 6-21 and 6-22. The scalloping seen in this image is similar to that seen in patients with celiac disease. Both patients had flat small intestinal mucosal biopsies with total loss of villi. Consequently, the scalloping lesion may be a nonspecific finding in severe small intestinal enteropathies. (*Courtesy of* Robert Kruger, MD, Children's Hospital, Omaha, NE.)

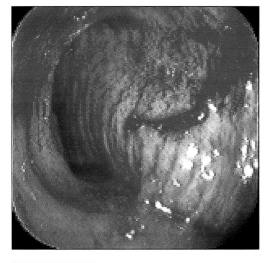

FIGURE 6-24.

Endoscopic image of the small intestine of a patient with short-bowel syndrome. This particular patient has bacterial overgrowth. Bacterial overgrowth is a common complication in patients with short-bowel syndrome who frequently have absence of the ileocecal valve, dilated small intestine, poor motility, and subsequent bacterial proliferation. The mucosa is friable and hemorrhagic. Although this disorder frequently responds to antibiotic therapy, treatment with anti-inflammatory agents, such as sulfasalazine or even corticosteroids, may be needed to control the inflammatory response.

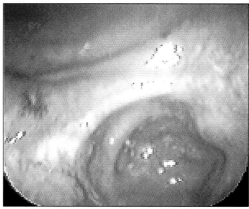

FIGURE 6-25.

Endoscopic image of the distal small intestine of a patient with short-bowel syndrome and small intestinal bacterial overgrowth. In addition to the conditions seen in Figure 6-24, discreet ulcerations are common in these patients. Treatment is similar. In some instances, deep ulcerations, especially located near the anastomosis, may require surgical resection to stop hemorrhage.

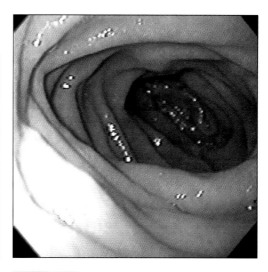

FIGURE 6-26.

Endoscopic image of the proximal small intestine of a patient with short-bowel syndrome. Note the dilated small intestine. Dilatation in patients with short-bowel syndrome is common after massive resection and is considered to be a compensatory process designed to increase absorptive surface area. Because peristalsis is impaired by intestinal dilatation, bacterial overgrowth commonly results. In this patient, aggressive use of antibiotic therapy and periodic enteral flushes have resulted in resolution of a previously existing enteritis. (*Courtesy of* Claire Wilson, MD, Honolulu, HI.)

Intestinal transplants

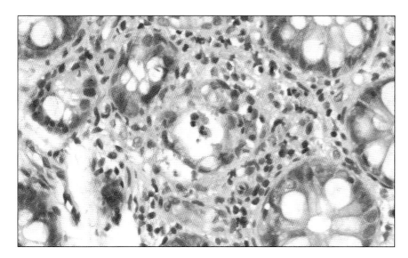

FIGURE 6-27.

Histologic specimen showing rejection in the small intestine following intestinal transplant. Intestinal transplantation is now becoming possible for the treatment of short-bowel syndrome and certain other disorders associated with diarrhea. Most intestinal transplants have been performed for end-stage parenteral nutrition-induced liver disease and have involved transplantation of both liver and small intestine. Smaller numbers of isolated intestinal transplants have also been performed. The most common causes of graft loss following intestinal transplantation include rejection, infection, and lymphoproliferative disease. Shown is a histologic specimen from a patient with mild graft rejection. The hallmark is crypt destruction, which can be seen in the center of the figure. Nonspecific inflammatory changes are also present. (*Courtesy of* Rodney Markin, MD, University of Nebraska, Omaha, NE.)

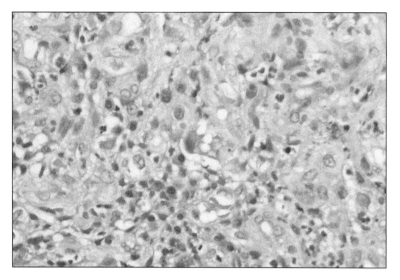

FIGURE 6-28.

Histologic specimen showing enteritis caused by cytomegalovirus (CMV) after intestinal transplant. This patient has CMV enteritis, another complication of intestinal transplantation. The cytomegalic inclusion bodies seen in the center of this figure are typical. (*Courtesy of* Rodney Markin, MD, University of Nebraska, Omaha, NE.)

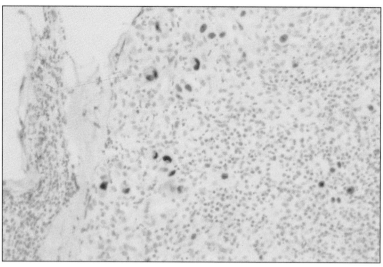

FIGURE 6-29.

Immunoperoxidase stain with cytomegalovirus (CMV) enteritis following intestinal transplantation of the same patient from in Figure 6-28. Here, the immunoperoxidase stain demonstrates the presence of CMV within the cells in the lamina propria. CMV-derived enteritis occurs primarily in patients who are immunosuppressed. The marked degree of immunosuppression needed for small intestinal transplantation creates an opportunity for CMV to invade the small bowel. (*Courtesy of* Rodney Markin, MD, University of Nebraska, Omaha, NE.)

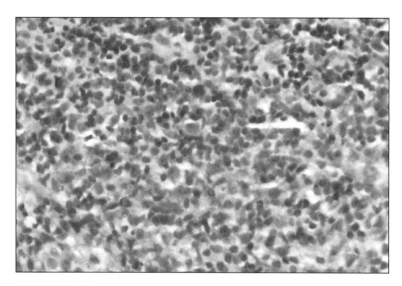

FIGURE 6-30.

A histologic specimen showing lymphoproliferative disease in the small intestine following small intestinal transplantation. Lymphoproliferative disease results from aggressive immunosuppression. Because transplantation of the small intestine requires greater immunosuppression than most other solid organ transplants, this complication is particularly common. In this case, densely packed lymphocytes are present in the lamina propria of a patient who underwent transplantation of the small intestine. This patient responded to reduction in immunosuppression, a characteristic feature of lymphoproliferative disease following transplantation. (*Courtesy of* Rodney Markin, MD, University of Nebraska, Omaha, NE.)

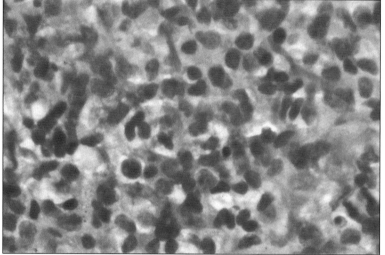

FIGURE 6-31.

Close-up view of lymphoproliferative disease following intestinal transplant. Note the dark staining nuclei in the lymphocytes. This complication of immunosuppression following intestinal transplantation appears to be an Epstein-Barr virus–driven lymphoma. (*Courtesy of* Rodney Markin, MD, University of Nebraska, Omaha, NE.)

INFLAMMATORY BOWEL DISEASE AND COLONIC DISEASE

Lymphoid hyperplasia

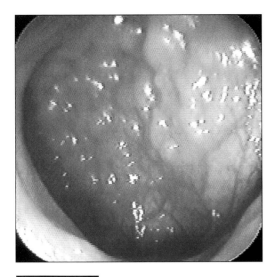

FIGURE 6-32.

Endoscopic image demonstrating lymphoid hyperplasia in the terminal ileum. Lymphoid hyperplasia is a common finding in the terminal ileum, especially in children and teenagers. Radiographically, it is often difficult to distinguish ileal lymphoid hyperplasia from Crohn's disease. Endoscopic biopsies now make this distinction possible because endoscopic intubation of the ileum is simple with today's colonoscopes.

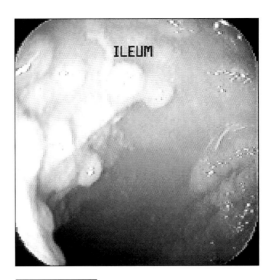

FIGURE 6-33.

Another example of ileal lymphoid hyperplasia. The lymphoid nodules are somewhat more prominent in this patient than the patient in Figure 6-32. This is a normal finding in children and teenagers and should not be confused with Crohn's disease or another pathologic process.

Crohn's disease of the ileum

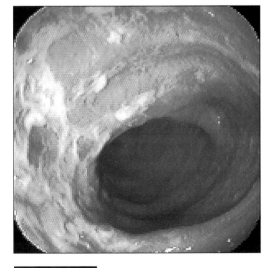

FIGURE 6-34.

Endoscopic image of Crohn's disease of the ileum. Compare Figure 6-33 with this image of the ileum of a child with early Crohn's disease. Here, friability of the mucosa with erythema and loss of ramifying vascular pattern are the most prominent features. Again, histologic confirmation of the diagnosis can be made endoscopically.

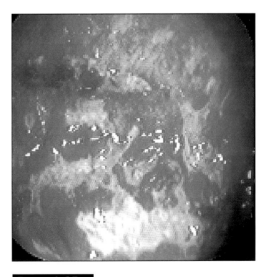

FIGURE 6-35.

Endoscopic image of different child with Crohn's disease of the ileum. Here, the disease is more advanced, the erythema is more intense, and irregular ulcerations, which are the endoscopic hallmark of Crohn's disease, are beginning to form.

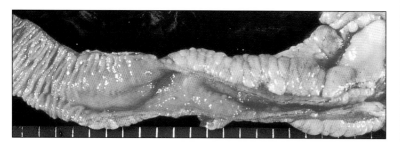

FIGURE 6-36.

Pathologic specimen from a child with Crohn's disease. This is a segment of the ileum, the most likely portion of the small intestine to be involved in Crohn's disease. As the disease progresses, transmural involvement with thickening of the bowel wall, scarring, and formation of stricture results. Surgery is often necessitated at this point to relieve symptoms of partial obstruction of the small intestine. The pathologic specimen demonstrates accumulation of fat in the mesentery that often accompanies advanced Crohn's disease. This finding can be very helpful in making the diagnosis at the time of laparotomy. (*Courtesy of* Robert Kruger, MD, Childrens Hospital, Omaha, NE.)

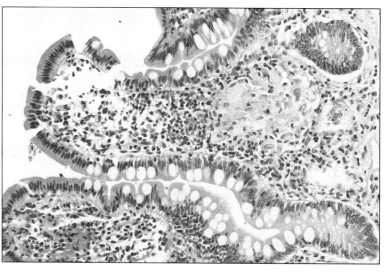

FIGURE 6-37.

A biopsy specimen from a patient with Crohn's disease. Note the granuloma present in the lamina propria. Granulomas are considered diagnostic for Crohn's disease in an appropriate clinical setting. They are not always present, however, and the chances of finding one with only limited sampling is not very good. The remainder of the changes with Crohn's disease are nonspecific and consist of mixed cell infiltrates, epithelial damage, and inflammation of various severity.

Colitis

Ulcerative colitis

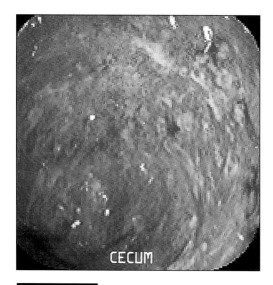

FIGURE 6-38.

Endoscopic image of the proximal colon of a patient with ulcerative colitis. This is a moderate disease state. The mucosa is friable. Ramifying vessels are not seen, although the mucosa is smooth. The lesion is continuous, and if the cecum is involved, the entire colon appears abnormal, at least histologically. The inflammatory changes are usually more severe in the distal colon.

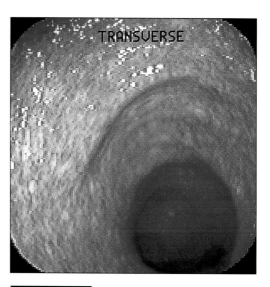

FIGURE 6-39.

Endoscopic image of the transverse colon of a patient with ulcerative colitis. This patient has more severe disease than the patient in Figure 6-38. The triangular appearance of the transverse colon is somewhat indistinct. The mucosa appears hemorrhagic, but still flat. Ramifying vessels are not seen. No normal mucosa is present.

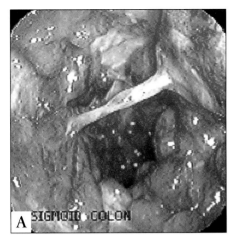

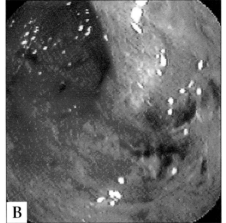

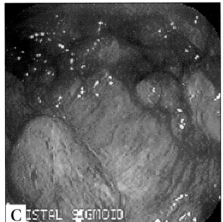

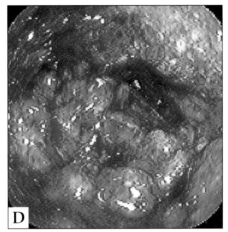

FIGURE 6-40.

A–D, Endoscopic images from a patient with severe ulcerative colitis. This is a debilitating disease. Chronic inflammation and scarring have resulted in formation of pseudopolyps. Patients with severe disease are more difficult to control medically and frequently require colectomy. Complications, such as severe iron deficiency anemia and hypoproteinemia, as well as fluid and electrolyte abnormalities, are common in patients with severe ulcerative colitis.

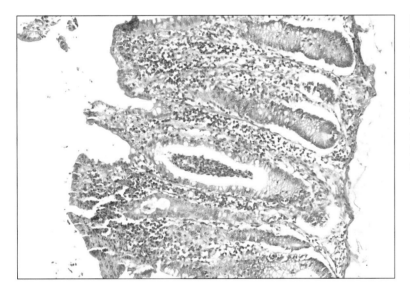

FIGURE 6-41.

Mucosal biopsy specimen from a patient with ulcerative colitis. An intense inflammatory infiltrate is typical. Crypt abscesses may occur in both Crohn's disease and ulcerative colitis but tend to be more prominent in ulcerative colitis. Multiple crypts filled with neutrophils are therefore more suggestive of ulcerative colitis. Granulomas are absent. Inflammation is limited to the mucosa with no extension into the deeper layers.

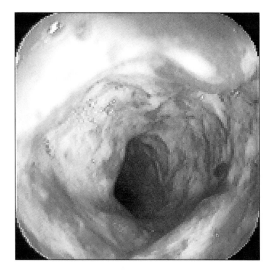

FIGURE 6-42.

Endoscopic image of a patient with pseudomembranous colitis. Note that the pseudo-membranes adhere to the mucosa. This particular patient had ulcerative colitis. It is important to remember that although pseudomembranous colitis is considered to be a hallmark of *Clostridium difficile*, it may be associated with other forms of colitis, as in this case of ulcerative colitis. It also may occur with disorders resulting from other infectious organisms, such as shigellosis. (*Courtesy of* Stuart S. Kaufman, MD, Creighton University, Omaha, NE.)

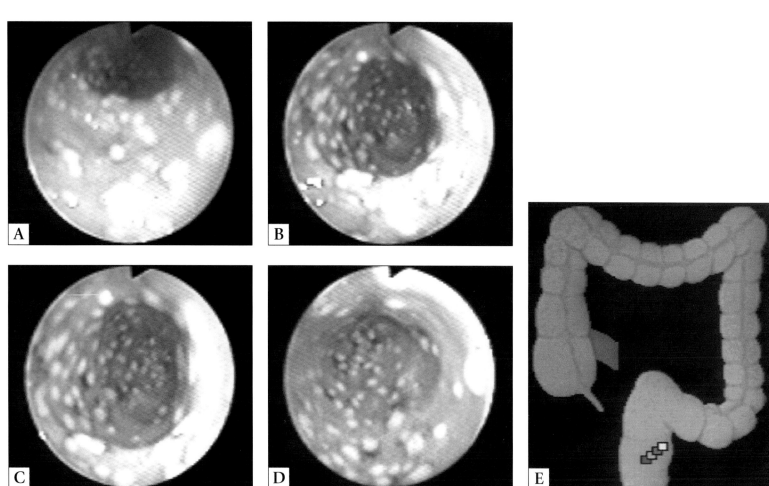

FIGURE 6-43.

A–D, Endoscopic images of pseudomembranous colitis in a child receiving antibiotic therapy. This particular patient had antibiotic-induced diarrhea due to overgrowth of *Clostridium difficile*. Although *C. difficile* is commonly associated with pseudomembranous colitis, the majority of patients with diarrhea caused by *C. difficile* do not have pseudomembranous colitis. When pseudomembranes are seen and there is a history of antibiotic exposure, however, *C. difficile* should certainly be considered at the top of the differential diagnosis. Patchy yellow plaques that adhere to the mucosa are present and are difficult to remove. The mucosa is usually quite friable. It is also important to remember, as shown in Figure 6-42, that pseudo-membranous colitis may result from a variety of pathogens other than *C. difficile*. Color codes in **E**: red—location of **A**; green—location of **B**; purple—location of **C**; yellow—location of **D**. (*Courtesy of* Thomas Rossi, MD, Buffalo, NY.)

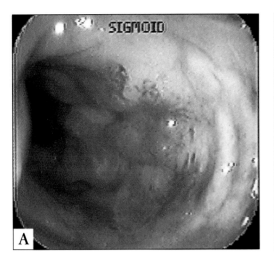
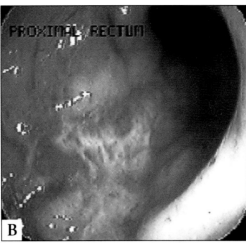
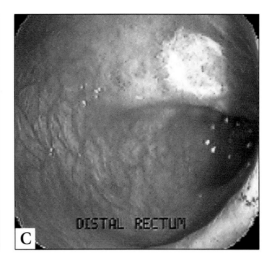

FIGURE 6-44.

A–C, Endoscopic images of the sigmoid colon of a patient with Crohn's disease. An isolated ulcer is shown in the distal rectum. More proximally, linear ulcerations and patchy inflammation are seen. All of these features are characteristic of Crohn's disease. The lesion is typically patchy with areas of involvement interspersed with other areas of normal-appearing mucosa. Ulcerations and involvement deep to the mucosa occur. Compare these images with the earlier images of the patients with ulcerative colitis.

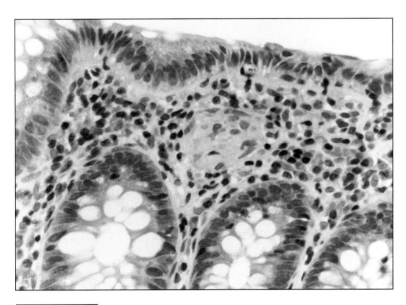

FIGURE 6-45.

Histologic specimen of Crohn's disease of the colon. Here, a granuloma is seen in the lamina propria. Although granulomas are usually not identified in great numbers, finding one in a patient with inflammatory bowel disease helps firmly establish the diagnosis of Crohn's disease. (*Courtesy of* Robert Kruger, MD, Children's Hospital, Omaha, NE.)

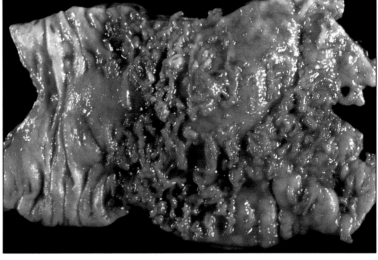

FIGURE 6-46.

Colonic specimen from a patient with Crohn's disease. In this gross specimen, the scarring, pseudopolyp formation, and loss of epithelial surface area can be seen. Adjacent to chronically involved tissue is a segment of normal-appearing colon, demonstrating one classic feature of Crohn's disease of the colon: the skip lesion. Severely abnormal areas can be seen adjacent to normal-appearing colon. (*Courtesy of* Robert Kruger, MD, Children's Hospital, Omaha, NE.)

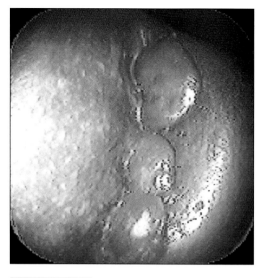

FIGURE 6-47.

Patient with Crohn's disease of the anus. Perianal skin tags and fistulas are quite common. Medical management is often difficult, requiring aggressive immunosuppression and the adjunctive use of metronidazole. Such lesions are usually not seen with ulcerative colitis.

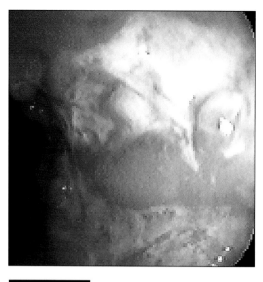

FIGURE 6-48.

Endoscopic image of a colon ulcer in Crohn's disease. During the early stages, Crohn's disease appears much like ulcerative colitis endoscopically. As the disease progresses, more distinct differentiating features occur. Shown is a deep ulcer with irregular borders characteristic of Crohn's disease in the colon. Although the presence of granulomas on biopsy confirms the diagnosis, the presence of this type of lesion endoscopically in a patient with symptoms of chronic inflammatory bowel disease is nearly diagnostic of Crohn's disease.

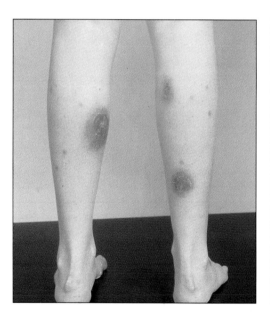

FIGURE 6-49.

Pyoderma gangrenosum in Crohn's disease. Not all of the inflammation in inflammatory bowel disease occurs in the gastrointestinal tract. A small percentage of patients with ulcerative colitis or Crohn's disease develops extraintestinal manifestations of the disease, including arthritis, uveitis, or, as in this patient, skin lesions. Erythema nodosum and pyoderma gangrenosum are most common. Here, the deep ulcerated lesions of pyoderma gangrenosum on the legs are shown. (*Courtesy of* David R. Mack, MD, University of Nebraska, Omaha, NE.)

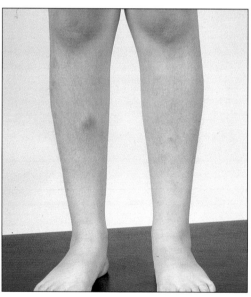

FIGURE 6-50.

Patient with erythema nodosum. This disorder consists of nodular erythematous lesions that are usually on the anterior surface of the legs in patients with inflammatory bowel disease. Unlike pyoderma gangrenosum, the skin is not broken by these lesions.

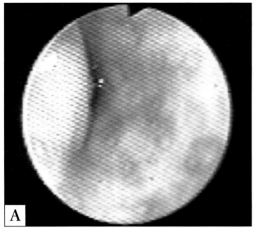

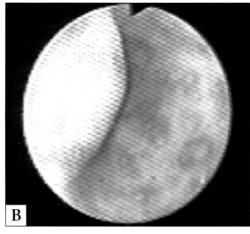

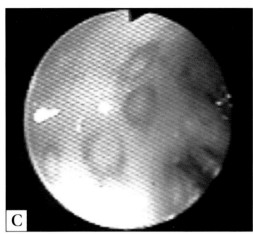

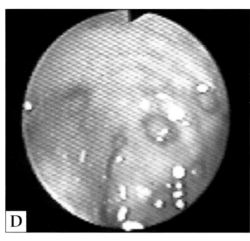

FIGURE 6-51.

A–D, Endoscopic images of lymphoid hyperplasia in an infant. Lymphoid hyperplasia in the colon is a common anatomic variant in infants and children. It often presents with loose, or occasionally bloody, stools. Although the lesion may accompany colitis in infants with milk-protein intolerance, histologically, the intervening mucosa is normal in lymphoid hyperplasia and abnormal in milk protein–induced colitis. The condition is self-limited and requires no treatment. It usually regresses by 4 or 5 years of age. (*Courtesy of* Thomas Rossi, MD, Buffalo, NY.)

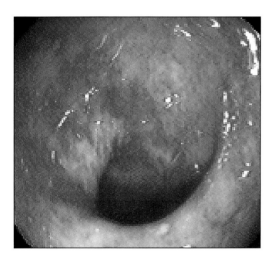

FIGURE 6-52.

Endoscopic image of infectious colitis in a 7-year-old girl. This particular child had colitis caused by *Escherichia coli* 0157H7. Other bacterial organisms, such as *Shigella, Salmonella,* and *Campylobacter jejuni,* may appear indistinguishable. The patchy, erythematous, and occasionally hemorrhagic mucosa is typical and not significantly different from that seen in early ulcerative colitis. Consequently, children presenting with relatively sudden bloody diarrhea should always be evaluated for infectious colitis before the diagnosis of inflammatory bowel disease is entertained.

Chapter 7

Inflammatory Bowel Disease in Pediatrics

ANUPAMA CHAWLA
FREDRIC DAUM

Inflammatory bowel disease (IBD) refers to two distinct diseases, Crohn's disease and ulcerative colitis, both of which cause chronic inflammation of the digestive tract. Crohn's disease is a transmural process that affects any part of the gastrointestinal tract, whereas ulcerative colitis results in inflammation limited to the mucosa and submucosa of the colon.

Epidemiologic data for children and adolescents with Crohn's disease and ulcerative colitis are limited. From a census in 1971, 45% of all newly diagnosed cases of both Crohn's disease and ulcerative colitis occurred in patients less than 20 years of age, the preponderance of which are teenagers [1]. In a study from Scandinavia, the age-specific incidence of Crohn's disease was reported to be as high as 16 per 100,000 in adolescents 15 to 19 years of age. By contrast, an incidence of only 2.5 per 100,000 was noted in children under 15 years of age [2]. Whereas the incidence of ulcerative colitis appears to have remained relatively stable over the years, the incidence of Crohn's disease inexplicably appears to have dramatically increased worldwide. One recent report from Scotland recorded a more than threefold rise in pediatric Crohn's disease incidence (0.6/100,000 in 1968 vs 2.3/100,000 in 1983) [3]. As these diseases are rarely fatal, pediatric prevalence rates of about 11 per 100,000 have been estimated [4].

Children with Crohn's disease are three times less likely to have been breast-fed and three times more likely to have developed a diarrheal illness during infancy than control patients [5,6]. By contrast, the presence or absence of a history of breastfeeding is no different in children with ulcerative colitis than in control patients, although children with ulcerative colitis also have an increased likelihood of having had a diarrheal illness during infancy [7].

Inherited factors are frequently, but not universally, associated with the development of IBD. The proportion of patients with a positive family history for IBD is about 10% to 20%. However, in probands of families who develop IBD before 20 years of age, the proportion with a positive family history is as high as 34% for patients with ulcerative colitis and 39% for those with Crohn's disease [8]. There is also a higher concordance rate for monozygotic than dizygotic twins, especially in patients with Crohn's disease.

A consensus exists that the immune system is responsible for tissue damage in IBD [9–14]. Increasing evidence indicates the presence of hyperactivation of the mucosal immune system in IBD, which may be the result of some fundamental defect in mucosal immune regulation [9,11]. Unchecked immune reactivity leads to a cascade of events including lymphocyte proliferation, cytokine release, and secondary recruitment of auxiliary effector cells such as neutrophils.

Although Crohn's disease and ulcerative colitis represent distinct pathologic entities, the diseases are frequently indistinguishable clinically. Symptoms of either Crohn's disease or ulcerative colitis can appear suddenly or insidiously. The onset may be acute mimicking enteric gastrointestinal infection, or symptoms may wax and wane for months before diagnosis. Occasionally, gastrointestinal symptoms may be absent and the diagnosis made during the evaluation of an extraintestinal symptom or sign such as arthritis, fever of unknown origin, or short stature. Severe cramps and watery bloody diarrhea often occur with extensive colonic involvement. By contrast, in patients with proctosigmoiditis, weight loss and systemic symptoms are frequently absent. Active proctitis usually results in tenesmus and urgency but may be occasionally manifested by constipation. Patients with Crohn's disease of the small bowel commonly experience cramps with various degrees of diarrhea. Stools are frequently positive for occult blood; severe bleeding from small-bowel disease, although uncommon, has been described [15–17]. Dyspeptic symptoms may arise from Crohn's disease affecting the esophagus, stomach, or duodenum.

Extraintestinal manifestations are seen in both Crohn's disease and ulcerative colitis. Transient arthralgias are common, but arthritis occurs infrequently. Rashes including erythema nodosum, vasculitic skin changes (similar to those found in Henoch-Schönlein purpura), and pyoderma gangrenosum have been described. Other extraintestinal manifestations include uveitis, episcleritis, mouth sores, primary sclerosing cholangitis, and other hepatobiliary abnormalities.

Chronic perianal fissures and tags are present in approximately 50% of children and adolescents with Crohn's disease [18]. Less frequently seen are perianal fistulas and abscesses (15% of children with Crohn's disease).

IBD in children is further complicated by a marked effect on growth and sexual development. If IBD develops before completion of the adolescent growth spurt, the effect can be dramatic and potentially irreversible. Although patients with Crohn's disease are at greater risk for growth problems, those with ulcerative colitis can also be affected. Inadequate nutritional intake [19], continuing disease activity, and use of corticosteroids are the primary factors for permanent growth failure documented in 20% to 30% of young adults whose onset of IBD occurred prior to puberty [20,21].

Evaluation requires a thorough history, physical examination, and laboratory tests. Growth records for many years before the onset of a patient's symptoms are crucial because long-standing growth suppression may not be evident by evaluation of a patient's current weight for height proportion. Contrast radiography of the gastrointestinal tract is helpful to identify changes suggestive of IBD and to assess the extent of disease. Endoscopy of the colon and upper gastrointestinal tract allows both visualization and biopsy sampling of the mucosa. In the untreated patient, diffuse inflammation and inflammation extending proximally from the anal verge favor the diagnosis of ulcerative colitis, whereas patchy inflammation, the presence of small aphthous ulcerations, and distinct skip lesions are more consistent with Crohn's colitis.

The pharmacologic and nutritional therapies of both Crohn's disease and ulcerative colitis remain primarily supportive. Treatment aims include the suppression of incapacitating symptoms, the promotion of normal growth and sexual development, the control of unavoidable complications, and the avoidance of excessive or inappropriate therapy. Because symptoms at times cannot be completely eliminated, treatment requires a careful balance between sufficient intervention to ensure normal daily functioning, and avoidance of overtreatment. While treating the physical illness, one must always keep in mind the psychosocial burden of IBD on children. In one study, 60% of children and adolescents with either Crohn's disease or ulcerative colitis manifested identifiable psychiatric disorders, the most common being depression [22]. With proper team management, which includes a pediatric gastroenterologist, psychotherapist, nurse clinician, and the support of other parents and children, the family and patient learn to cope and, it is hoped, to live productive lives with minimal morbidity.

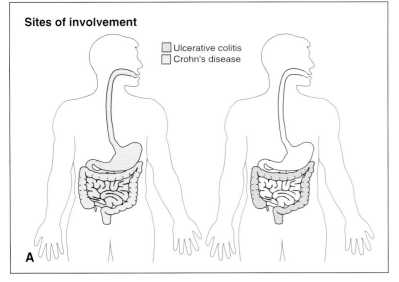

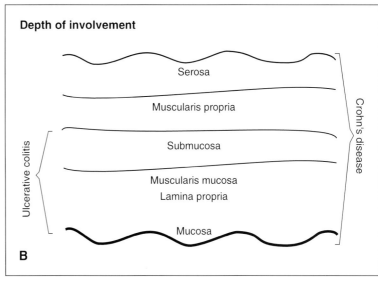

FIGURE 7-1.

Inflammatory bowel disease comprises two distinct diseases—ulcerative colitis and Crohn's disease. In both, there is chronic inflammation of the gastrointestinal tract. **A**, Although ulcerative colitis involves only the colon, Crohn's disease can involve any part of the gastrointestinal tract from the mouth to the anus, including the perianal region. In Crohn's disease, ileocolonic involvement is the most common. In ulcerative colitis presenting in adults, proctitis is the most common initial presentation (46.5%), 23% presenting with more extensive left-sided colitis and about 10% to 15% with total colitis. The extent of inflammation in children at presentation is still uncertain. Of patients with proctitis, 50% to 60% progress to left-sided or total colitis [23]. **B**, In Crohn's disease, the inflammation is transmural, whereas in ulcerative colitis the inflammation is limited to the mucosa and submucosa.

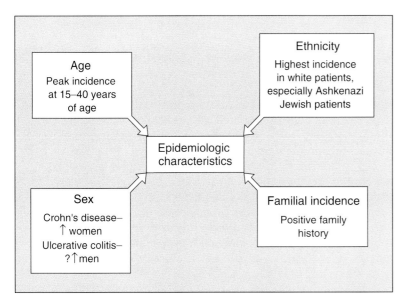

FIGURE 7-2.

Epidemiologic characteristics of inflammatory bowel disease (IBD). Peak incidence occurs between 20 to 40 years of age with a second peak later than 60 years of age. In children, the highest incidence is in the second decade of life, but up to 40% of children are diagnosed under 13 years of age. In Crohn's disease, female predominance is consistently reported. Conversely, there may be a slight predominance in males in ulcerative colitis.

Familial aggregation is a feature of IBD. The increased monozygotic twin concordance rates and the rarity of IBD in spouses suggest a genetic component. Positive family history is seen in 10% to 20% of cases [24,25]. However, when probands of patients developing IBD before 20 years of age are studied, the proportion of patients with a positive family history is as high as 34% for ulcerative colitis and 39% for Crohn's disease [8]. Highest incidence is reported in white, especially Ashkenazi Jewish, patients. Black and Asian patients have lower incidence.

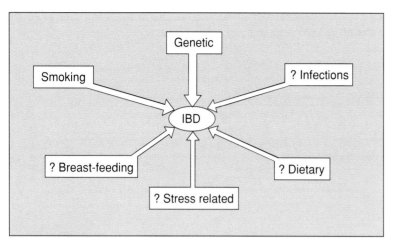

FIGURE 7-3.

Pathogenesis of inflammatory bowel disease (IBD). There are several theories as to the pathogenesis of IBD. It is clear that genetic factors play a role. The role of dietary antigens remains unresolved. Cow's milk–protein sensitivity during infancy has been noted in patients with IBD [26]. Studies have shown that children with Crohn's disease are three times less likely to have been breast-fed and three times more likely to have had a diarrheal illness during infancy [5]. Patients with ulcerative colitis were three times more likely to have had diarrheal diseases during infancy than their unaffected siblings [7]. Breast-feeding was not associated with decreased risk of ulcerative colitis. Studies have suggested smoking may decrease the risk of ulcerative colitis but increase the risk for Crohn's disease [27–29]. Although few data suggest that psychosocial factors are causative in IBD, children with IBD often exhibit increased symptomatology when stressed.

FIGURE 7-4.

Evidence for genetic predisposition. Several studies provide evidence that ulcerative colitis and Crohn's disease are associated with genetic predisposition. There is a higher incidence in offspring as well as first- and second-degree relatives. Spouses do not seem to be at greater risk. Higher concordance rates for monozygotic twins than dizygotic twins have been documented in both Crohn's disease and ulcerative colitis.

Inflammatory bowel disease is associated with well-defined genetic syndromes: Turner's syndrome [30–33], Hermansky-Pudlak syndrome [34–36], and glycogen storage disease type 1b [37–39]. Antineutrophil cytoplasmic antibodies (ANCAs) are seen more often in pediatric ulcerative colitis (50% to 80% of cases) [40–43] and are also present in healthy relatives of patients with ulcerative colitis [44].

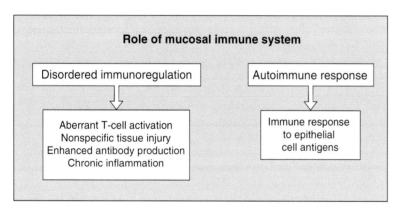

FIGURE 7-5.

Role of mucosal immune system. Two potential mechanisms for the involvement of the gut-associated lymphoid tissue in the pathogenesis of inflammatory bowel disease are postulated. First, disordered immunoregulation leads to immune activation of the T cells [45], leading to nonspecific tissue injury, enhanced antibody production, and chronic inflammation. The activated T cells are postulated to cause tissue injury by the production of lymphokines and cytokines. Second, an autoimmune process has been postulated by which specific immune reponse is directed against epithelial cell antigens. Antibodies to colonic epithelial cells have been reported in patients with Crohn's disease and patients with ulcerative colitis [46–48].

TABLE 7-1. DIFFERENTIATION BETWEEN ULCERATIVE COLITIS AND CROHN'S DISEASE

	ULCERATIVE COLITIS	CROHN'S DISEASE
Site of disease	Colon only	Any part of gastrointestinal tract
Symptoms		
Bleeding	+++	+
Diarrhea	+++	++
Abdominal pain	++	+++
Growth failure	+	+++
Tenesmus	+++	±
Perianal disease	-	+
Endoscopic findings		
Rectal involvement	+++	+
Inflammation	Continuous	Discontinuous
	Diffuse erythema	Patchy lesions
	Ulceration in inflamed mucosa	Discrete ulcers in normal mucosa
Complications		
Fistulas	Exceedingly uncommon (? Crohn's)	Frequent
Strictures	Uncommon (? malignancy)	Common
Cancer risk (> 10 years)	Increased	Increased

TABLE 7-1.

Differentiation of ulcerative colitis and Crohn's disease. It is not always easy to differentiate ulcerative colitis from Crohn's disease. Bloody diarrhea is more common with ulcerative colitis but can occur in Crohn's disease. Tenesmus is more often seen in ulcerative colitis because of the rectal involvement. Growth failure and perianal disease are more typical of Crohn's disease. Endoscopy is an important diagnostic tool. In ulcerative colitis, the mucosa is diffusely involved with superficial ulceration of inflamed mucosa. In Crohn's disease, focal aphthous or deep linear ulcers with normal surrounding mucosa are more characteristic. Fistulas, abscesses, and inflammatory masses [49,50] are characteristic of Crohn's disease. Strictures are more common in Crohn's disease. The presence of a colonic stricture in ulcerative colitis warrants thorough evaluation for a malignancy. Dysplasia and adenocarcinoma are seen with increasing frequency in both ulcerative colitis and Crohn's colitis, especially after 10 years of disease. Adenocarcinoma of the small intestine has also been documented in long-standing Crohn's disease.

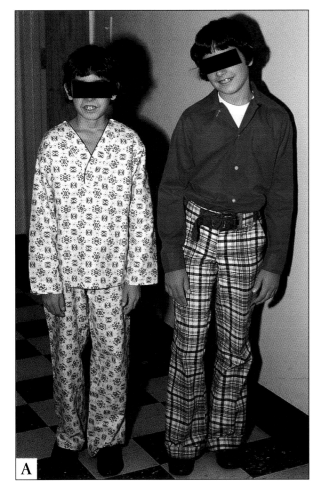

FIGURE 7-6.

Growth failure. **A,** Monozygotic twins at 12 years of age. The patient on the left was 3 inches shorter and 15 pounds lighter at presentation than his monozygotic twin brother.

(*continued on next page*)

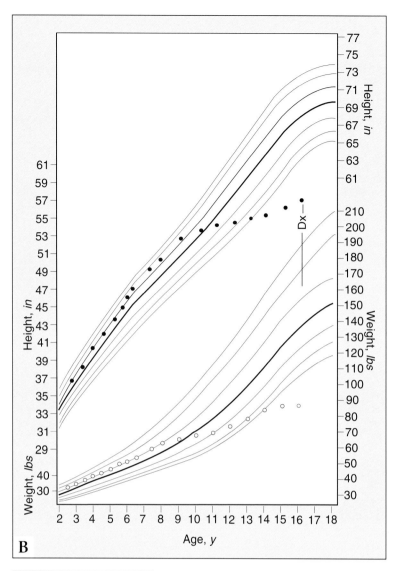

B

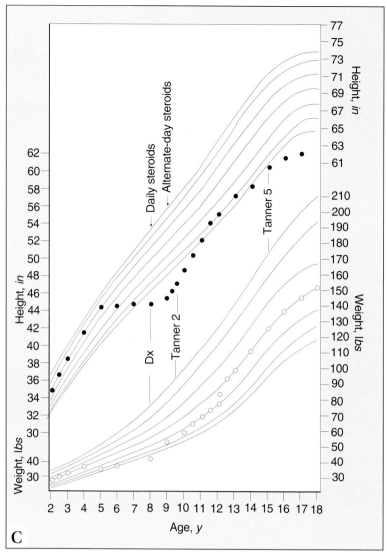

C

FIGURE 7-6. (CONTINUED)

B, Weight and height gain can slow down years before there are any gastrointestinal symptoms. This growth chart presents a boy diagnosed at 16 years of age with minimal diarrhea and no bleeding. He presented with abdominal pain, growth failure, and delayed sexual development. His growth chart showed slowing of weight and height gain for 6 to 7 years before he was diagnosed to have Crohn's disease. This slowing of growth may not be apparent unless these growth charts are maintained. This child did gain both weight and height every year, but at a slower rate, thus reaching lower percentile levels. **C**, Growth failure can be secondary not only to disease activity and poor nutrition as shown in *panel B*, but also to iatrogenic causes.

Daily use of corticosteroids can suppress linear growth. A regimen of steroids taken every other day has been shown to have a relative growth-sparing effect [51]. This growth chart also shows slowing of weight and height gain for 3 to 4 years before diagnosis. Daily steroid therapy was initiated on diagnosis and continued for 12 months. Daily steroids were then tapered to alternate-day steroids. The child showed rapid growth and sexual maturation. Catch-up growth was not achieved, however, despite good weight gain and laboratory tests consistent with suppression of disease activity. This failure to achieve catch-up height may at least in part be explained as a side effect of chronic steroid therapy.

TABLE 7-2. NUTRITIONAL EVALUATION

EVALUATION	MEANS OF EVALUATION
Decreased intake	Calorie counts
Malabsorption	72-hour fecal fat; serum B_{12} and folate
Increased losses caused by inflammation	Fecal α-1-antitrypsin, serum albumin
Increased requirements	Indirect calorimetry

TABLE 7-2.

Nutritional evaluation. Poor nutritional status is well-documented in inflammatory bowel disease (IBD); several factors play a role. Poor appetite is a common symptom, especially in Crohn's disease. Increased requirements caused by hypercatabolic states (*eg,* fever and inflammation) and growth in children place added demands on these patients. Indirect calorimetry [52] provides an assessment of the energy requirements, which may be more accurate than needs calculated from a patient's height, weight, and age.

Maldigestion and malabsorption are infrequent contributory factors to poor nutritional status. Quantitative stool fat analysis provides the most sensitive marker of malabsorption [53], whereas stool carbohydrate and stool nitrogen studies [54] provide a wider assessment of malabsorption. True iron deficiency anemia or impaired use of iron is usually responsible for the anemia. Vitamin B_{12} and folate deficiencies rarely cause anemia in children with IBD [55,56]. The hypoalbuminemia that occurs in 60% of children with Crohn's disease [57] is primarily caused by enteric protein losses and not undernutrition. A fecal α-1-antitrypsin concentration provides an indicator of protein loss and disease activity.

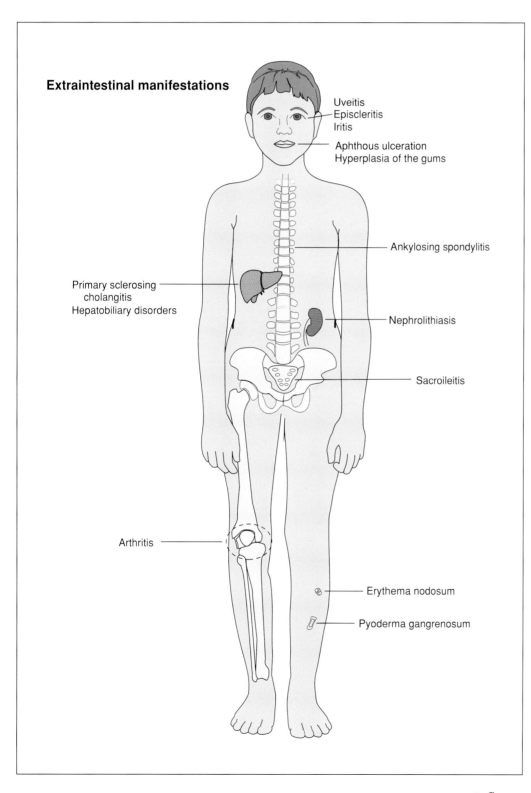

Extraintestinal manifestations

- Uveitis
- Episcleritis
- Iritis
- Aphthous ulceration
- Hyperplasia of the gums
- Ankylosing spondylitis
- Primary sclerosing cholangitis
- Hepatobiliary disorders
- Nephrolithiasis
- Sacroileitis
- Arthritis
- Erythema nodosum
- Pyoderma gangrenosum

FIGURE 7-7.

Extraintestinal manifestations (EIMs). EIMs occur frequently in inflammatory bowel disease and may precede overt bowel symptoms [58–61]. Primary EIMs are those that seem to share the pathogenesis of the disease involving the skin, eyes, liver, joints, and mucous membranes. Secondary EIMs are those secondary to long-standing disease (*eg,* kidney stones, obstructive uropathy, and gallstones). Secondary EIMs appear to occur more often in patients with Crohn's disease.

Arthralgias are probably the most common EIM in inflammatory bowel disease. Arthritis is uncommon. When arthritis occurs, it presents most commonly as peripheral arthritis, is asymmetric, and involves the lower extremity joints. Axial arthropathies consisting of sacroileitis with ankylosing spondylitis occur in patients with inflammatory bowel disease 10 to 30 times more often than in the general population [62,63]. Severity of peripheral arthritis correlates with the severity of inflammatory bowel disease, whereas the symptoms of axial arthropathies do not. Axial arthropathies are rarely seen in childhood.

Dermal manifestations associated with inflammatory bowel disease are also frequently seen; the most frequent are erythema nodosum, vasculitic skin changes, and pyoderma gangrenosum [64]. Psoriasis is also seen with increased frequency in patients with Crohn's disease [65]. Ocular manifestations include uveitis, episcleritis, iritis, and marginal corneal ulcerations. Crohn's disease patients with disease limited to the large bowel have a higher incidence of eye abnormalities [66–68].

A relatively common hepatobiliary disorder seen in association with inflammatory bowel disease is sclerosing cholangitis [69,70]. Sclerosing cholangitis can occur alone or in association with inflammatory bowel disease. It is more frequently seen in association with ulcerative colitis than with Crohn's disease [71,72]. Incidence of inflammatory bowel disease in sclerosing cholangitis is reported to be from 25% to 74% [73,74]. Sclerosing cholangitis is seen in 1% to 4% of patients with inflammatory bowel disease.

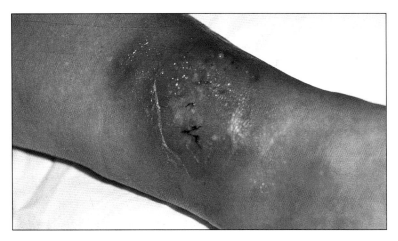

FIGURE 7-8.

Pyoderma gangrenosum. Pyoderma gangrenosum is a chronic ulcerating skin disorder seen in 20% to 50% of patients who have no associated organic illness, 2% to 12% of patients with ulcerative colitis, and 1% to 2% of patients with Crohn's disease [75–78]. The classic lesion often precipitated by trauma is an ulcer with irregular, undermined margins. The base contains necrotic exudate and the skin around the lesion is erythematous. Multiple lesions may be present, especially when pyoderma occurs adjacent to an ileostomy. Ulcerative colitis and Crohn's disease are the diseases most commonly associated with pyoderma gangrenosum, but it is also seen in patients with arthritis, multiple myeloma, and myelocytic and hairy-cell leukemia. Cyclosporine is the drug of choice [79,80].

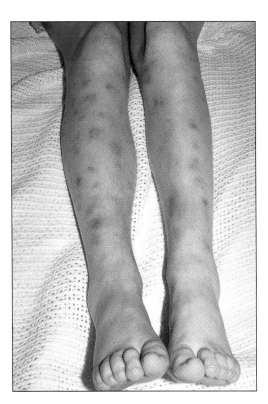

FIGURE 7-9.

Erythema nodosum. Erythema nodosum is the most common dermatologic manifestation of inflammatory bowel disease [81]. The incidence of erythema nodosum ranges from 0.5% to 9% among patients with ulcerative colitis and 2% to 15% among patients with Crohn's disease [82,83]. Erythema nodosum often appears with active disease.

The lesions, usually multiple, are characterized by very tender, warm, red subcutaneous nodules on the pretibial region of the lower extremities. Erythema nodosum has been noted with pregnancy, use of oral contraceptives, and in association with several systemic conditions, including streptococcal infection, tuberculosis, sarcoidosis, viral illness, and certain drug eruptions [84–87]. The nodules of erythema nodosum associated with inflammatory bowel disease often respond rapidly to treatment of the bowel disease, especially if corticosteroids are prescribed.

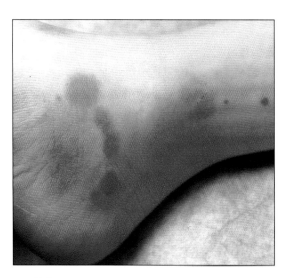

FIGURE 7-10.

Vasculitic lesion. Vasculitic lesions present as macular, erythematous, tender lesions that are often associated with edema of the site and are mistakenly diagnosed as cellulitis. Histologic findings are consistent with vasculitis. These lesions resolve with systemic steroid therapy.

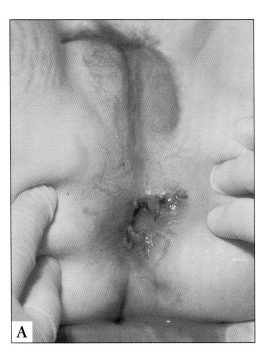

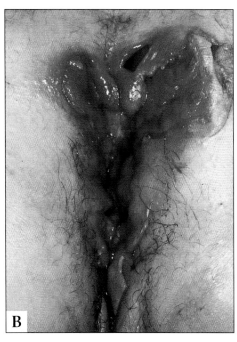

FIGURE 7-11.

Perianal disease. Almost 50% of children with Crohn's disease have perianal disease [88,89], mostly related to skin tags, fissures, fistulas, and abscesses. Poor growth and perianal disease may be the only presenting features in adolescents with Crohn's disease. Highly destructive perianal disease occurs but is unusual, and black children are possibly at an increased risk. Inflammation may be limited to the left colon in children with these severe lesions.

A, Fissures and a fistulous opening in a patient with Crohn's disease. **B,** Highly destructive perianal disease; multiple fistulous tracts and extensive destruction of the perianal area are pictured. Metronidazole, 6-mercaptopurine, and ciprofloxacin may be effective in the treatment of perianal lesions, but the relapse rate is significant [90] after discontinuation of treatment. Cyclosporine may also prove to be of benefit.

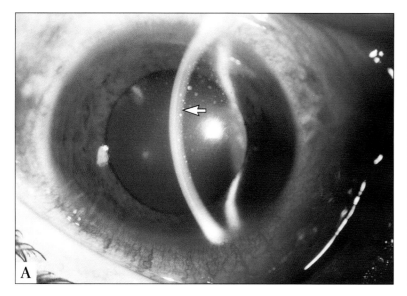
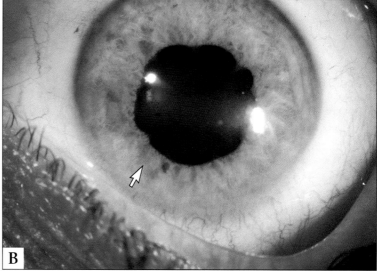

FIGURE 7-12.

Ophthalmologic findings. A multiplicity of eye problems are seen in both Crohn's disease (5%–10%) and ulcerative colitis (5%), including episcleritis and scleritis, optic neuritis and uveitis. Iritis and iridocyclitis are types of uveitis seen in inflammatory bowel disease. **A**, Iridocyclitis in one or both eyes is the most common finding in patients with ulcerative colitis. Characteristic peripheral keratitic precipitation on the cornea is seen on slit-lamp examination (*arrow*). **B**, Patient with Crohn's disease with acute iritis and typical posterior synechiae (*arrow*) reflecting inflammatory adhesions of the iris to the lens capsule. (*Courtesy* of Jeffrey L. Willig, MD, Manhasset, NY.)

TABLE 7-3. SCREENING DIAGNOSTIC TESTS FOR INFLAMMATORY BOWEL DISEASE

LABORATORY TEST

BLOOD	STOOL
CBC, differential, ESR, platelets	Leukocytes
Serum albumin, alkaline phosphatase	Bacterial culture
Liver tests	*Clostridium difficile* toxin
Vitamin B$_{12}$, folate	Ova and parasite
Serum iron, TIBC, ferritin	α-1 antitrypsin
? ANCA	72 Fecal fat

RADIOLOGIC STUDIES	ENDOSCOPIC EVALUATION
Gastrointestinal contrast studies	Upper and lower endoscopies
Bone age	Histologic evaluation of biopsies

TABLE 7-3.

Screening and diagnostic tests for inflammatory bowel disease. The diagnosis is based on clinical presentation, hematologic and biochemical profile, radiologic studies, endoscopic findings, and histology. Laboratory tests are not diagnostic but help rule out infectious causes and provide parameters to assess disease activity. A complete blood count will detect leukocytosis, with or without an increase in bands, and anemia. The erythrocyte sedimentation rate (ESR) is elevated in over two thirds of patients. Serum total protein and albumin may be low as a consequence of enteric losses and undernutrition. Serum vitamin B$_{12}$ and cholesterol concentrations may be low secondary to ileal malabsorption. This low level is especially pronounced with ileal resection and proximal recurrence of disease. Increased fecal α-1 antitrypsin concentrations may be the best parameter of assessing intestinal inflammation. Fresh stool should also be obtained for blood, leukocytes, and infectious pathogens, especially *Yersinia enterocolitica*, which may mimic Crohn's ileitis. Any of the enteric infections may either simulate or be superimposed on inflammatory bowel disease. Antineutrophil cytoplasmic antibodies (ANCAs) are detected in 66% of pediatric patients with ulcerative colitis and in 19% with Crohn's disease [91]. CBC—complete blood count; TIBC—total iron binding capacity.

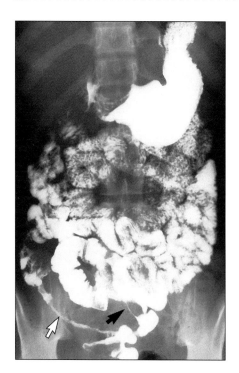

FIGURE 7-13.

Distal ileal Crohn's disease. Long segments of distal and terminal ileal (*open arrow*) Crohn's disease demonstrating narrowing (string sign) of the lumen and marked separation from surrounding loops. Radiographs of the ileum are best obtained using compression by a paddle. On compression films, a sinus tract (*closed arrow*) arising from the involved segment of distal ileum is clearly visualized. The rest of the small bowel appears normal. Upper gastrointestinal and small-bowel follow-through imaging series with barium are very helpful in the study of Crohn's disease of the esophagus, stomach, and small intestine.

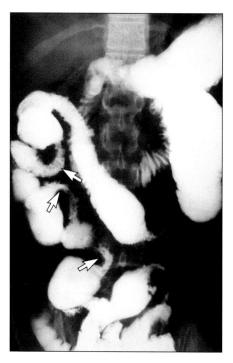

FIGURE 7-14.

Crohn's disease of the small bowel with multiple strictures. Upper gastrointestinal and small-bowel follow-through imaging series with barium. Multiple stenotic segments (*arrows*) of small bowel are seen with dilatation of the proximal bowel. This is usually associated with long-standing disease and clinical symptoms and signs of partial small-intestinal obstruction. Hyperplasia of the muscularis mucosa and fibrosis in diseased segments results in these stenotic lesions.

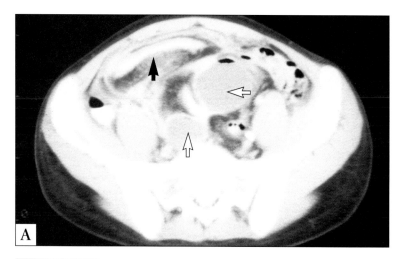

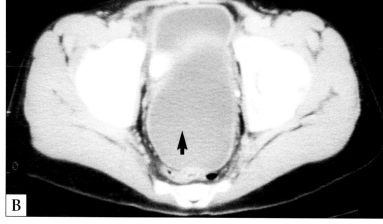

FIGURE 7-15.

Crohn's disease with large pelvic abscess: computed tomography (CT). **A**, Terminal ileum is involved. A markedly thickened loop of small-bowel wall with separation of bowel loops is identified in the right lower quadrant (*closed arrow*). **B**, Large thick-walled pelvic abscess (*closed arrow*) (11 × 8.3 cm) is seen in the rectovesical space extending superiorly into two components, (*open arrows* in

Panel A). Mild to moderate right hydronephrosis and hydroureter were visualized in higher abdominal cuts. This abscess was drained rectally. The diseased ileocecal segment was resected after a 4-week course of antibiotics and corticosteroids. Multiple sinus tracts were noted in the diseased segment. Hydronephrosis resolved on follow-up CT scan 4 weeks later.

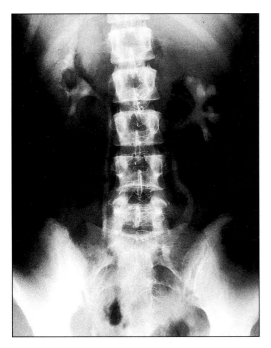

FIGURE 7-16.

Obstructive uropathy with Crohn's disease. Intravenous pyelogram. Obstructive uropathy caused by a noncalcified right distal ureteral calculus is illustrated. The patient had undergone ileocecal resection and an ileostomy. Renal stones, often composed of oxalate, occur in 6% to 10% of patients with Crohn's disease [92], particularly in those patients with extensive ileal disease or resection. Normally, calcium binds oxalate in the intestinal lumen to form an insoluble, nonabsorbable complex. In patients with ileal dysfunction with fat malabsorption, however, calcium binds to luminal free fatty acids, thereby permitting oxalate to remain soluble. Free oxalate is absorbed in much greater amounts than oxalate bound to calcium [93]. Obstructive uropathy may also be seen in patients with Crohn's disease with an inflammatory right lower quadrant mass or abscess.

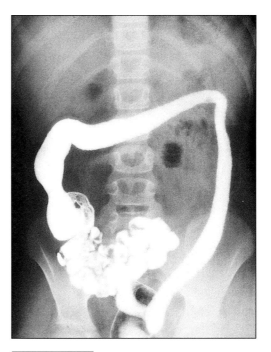

FIGURE 7-17.

Long-standing inflammatory bowel disease of the colon. Barium enema. Absent haustral markings, marked foreshortening of the bowel, and diffuse marginal ulceration are present. This figure shows findings more characteristic of ulcerative colitis with pancolitis but they may also be seen in patients with Crohn's colitis.

■ ENDOSCOPIC EVALUATION

Crohn's colitis

TABLE 7-4. CROHN'S VERSUS ULCERATIVE COLITIS

CROHN'S COLITIS	ULCERATIVE COLITIS
Rectum spared in 20% to 30% of children	Rectum almost always involved
Inflammation	Inflammation
Patchy	Continuous
Early	Early
Aphthous ulcers in normal mucosa	Granular mucosa
	Friable mucosa
Late	Late
Linear deep ulcers in normal mucosa	Diffusely inflamed mucosa with ulceration
Pseudopolyps	Pseudopolyps
Sinuses, fistulas, and strictures	Strictures (rule out malignancy)

TABLE 7-4.

Crohn's colitis versus ulcerative colitis. Despite the differences enumerated in 10% of cases, it still is impossible to distinguish between Crohn's colitis and ulcerative colitis. Endoscopic biopsies, which only include the mucosa and muscularis mucosa, often do not distinguish between the two conditions. Rectal sparing, patchy involvement, and aphthous ulceration, features that are considered pathognomonic of Crohn's disease, have been seen in endoscopic and surgical specimens of ulcerative colitis [94]. Inflammatory infiltration of mucosa and submucosa associated with crypt distortion, crypt abscesses, and Paneth's cell metaplasia can be seen in both. However, in Crohn's disease, granulomas may be present in up to 28% of rectal biopsies if serially sectioned [95,96], a feature not seen in ulcerative colitis.

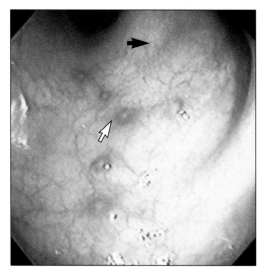

Figure 7-18.

Crohn's colitis—aphthous ulceration. Aphthous ulcers are tiny, pinpoint lesions with exudate (*open arrow*) surrounded by an erythematous margin. Microscopically, these are tiny foci of mucosal ulceration often overlying enlarged lymphoid follicles. Normal mucosa (*closed arrow*) is seen adjacent to the inflamed mucosa.

Aphthous ulcers may be the earliest recognizable lesion of Crohn's disease, but infiltration by lymphocytes, polymorphonuclear cells, and plasma cells probably precedes the development of the aphthous ulcer [97]. Aphthous ulcers can occur anywhere from the mouth to the anal area. These lesions may also be seen by air-contrast barium enema.

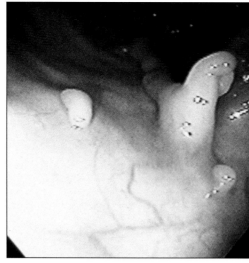

Figure 7-19.

Pseudopolyps. Pseudopolyps are seen in long-standing ulcerative colitis and Crohn's colitis. Endoscopically, these are polypoid mucosal projections. Pseudopolyps are not pathognomonic of inflammatory bowel disease because they may also be seen in other chronic inflammatory conditions such as amebiasis and infections caused by *Strongyloides* parasites. These polyps represent regenerative mounds of epithelium [98]. Most commonly, they are small and multiple, occurring throughout the colon. On occasion they may be so large or clustered as to cause obstructive symptoms [99–105]. They do not have greater malignant potential than the rest of the colonic mucosa [104,105]. Pseudopolyps may persist in quiescent colitis.

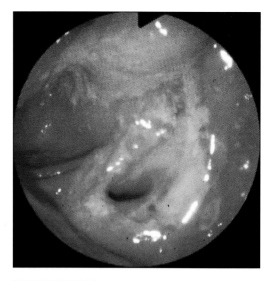

Figure 7-20.

Crohn's colitis—fistulous tract. Fistulous tracts are characteristic of long-standing Crohn's disease [49,50]. Endoscopically, the orifice is fixed and may be filled with exudate. Initially, there is formation of a fissure or sinus tract by extension of the mucosal ulcer into deeper layers of the bowel wall. A fistula is formed when a sinus tract communicates with other segments of bowel, bladder, vagina, or skin (*ie,* an epithelial-lined surface).

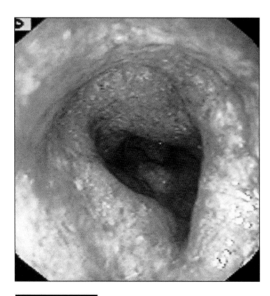

Figure 7-21.

Ulcerative colitis—diffuse hemorrhage. Diffusely involved, friable, granular mucosa is characteristic of ulcerative colitis. Diffuse edema with small superficial erosions gives the mucosa a coarse granular appearance. These changes may be limited to the rectum [106] or extend proximally in continuity. Therefore, in the untreated patient, if the right colon is diseased and the left colon is spared, the diagnosis of ulcerative colitis is less likely.

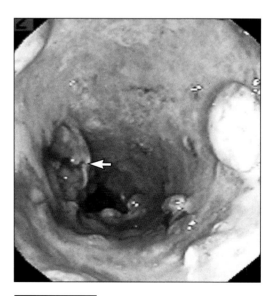

Figure 7-22.

Ulcerative colitis—mass lesion. Adenomatous polyps are extremely rare in the pediatric population. Endoscopically, adenomas (*arrow*) are indistinguishable from pseudopolyps. Adenocarcinoma is a well-known complication of ulcerative colitis; an increased incidence is also being reported in Crohn's disease [108]. Consensus is that in disease present over 10 years and with pancolitic involvement, there is a greater risk of colon cancer, even in the pediatric population [109].

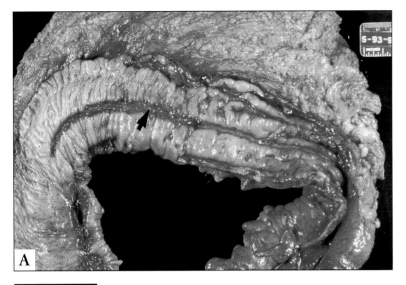

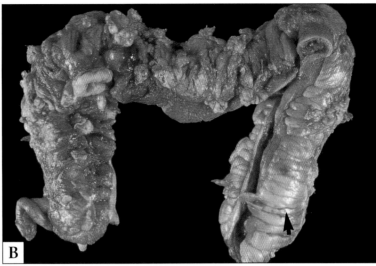

FIGURE 7-23.

Crohn's colitis—linear ulceration. **A**, Macroscopic appearance of the colon in a patient with Crohn's colitis. Longitudinal ulceration (*arrow*) with edematous mucosa and cobblestone appearance. Earliest manifestation of Crohn's disease is the aphthous ulcer. As Crohn's disease progresses, aphthous ulcers enlarge and coalesce, often producing elongated, longitudinal ulcers along the long axis of the bowel. Creeping fat is noted in the right lower corner of the specimen. **B**, Marked creeping of fat is noted over the serosal surface of the colon (*arrow*). Pericolic adipose tissue is wrapped around the entire circumference. (*Courtesy of* E. Kahn, Manhasset, NY.)

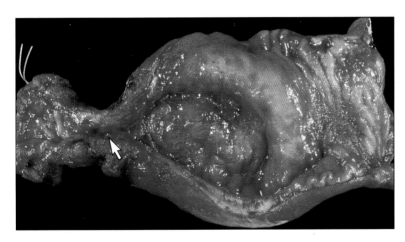

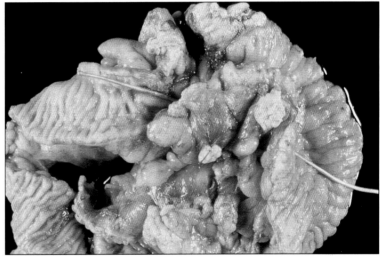

FIGURE 7-24.

Crohn's ileitis—stenosis. Stenosis of the distal portion of the specimen (*arrow*) associated with marked thickening of the bowel wall and proximal dilatation with mucosal ulceration. Classically, such patients present with symptoms of obstruction and a "string sign" radiologically. Histologic sections of the strictured intestine demonstrate muscularis mucosa, markedly expanded by hyperplasia of the smooth muscle cells and the presence of large amounts of collagen. The muscularis propria is also expanded. (*Courtesy of* E. Kahn, Manhasset, NY.)

FIGURE 7-25.

Crohn's ileitis—fistula. The probe indicates an ileoileal fistula. Fistulas arise as a result of the extension of an aphthous ulcer through the serosal surface and are commonly associated with stricture formation [49]. The penetrating ulcer may end blindly in the serosa as a fissure or form a fistula that communicates with other portions of bowel or even the bladder, vagina, or skin. Fistulas are lined with chronically inflamed granulation tissue, with purulent exudate on the surface, and a deeper zone of fibrosis. (*Courtesy of* E. Kahn, Manhasset, NY.)

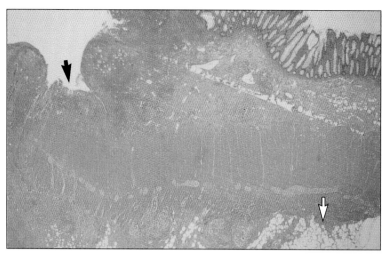

FIGURE 7-26.

Crohn's colitis—transmural inflammation. Ulceration extends into the muscularis propria (*closed arrow*). Transmural inflammation with involvement of pericolic fat (*open arrow*) is noted. Transmural inflammation is characteristic of Crohn's disease. Lymphoid aggregates are present in the submucosa and the subserosa. Frequently, serosal lymphoid aggregates extend into the mesenteric fat. Inflammation results in mesenteric fat wrapping itself around the serosal surface of the bowel. (Hematoxylin and eosin, original magnification × 50.) (*Courtesy of* E. Kahn, Manhasset, NY.)

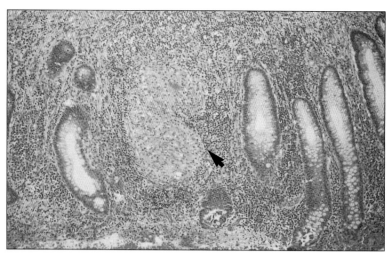

FIGURE 7-27.

Crohn's colitis—granulomatous colitis. Noncaseating granuloma in the lamina propria composed of epithelioid cells and lymphocytes (*arrow*). Granulomas are characteristic of Crohn's disease and are not seen in ulcerative colitis. Studies report up to 30% positivity for granulomas in rectal biopsies [109,110]. In pediatric Crohn's disease, the incidence of granuloma is said to be twice that in adults [111]. In pediatric Crohn's disease, rectosigmoid granulomas have been associated with a poorer prognosis [112]. (Hematoxylin and eosin, original magnification × 50.) (*Courtesy of* E. Kahn, Manhasset, NY.)

FIGURE 7-28.

Crohn's colitis—patchy inflammation. The inflammation in Crohn's disease is usally patchy as noted in this biopsy specimen. Patchy active inflammation is characterized by cryptitis and crypt abscess formation composed of polymorphonuclear cells and plasma cells. The same biopsy specimen shows normal, uninvolved mucosa and lamina propria (*open arrow*) adjacent to the inflamed mucosa (*closed arrow*). (Hematoxylin and eosin stain, original magnification × 50) (*Courtesy of* E. Kahn, Manhasset, NY.)

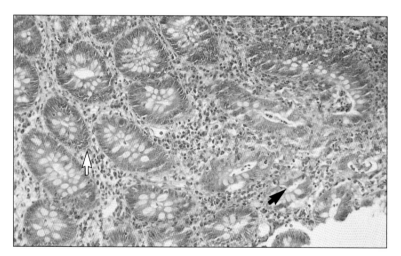

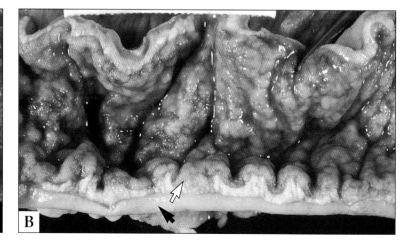

FIGURE 7-29.

Ulcerative colitis—diffuse colitis. **A,** Diffuse colonic mucosal ulceration. Tan areas (*open arrow*) correspond to areas of ulceration, pinkish areas (*closed arrow*) to inflamed mucosa. The mucosal surface is granular, friable, and ulcerated. The involvement is continuous, contrasting with the patchy involvement in Crohn's disease. **B,** Thickened mucosa and submucosa (*open arrow*) with uninvolved muscularis propria seen as a sharply well-defined layer (*closed arrow*). Involvement of only the mucosa and submucosa is characteristic of ulcerative colitis contrasted with the transmural inflammation that is characteristic of Crohn's disease. (*Courtesy of* E. Kahn, Manhasset, NY.)

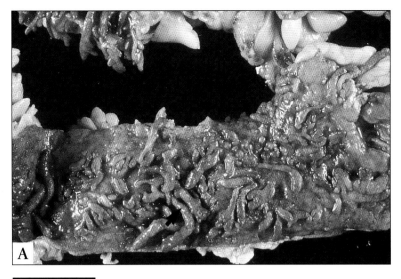
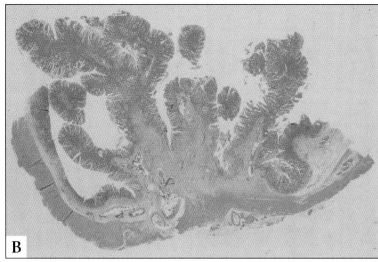

FIGURE 7-30.

Ulcerative colitis—pseudopolyps. **A,** Pseudopolyps are common to all forms of chronic colitis, including ulcerative colitis, and appear as diffuse polypoid mucosal projections. Pseudopolyps appear as densely placed finger-like projections (*arrow*). **B,** Microscopically, a pseudopolyp is composed of mucosa and muscularis mucosae with various degrees of inflammation. Pseudopolyps can persist even when inflammation has abated, and the surface may show the typical changes of healed mucosa. (Hematoxylin and eosin, original magnification × 50.) (*Courtesy of* E. Kahn, Manhasset, NY.)

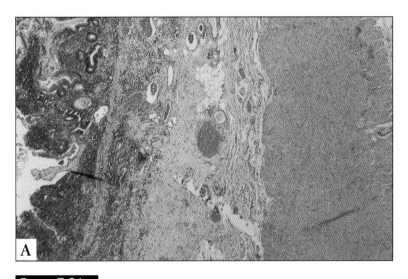
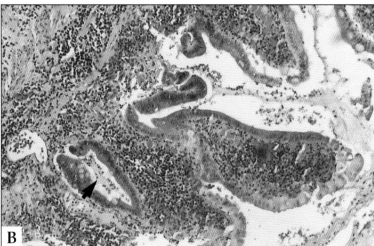

FIGURE 7-31.

Ulcerative colitis—histology. **A,** Inflammation is limited to the mucosa and submucosa in ulcerative colitis in contrast to Crohn's disease, where the inflammation is transmural as seen in Fig. 7-26. In ulcerative colitis, the muscularis propria is intact and not inflamed. **B,** High-power view of the inflamed mucosa in ulcerative colitis demonstrates diffuse inflammation contrasted with the usual patchy inflammation in Crohn's disease (*see* Fig. 7-28). A characteristic, but not pathognomonic, finding in ulcerative colitis is the presence of crypt abscesses (*arrow*). Goblet cell depletion is also well documented in ulcerative colitis but may also be seen in Crohn's colitis. (Hematoxylin and eosin stain, original magnification × 50.) (*Courtesy of* E. Kahn, Manhasset, NY.)

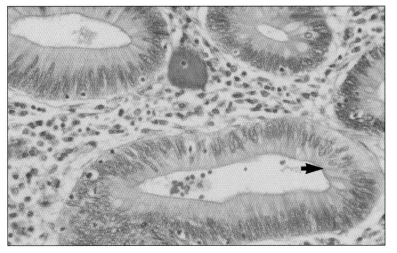

FIGURE 7-32.

Low-grade dysplasia. Low-grade dysplasia is characterized by stratification of the nuclei in the epithelial cells with basal distribution of the nuclei (*arrow*). Low-grade epithelial dysplasia shows a premalignant mucosal change [113]; the glandular pattern is generally preserved. Low-grade dysplasia seen with significant inflammation is called *indefinite dysplasia* and may disappear after appropriate treatment. (Hematoxylin and eosin stain, original magnification × 50.) (*Courtesy of* E. Kahn, Manhasset, NY.)

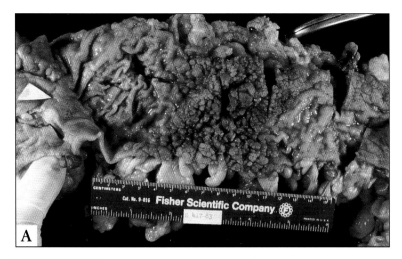 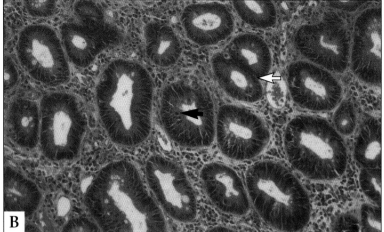

FIGURE 7-33.

High-grade dysplasia. **A,** Thickened velvety appearance of the mucosa forming a mass lesion. Grossly and endoscopically, high-grade dysplasia is difficult to differentiate from early infiltrating adenocarcinoma. The recognition of high-grade dysplasia in a patient with long-standing inflammatory bowel disease should be regarded as an indication for colectomy. **B,** High-grade dysplasia marked with a distorted and crowded crypt pattern (*open arrow*) associated with nuclear stratification extending to the crypt lumen (*closed arrow*). (Hematoxylin and eosin stain, original magnification × 50.) (*Courtesy of* E. Kahn, Manhasset, NY).

■ PHARMACOTHERAPY

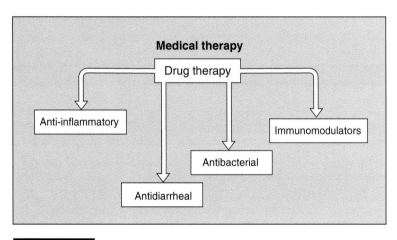

Medical therapy

Drug therapy

Anti-inflammatory

Immunomodulators

Antibacterial

Antidiarrheal

FIGURE 7-34.

Drugs used to treat inflammatory bowel disease can be classified into three groups: anti-inflammatory agents, antibacterial agents, and immunomodulators. Antidiarrheal agents are also used occasionally for symptomatic relief. Inflammatory agents sulfasalazine, mesalamine (5-aminosalicylic acid), and glucocorticoids are commonly used for treatment of mild to moderate ulcerative colitis and Crohn's colitis [114–117].

Although antibacterial agents have little if any role in the primary treatment of ulcerative colitis, the role of antibiotics in the treatment of Crohn's disease remains more controversial. Metronidazole is the most commonly used antibiotic for primary therapy for small-bowel Crohn's disease and may be as effective as sulfasalazine. Some studies have shown that metronidazole may have immunomodulatory effects [118]. Peripheral neuropathy has been reported [119] after 4 to 11 months of treatment. Although the paresthesias and dysesthesias were reversible, the frequency of these symptoms has limited acceptance of this therapy. In bacterial overgrowth of the small bowel, antibacterial therapy is indicated as adjunct therapy to other primary treatment modalities. Drugs with primarily immunosuppressive or immunomodulative activity have proven to be effective, rendering further support to the theory that the immune system plays a significant role in mediating the tissue injury in these conditions [120,121].

TABLE 7-5. DRUG THERAPY—AMINOSALICYLATE PREPARATIONS

DRUG	FORMULATION	SITE/ACTIVATION
ORAL		
Sulfasalazine	Sulfapyridine linked to 5-ASA by azo bond	Colon; bacterial cleavage of azo bond
Rowasa (Solvay Pharmaceuticals, Marietta, GA)	5-ASA coated with acrylic resin L 100	Distal ileum and colon; pH > 6
Asacol (Proctor & Gamble, Cincinnati, OH)	5-ASA coated with acrylic resins	Distal ileum and colon; pH > 6
Pentasa (Marion Merrell Dow, Kansas City, MO)	5-ASA in ethyl cellulose microgranules	Small intestine; time release
Dipentum (Kabi Pharmacia, Piscataway, NJ)	5-ASA dimer linked by azo bond	Colon; bacterial cleavage of azo bond
RECTAL		
Foam	5-ASA	Rectum/sigmoid
Enemas	5-ASA suspension	Rectum/sigmoid and left colon
Suppositories	5-ASA	Rectum/sigmoid
		? Left colon

TABLE 7-5.

Aminosalicylate preparations. Sulfasalazine has been used for almost 50 years in the treatment of inflammatory bowel disease. It is used in mild to moderate ulcerative colitis and Crohn's colitis. Intolerance and allergic reactions have limited its use [122]. Sulfasalazine interferes with the absorption of folic acid, thus requiring folic acid supplementation. Most of the drug's toxicity has been attributed to the sulfa portion, which serves as a vehicle for transport of 5-aminosalicylic acid (5-ASA) to the colon. Because of possible toxicity, mesalamine preparations have been formulated using a variety of carrier systems. Various vehicles used require bacterial cleavage, a pH higher than 6, or are time-released, therefore making the active ingredient available in the distal ileum and/or colon. Eighty percent to 90% of patients intolerant or allergic to sulfasalazine can tolerate the newer agents [123].

Rectal 5-ASA therapy has proven to be efficacious in patients with distal ulcerative colitis. A dosage of 2 to 4 g per day of 5-ASA in enema form has been shown to achieve a 93% clinical and sigmoidoscopic remission rate [124,125]. 5-ASA in suppository form given in doses of 200 mg to 1 g, 2 to 3 times daily, has also proven to be effective in patients with proctitis and distal colitis [126,127]. Recently, a foam preparation has also become available.

Mode of action of these 5-ASA preparations remains unclear. 5-ASA has an inhibitory effect on the lipoxygenase pathway of arachidonic-acid metabolism and thus decreases the production of leukotrienes that cause the inflammation inherent in inflammatory bowel disease [128]. 5-ASA has also been shown to be an effective scavenger of oxygen-derived free radicals implicated in the pathogenesis of a variety of inflammatory states [129].

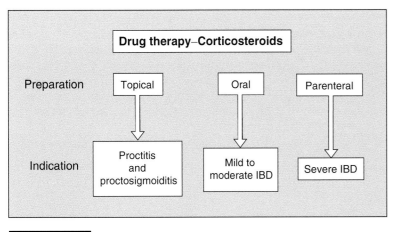

FIGURE 7-35.

Corticosteroids. Topical preparations are often used in children with mildly active ulcerative colitis or Crohn's colitis with symptoms predominantly of distal left-sided colitis (tenesmus and urgency). In the asymptomatic child, rectosigmoid pathology is not an indication in itself for corticosteroid therapy [130]. For the moderately ill child with inflammatory bowel disease (IBD), oral prednisone is effective in a dose ranging from 0.2 to 2 mg/kg per day (to a maximum of 50 to 75 mg/d). For more severe symptoms, intravenous hydrocortisone is the treatment of choice (0.2 to 1.0 mg/kg/dose every 6 hours). It is unclear whether steroids have a role in maintenance therapy. There are no dose-dependent studies

based on clinical, laboratory, endoscopic, or histologic data to indicate the daily dosage required to induce remission.

In children treated with steroids, there are two side effects that are of great concern: cosmetic side effects and linear growth suppression. The cosmetic side effects of steroids are very disturbing, especially to adolescent patients. These include a moonlike facies, acne, hirsutism, and striae. In children with IBD, it has been shown that daily steroid therapy for 7 days can decrease serum procollagen levels, a biochemical marker for linear bone growth [131]. Steroids taken every second day have been shown to be beneficial in limiting these effects while maintaining reduced disease activity [132].

Rectal enemas and foam preparations, although efficacious, may lead to considerable absorption and systemic side effects. Glucocorticoid derivatives have been developed that act locally on the mucosa but have little or no systemic activity. Beclomethasone dipropionate [133], tixocortol pivalate [134,135], budesonide [136,138], and fluticasone propionate [139] have proven to be effective topical therapies that do not severely depress plasma cortisol levels. They all undergo a rapid first-pass metabolism in the liver, thereby limiting their systemic side effects. Oral budesonide has led to remission in 50% to 60% of patients with Crohn's disease. Fluticasone propionate is poorly absorbed (<50%) and whatever is absorbed is rapidly metabolized during its first pass through the liver, thus making it more attractive for the treatment of small-bowel Crohn's disease. These newer steroids have been used only rarely in the pediatric population, and their efficacy has not yet been determined.

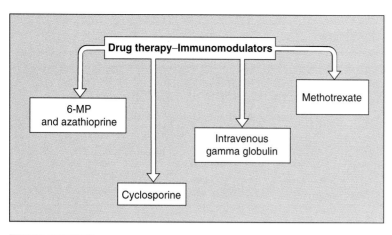

FIGURE 7-36.

Immunomodulators. Azathioprine and 6-mercaptopurine (6-MP) (a major metabolite of azathioprine) both appear effective in the treatment of Crohn's disease and ulcerative colitis. 6-MP is being used increasingly in adolescents with steroid-dependent and intractable Crohn's disease. Clinical trials in adults with Crohn's disease have demonstrated marked improvement in symptoms and lessened disease activity when these agents have been used for at least 3 to 6 months [140]. Data from clinical experience in adolescents with intractable Crohn's disease indicate that two thirds of these patients experienced remission of disease and that 80% were able to discontinue corticosteroid treatment completely when 6-MP was used for at least 1 year [141].

In limited observations, cyclosporine [142,143] has been effective pharmacotherapeutically in about 40% to 50% of children with acute fulminant ulcerative colitis. Further data are needed to determine the actual efficacy of cyclosporine in both the short-term and long-term treatment of children with ulcerative colitis. Cyclosporine has little role in the treatment of Crohn's disease, but it may be effective in the treatment of fistulas complicating Crohn's disease [144].

Intravenous gamma globulin therapy is an alternative medical therapy proposed for Crohn's disease and ulcerative colitis. Experience indicates that selected patients with intractable Crohn's disease may respond favorably to intravenous gamma globulin infusion [145]. There are no data to indicate the efficacy or adverse side effects of methotrexate in children with inflammatory bowel disease.

■ SURGICAL MANAGEMENT

TABLE 7-6. SURGICAL MANAGEMENT— ULCERATIVE COLITIS (CURATIVE)

INDICATIONS

ACUTE	ELECTIVE
Fulminant colitis	Intractable symptoms
Exsanguinating hemorrhage	Steroid dependency
? Toxic megacolon	Stricture (? malignancy)
Free perforation	Premalignant changes
	Colonic malignancy

TABLE 7-6.

Ulcerative colitis. About 50% of patients with ulcerative colitis come to elective surgery within the first 10 years of their illness because of intractable symptoms, steroid dependency, and significant morbidity. Growth failure alone is no longer considered an indication for surgery in ulcerative colitis. Normal growth and sexual maturation can usually be achieved if the child receives adequate calories and is not taking high doses of steroids. Increments in height velocity and catch-up growth often occur if surgery is performed early in puberty [146].

Only 10% to 15% of patients with ulcerative colitis present initially with symptoms requiring emergency surgical intervention. The acute indications include massive hemorrhage, free perforation, and possibly toxic megacolon, all of which are unusual in the pediatric population.

Massive hemorrhage in ulcerative colitis occurs in less than 1% of patients [147]. Pancolitis with a clinically severe attack can present with perforation. Acute toxic megacolon in the past has been described in about 6% of adults with ulcerative colitis [148], but appears to occur much less frequently at this time. Toxic megacolon may be treated medically in some patients, so that surgery may be performed electively or deferred indefinitely.

Prophylactic surgery for colonic carcinoma in adolescents who have had ulcerative colitis for more than 10 years remains controversial. The presence of dysplasia in the setting of noninflamed tissue, positive flow cytometry [149], or malignancy are indications for colectomy. Some clinicians think that positive flow cytometry and/or low-grade dysplasia warrant close surveillance by colonoscopy and biopsies, whereas others recommend surgery because even multiple surveillance biopsies may miss dysplasia or adenocarcinoma.

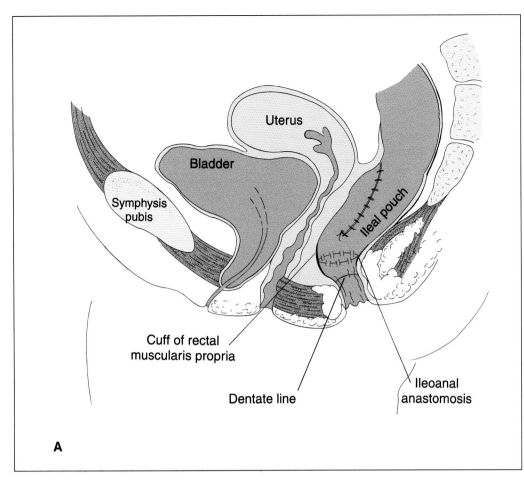

A

Uterus

Bladder

Symphysis pubis

Ileal pouch

Cuff of rectal muscularis propria

Dentate line

Ileoanal anastomosis

FIGURE 7-37.

Ulcerative colitis. Total proctocolectomy with a Brooke ileostomy was previously the surgical treatment of choice for ulcerative colitis. It is curative but leaves the patient with a permanent ostomy. Patients may develop bladder and sexual dysfunction associated with parasympathetic nerve injury.

At present, a subtotal colectomy with a mucosal proctectomy with ileorectal pull-through and anal anastomosis is the most popular procedure, especially in adolescents and young adults (**A**) [150]. The cuff of rectal muscularis propria is created by stripping the mucosa and submucosa of the rectum to the proximal end of the columns of Morgagni. The distal end of the ileum is anastomosed to the distal end of the stripped rectal cuff. Theoretically, about a centimeter of rectal mucosa may be left behind with potential of eventual malignant transformation. Some surgeons prefer a subtotal colectomy with ileoanal anastomosis, in which 1 cm of the anal mucosa is left intact (**B**).

(*continued on next page*)

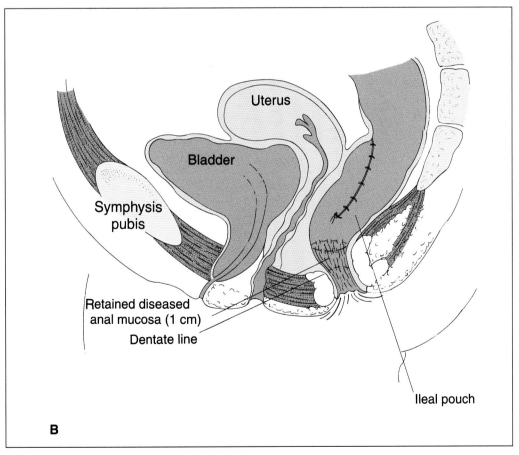

B

Uterus

Bladder

Symphysis pubis

Retained diseased anal mucosa (1 cm)

Dentate line

Ileal pouch

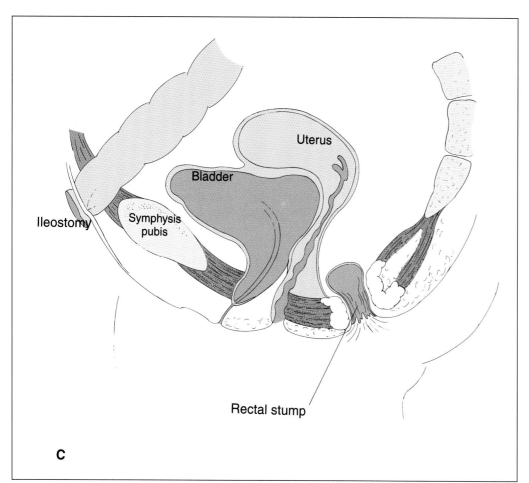

Ileostomy

Symphysis pubis

Bladder

Uterus

Rectal stump

C

FIGURE 7-37. (*CONTINUED*)

In children, initial surgery usually includes a subtotal colectomy, ileostomy, and retention of the rectal stump (**C**), with the pull-through done at a later time. This approach allows a definitive diagnosis of ulcerative colitis by examination of the subtotal colectomy specimen by the pathologist.

TABLE 7-7. SURGICAL MANAGEMENT— CROHN'S DISEASE (PALLIATIVE)

INDICATIONS

ACUTE	ELECTIVE
Perforation	Obstruction
Exsanguinating hemorrhage (rare)	Intractable symptoms
Perianal abscess ± systemic toxicity	Premalignant changes
? Toxic megacolon	Malignancy

TABLE 7-7.

Crohn's disease. In Crohn's disease, surgery is palliative but not curative. Therefore, surgery is performed to treat complications. Most surgical procedures are done on an elective basis because acute complications in Crohn's disease occur infrequently and are often initially managed medically. Of patients with small-intestinal disease, 80% to 90% will eventually require surgery for complications [151]. Obstruction is the most common reason for surgery.

Growth retardation in the setting of limited small-bowel involvement and intractable symptoms requiring steroids may improve with a resection of the diseased segment. Reports of cancer in adults with long-standing disease of the small intestine and colon are appearing with increased frequency [152].

TABLE 7-8. SURGICAL OPTIONS— CROHN'S DISEASE

SURGICAL OPTIONS

Partial intestinal resection
Strictureplasty
Colonic resection with ileostomy
    Subtotal colectomy with retention of rectal stump
    Total proctocolectomy
Incision and drainage of perianal abscess

TABLE 7-8.

Crohn's disease. Partial small-intestinal resection is the most common surgical procedure in Crohn's disease. Strictured areas may require resection, but strictureplasty now offers an alternative that can obviate the loss of small bowel, thus preserving a more normal nutritional status. Nonetheless, strictures are almost always noted in areas of inflammation, the patient usually continues to require anti-inflammatory therapy, and there is the likelihood of subsequent surgery for new strictures.

Of patients with Crohn's disease, 10% to 15% have findings limited to the colon. Refractory colitis is effectively managed by subtotal or total colectomy with ileostomy. If the rectal stump is retained, surveillance for dysplasia and malignancy should be initiated after 8 to 10 years of disease. Incision and drainage of a perianal abscess is indicated if the abscess is painful and fluctuant with or without systemic toxicity. For intra-abdominal abscesses, percutaneous drainage may be indicated if the abscess causes severe abdominal pain, obstructive symptoms, or systemic toxicity.

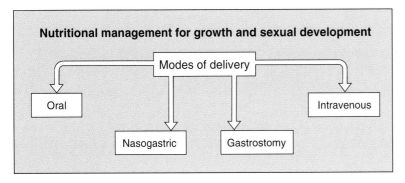

FIGURE 7-38.

Nutritional management for growth and sexual development. Calorie malnutrition and nutrient deficiency are problems in children with inflammatory bowel disease (IBD), especially Crohn's disease. Decreased intake, increased losses, and increased requirements all contribute to the malnutrition. IBD-induced malnutrition can lead to growth failure. If adequate nutrition is provided, about 70% of children will have catch-up growth [153]. Means of assessment of malnutrition are outlined in Table 7-2.

Enteral and parenteral nutrition have been prescribed as primary therapies for patients with inflammatory bowel disease [154–157] but are used mainly for nutritional support. If the gut can be used, most pediatric gastroenterologists prefer enteral nutrition. Children with inflammatory bowel disease often require 80 to 90 kcal and 3 to 3.4 g of protein per kilogram of ideal body weight per day to achieve their ultimate height potential [158], about 30% to 50% more than an age-comparable healthy adolescent. Although improved weight and height can be achieved by supplementing with an oral liquid formula, often the unacceptable taste and early satiety make this approach less feasible. Long-term nocturnal or short-term intermittent continuous nasogastric infusions of either nonelemental [159] or elemental [160] formulas have improved growth. After optimal nutritional support is established, increments in height may not occur for 3 to 6 months after weight gain. A percutaneous endoscopic gastrostomy button may be more acceptable than a nightly nasogastric tube as an alternative means of providing enteral nutrition in children with Crohn's disease [161]. Use of high-calorie intravenous infusions [162] during sleep is another alternative to deliver increased calories. This approach is more expensive and riskier than tube feedings, occasionally leading to infection and hepatobiliary dysfunction.

PSYCHOSOCIAL CONSEQUENCES

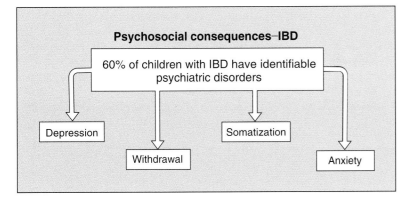

FIGURE 7-39.

Psychosocial consequences—inflammatory bowel disease (IBD). Comorbid psychiatric illnesses have been reported in children and adolescents with IBD. In one study, 60% of children and adolescents with either Crohn's disease or ulcerative colitis had an identifiable psychiatric disorder [162]. Adolescents with IBD have psychologic styles characterized by depression, anxiety, withdrawal, and frequent somatization. These traits appear to be at least in part the sequelae of having chronic intestinal disease. Studies have shown these adolescents have abnormal coping skills in dealing with stressful life events [164].

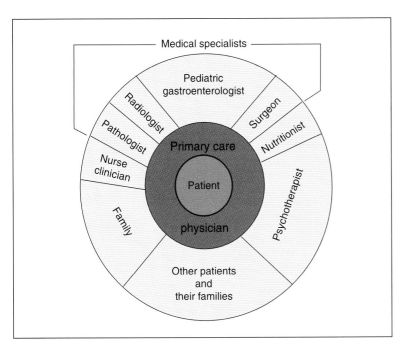

FIGURE 7-40.

Team approach. To care for this group of chronically ill children and their families adequately, a team approach is essential. A comprehensive team consists of a primary-care physician, a pediatric gastroenterologist, a pediatric psychotherapist, a nurse clinician, a pediatric nutritionist, and a pathologist with special interest in the gastrointestinal tract. Pediatric surgeons and radiologists are essential consultants.

Children and adolescents with similar experiences provide immense psychologic support for the newly diagnosed patient. Seminars about self-image, quality of life, sexuality, and marriage are very helpful. Easy access to the gastroenterologist and the constant support of the team helps these children learn to cope with their disease and lead happy, productive lives with minimal disruption of their daily activities.

▮ REFERENCES

1. Rogers BH, Clark LM, Kirsner JB: The epidemiologic and demographic characteristics of inflammatory bowel disease: An analysis of a computerized file of 1400 patients. *J Chronic Dis* 1971, 24:743–773.

2. Olafsdottir EJ, Fluge G, Haug K: Chronic inflammatory bowel disease in children in western Norway. *J Pediatr Gastroenterol Nutr* 1989, 8:454–458.

3. Barton JR, Gillon S, Ferguson A: Incidence of inflammatory bowel disease in Scottish children between 1968 and 1983: Marginal fall in ulcerative colitis, three-fold rise in Crohn's disease. *Gut* 1989, 30:618–622.

4. Ferguson A, Rifkind EA, Doig CM: Prevalence of inflammatory bowel disease in British children. In *The Genetics and Epidemiology of Inflammatory Bowel Disease (Frontiers in Gastrointestinal Research 11)*. Edited by McConnell RB, Rozen P, Langman MJS, Gilat T. Basel: Karger; 1986.

5. Koletzko S, Sherman P, Corey M, *et al.*: Role of infant feeding practices in development of Crohn's disease in childhood. *Br J Med* 1989, 298:1617–1618.

6. Bergstrom O, Hellers G: Breast feeding during infancy in patients who later develop Crohn's disease. *Scand J Gastroenterol* 1983, 18:903–906.

7. Koletzko S, Griffiths A, Corey M, *et al.*: Infant feeding practices and ulcerative colitis in childhood. *Br J Med* 1991, 302:1580–1581.

8. Farmer RG: Study of family history among patients with inflammatory bowel disease. *Scand J Gastroenterol* (suppl 170) 1989, 24:64–65.

9. Shanahan F, Targan S: The immunology of inflammatory bowel disease. In *Modern Concepts in Gastroenterology*, vol. 2. Edited by Shaffer E, Thomson ABR. New York: Plenum; 1989: 291–310.

10. Shanahan F: Inflammatory bowel disease: Immunology of intestinal diseases. *Ann Intern Med* 1987; 106:853–870.

11. Strober W, James SP: The immunologic basis of inflammatory bowel disease. *J Clin Immunol* 1986, 6:414–432.

12. MacDermott RP, Stenson WF: The immunology of idiopathic inflammatory bowel disease. *Adv Immunol* 1988, 42:285–328.

13. MacDermott RP, Stenson WF: Inflammatory bowel disease. In *Immunology and Immunopathology of the Liver and Gastrointestinal Tract*. Edited by Targan S, Shanahan F. New York/Tokyo:Igaku-Shoin; 1990:459–486.

14. Elson CO: The immunology of inflammatory bowel disease. In *Inflammatory Bowel Disease* 3d ed. Edited by Kirsner J, Shorter R. Philadelphia: Lea & Febiger; 1988:97–164.

15. Rubin M, Herrington JL, Schneider R: Regional enteritis with major gastrointestinal hemorrhage as the initial manifestation. *Arch Intern Med* 1980, 140:217–219.

16. Strodel WE, Eckhauser FE, Simmons JL: Primary ulceration of the ileum. *Dis Colon Rectum* 1981, 23:183–185.

17. Sunaryo FP, Boyle JT, Ziegler MM, Heyman S: Primary nonspecific ileal ulceration as a cause of massive rectal bleeding. *Pediatrics* 1981, 68:247–250.

18. Markowitz J, Daum F, Aiges H, *et al.*: Perianal disease in children and adolescents with Crohn's disease. *Gastroenterology* 1984, 86:829–833.

19. Kelts DG, Grand RJ, Shen G, *et al.*: Nutritional basis of growth failure in children and adolescents with Crohn's disease. *Gastroenterology* 1979, 76:720–727.

20. Hildebrand H, Karlberg J, Kristiansson B: Longitudinal growth in children and adolescents with inflammatory bowel disease. *J Pediatr Gastroenterol Nutr* 1994, 18:165–173.

21. Kirschner BS: Growth and development in chronic inflammatory bowel disease. *Acta Pediatr Scand* (Suppl) 1990, 366:98–104.

22. Burke P, Meyer V, Kocoshis S, *et al.*: Depression and anxiety in pediatric inflammatory bowel disease and cystic fibrosis. *J Am Acad Child Adolesc Psychiatry* 1989, 28:948–951.

23. Perenboom RM, Rijk MC, Rikken GH, Van Tongeren JH: The course of illness in ulcerative colitis. *Ned Tijdschr Geneeskd* 1990, 134:438–442.

24. Roth MP, Petersen GM, McElree C, *et al.*: Familial empiric risk estimates of inflammatory bowel disease in Ashkenazi Jews. *Gastroenterology* 1989, 96:1016–1020.

25. Lashner BA, Evans AA, Kirsner JB, Hanauet SB: Prevalence and incidence of inflammatory bowel disease in family members. *Gastroenterology* 1986, 91:1396–1400.

26. Glassman MS, Newman LJ, Berezin S, Grybowski JD: Cow's milk protein sensitivity during infancy in patients with inflammatory bowel disease. *Am J Gastroenterol* 1990, 85:838–840.

27. Lindberg E, Tysk C, Andersson K, Jarnerot G: Smoking and inflammatory bowel disease. A control study. *Gut* 1988, 29:352–357.

28. Lorusso D, Leo S, Misciagna G, Guerra V: Cigarette smoking and ulcerative colitis: A case-control study. *Hepatogastroenterology* 1989, 36:202–204.

29. Tobin MV, Logan RF, Langman MJ, *et al*: Cigarette smoking and inflammatory bowel disease. *Gastroenterology*, 1987, 93:316–321.

30. Price WH: A high incidence of chronic inflammatory bowel disease in patients with Turner's syndrome. *J Med Genet* 1979, 16:263–266.

31. Arulanantham K, Kramer MS, Gryboski JD: The association of inflammatory bowel disease and X chromosomal abnormality. *Pediatrics* 1980, 66:63–67.

32. Keating JP, Ternberg JL, Packman R: Association of Crohn disease and Turner syndrome. *J Pediatr* 1978, 92:160–161.

33. Manzione NC, Kram M, Kram E, Das KM: Turner's syndrome and inflammatory bowel disease: A case report with immunologic studies. *Am J Gastroenterol* 1988, 83:1294–1297.

34. Schinella RA, Greco A, Cobert BL, *et al.* Hermansky-Pudlak syndrome with granulomatous colitis. *Ann Intern Med* 1980, 92:20–23.

35. Witkop CJ, Nunez-Babcock M, Rao GH, *et al.*: Albinism and Hermansky-Pudlak syndrome in Puerto Rico. *Assoc Med P R* 1990, 82:333–339.

36. Mahadeo R, Markowitz J, Fisher S, Daum F: Hermansy Pudlak syndrome with granulomatous colitis in children. *J Pediatr* 1991, 118:904–906.

37. Roe T, Schonfeld N, Thomas D, *et al.*: Regional enteritis and glycogen storage disease type Ib [**Letter**]. *Lancet* 1984, 1:1077.

38. Roe TF, Thomas DW, Gilsanz V, *et al.* Inflammatory bowel disease in glycogen storage disease type Ib. *J Pediatr* 1986, 109:55–59.

39. Couper R, Kapelushnik J, Griffths AM: Neutrophil dysfunction in glycogen storage disease Ib: association with Crohn's like colitis. *Gastroenterology* 1991, 100:549–554.

40. Winter HS, Lancers CJ, Winkelstein A, *et al.*: Anti-neutrophil cytoplasmic antibodies in children with ulcerative colitis. *J Pediatr* 1194, 125:707–711.

41. Saxon A, Shanahan F, Landers C, *et al.* A subset of antineutrophil anticytoplasmic antibodies is associated with inflammatory bowel disease. *J Allergy Clin Immunol* 1990, 86:202–210.

42. Duerr RH, Targan SR, Landers CJ, *et al.*: Anti-neutrophil cytoplasmic antibodies in ulcerative colitis. Comparison with other colitides/diarrhea illnesses. *Gastroenterology* 1991, 100:1590–1596.

43. Cambridge G, Rampton DS, Stevens TRJ, *et al.*: Anti-neutrophil antibodies in inflammatory bowel disease: prevalence and diagnostic role. *Gut* 1992, 33:668–674.

44. Shanahan F, Duerr RH, Rotter JI, *et al.*: Neutrophil autoantibodies in ulcerative colitis: Familial aggregation and genetic heterogeneity. *Gastroenterology* 1992, 103:456–461.

45. Shorter RG, Cardoza MR, ReMine SG, *et al.*: Modification of in vitro cytotoxicity of lymphocytes from patients with chronic ulcerative colitis or chronic granulomatous colitis for allogenic colonic epithelial cells. *Gastroenterology* 1970, 58:692–698.

46. Carlson HE, Lagercrantz R, Perlmann P: Immunological studies in ulcerative colitis, VIII. Antibodies to colon antigen in patients with ulcerative colitis. *Scand J Gastroenterol* 1977, 12:707–714.

47. Hibi T, Aiso S, Ishikawa M, *et al.*: Circulating antibodies to the surface antigens on colon epithelial cells in ulcerative colitis. *Clin Exp Immunol* 1983, 54:163–168.

48. Fiocchi C, Roche JK, Michener WM: High prevalence of antibodies to intestinal epithelial antigens in patients with inflammatory bowel disease. *Ann Intern Med* 1989, 110:786–794.

49. Kelly JK, Preshaw RM: Origin of fistulas in Crohn's disease. *J Clin Gastroenterol* 1989; 11:193–196.

50. Kelly JK, Siu TO: The strictures, sinuses, and fissures of Crohn's disease. *J Clin Gastroenterol* 1986, 8:594–598.

51. Issenman RM, Atkinson SA, Radoja C, Fraher L: Longitudinal assessment of growth, mineral metabolism, and bone mass in pediatric Crohn's disease. *J Pediatr Gastroenterol Nutr* 1993, 17:401–406.

52. Barot LR, Rombeau JL, Feurer ID, Mullen JL: Caloric requirements in patients with inflammatory bowel disease. *Ann Surg* 1982, 195:214–218.

53. Detsky ASM, McLaughlin JR, Baker JP, *et al.*: What is subjective global assessment of nutritional status? *JPEN J Parenter Enteral Nutr* 1987, 11:8–13.

54. Welch CS, Adams M, Wakefield EG: Metabolic studies in ulcerative colitis. *J Clin Invest* 1937, 16:161–168.

55. Dyer HH, Child JA, Mollin DL, *et al.*: Anemia in Crohn's disease. *Q J Med* 1972, 164:419–436.

56. Thompson ABR, Burst R, Mam A, *et al.*: Iron deficiency in inflammatory bowel disease: Diagnostic efficacy of serum ferritin. *Am J Dig Dis* 1978, 23:705–709.

57. Seidman EG: Nutritional management of inflammatory bowel disease. *Gastroenterol Clin North Am* 1989, 17:129–155.

58. Fiasse R, Lurhuma AZ, Favaro S, *et al.*: Circulating immune complexes and disease activity in Crohn's disease. *Gut* 1978, 19:611–617.

59. Jewell DP, Machennun I: Circulating immune complexes in inflammatory bowel disease. *Clin Exp Immunol* 1973, 14:219–226.

60. Doe WF, Booth CC, Brown DC: Evidence for complement-binding immune complexes in adult coeliac disease, Crohn's disease, and ulcerative colitis. *Lancet* 1973, 1:402–403.

61. Mayer I, Meyers S, Janowitz H: Cryoproteins in Crohn's disease: An etiology of extraintestinal manifestations. *J Clin Gastroenterol* 1981, 3 (suppl. 1):17.

62. Levine JB: The arthropathies of IBD: More than meets the eye. *IBD News* 1990, 11:1.

63. McEwen JC, Ling C, Kirsner JB: Arthritis accompanying ulcerative colitis. *Am J Med* 1962, 33:923–941.

64. Paller AS: Cutaneous changes associated with inflammatory bowel disease. *Pediatr Dermatol* 1986, 3:439–445.

65. Lee FI, Bellary SV, Francis C: Increased occurrence of psoriasis in patients with Crohn's disease and their relatives. *Am J Gastroenterol* 1990, 85:962–963.

66. Hopkins DJ, Horan E, Burton IL, *et al.*: Ocular disorders in a series of 332 patients with Crohn's disease. *Br J Ophthalmol* 1974, 58:732–737.

67. Calkins BM, Reed JF, *et al.*: The occurrence of extraintestinal complications in IBD patients by location of lesion and family history of IBD. *Lit Rev Ther Inflam Bowel Dis* 1990, 56:531.

68. Ellis PP, Gentry JH: Ocular complications of ulcerative colitis. *Am J Ophthalmol* 1964, 50:779–785.

69. LaRusso NF, Wiesner RH, Ludwig J, MacCarty RL: Primary sclerosing cholangitis. *N Engl J Med* 1984, 310:899–903.

70. Warren GH, Kern F: The biliary tract in inflammatory bowel disease. *Clin Gastroenterol* 1983, 12:255–268.

71. Helzberg JH, Petersen JM, Boyer JL: Improved survival with primary sclerosing cholangitis: A review of clinicopathologic features and comparison of symptomatic and asymptomatic patients. *Gastroenterology* 1987, 92:1869–1875.

72. White TT, Hart MJ: Primary sclerosing cholangitis. *Am J Surg* 1987, 153:439–443.

73. Wiesner RH, LaRusso NF: Clinicopathologic features of the syndrome of primary sclerosing cholangitis. *Gastroenterology* 1980, 79:200–206.

74. Kern F: Hepatobiliary disorders in inflammatory bowel disease. In *Progress in Liver Disease*. Edited by Popper H, Schaffner F. New York: Grune & Stratton; 1976, 5:575–589.

75. Thornton JR, Teague RH, Read AE: Pyoderma gangrenosum and ulcerative colitis. *Gut* 1980, 21:247–248.

76. Greenstein AJ, Janowitz HD, Sachar DB: The extraintestinal complication of Crohn's disease and ulcerative colitis: A study of 700 patients. *Medicine* 1976, 55:401–412.

77. Burgdorf W: Cutaneous manifestations of Crohn's disease. *J Am Acad Dermatol* 1981, 5:689–695.

78. Mir-Madjilessi SH, Taylor JS, Farmer RG: Clinical course and evolution of erythema nodosum and pyoderma gangrenosum in chronic ulcerative colitis: A study of 42 patients. *Am J Gastroenterol* 1985, 80:615–620.

79. Matis WL, Ellis CN, Griffiths CEM, Lazarus GS: Treatment of pyoderma gangrenosum with cyclosporine. *Arch Dermatol* 1992, 128:1060–1064.

80. Goldberg NS, Ottuso P, Petro J: Cyclosporine for pyoderma gangrenosum. *Plast Reconstr Surg* 1993, 91:91–93.

81. Johnson ML, Wilson HT: Skin lesions in ulcerative colitis. *Gut* 1969, 10:255–263.

82. Basler RSW: Ulcerative colitis and the skin. *Gut* 1980, 64:941–954.

83. Monsen U, Hellers G, Johansson C: Extracolonic diagnoses in ulcerative colitis; an epidemiologic study. *Am J Gastroenterol* 1990, 85:711–716.

84. Anderson PC: Erythema nodosum. In *Clinical Dermatology*. Edited by Demis DJ. Philadelphia: Harper & Row; 1990:1–8.

85. Moreno AJ, Weisman I, Kenney RL, *et al*: Concurrence of erythema multiforme and erythema nodosum. *Cutis* 1983, 31:275–278.

86. Lofgren S: Primary pulmonary sarcoidosis: Early signs and symptoms. *Acta Med Scand* 1992, 26:259–260.

87. Debois J, Vandepitte J, Degreef H, *et al*: Yersinia enterocolitica as a cause of erythema nodosum. *Dermatologica* 1978, 156:65.

88. Palder SB, Shanding B, Bilik R, *et al*: Perianal complications of pediatric crohn's disease. *Pediatr Surg* 1991, 26:513–515.

89. Markowitz J, Grancher K, Rosa J, *et al*: Highly destructive perianal disease in children with Crohn's Disease. *Pediatr Gastroenterol Nutr* 1995, 2:149–153.

90. Wolf JL: Ciprofloxacin may be useful in Crohn's disease [Abstract]. *Gastroenterology* 1990, 98A:A212.

91. Proujansky R, Fawcett PT, Gibney KM, *et al.*: Examination of anti-neutrophil cytoplasmic antibodies in childhood inflammatory bowel disease. *J Pediatr Gastroenterol Nutr* 1993, 17:193–197.

92. Gelzayd EA, Breuer RI, Kirsner JB: Nephrolithiasis in inflammatory bowel disease. *Am J Dig Dis* 1986, 13:1027–1034.

93. Chadwick VS, Modka K, Dowling RH: Mechanism for hyperoxaluria in patients with ileal dysfunctions. *N Engl J Med* 1973, 289:172–176.

94. Tanaka M, Riddell RH: The pathological diagnosis and differential dignosis of Crohn's disease. *Hepatogastroenterology* 1990, 37:18–31.

95. Surawicz CM, Meisel JL, Ylvisaker T, *et al.*: Rectal biopsy in the diagnosis of Crohn's disease: Value of multiple biopsies and serial sectioning. *Gastroenterology* 1981, 81:66–71.

96. Surawicz CM: Serial sectioning of a portion of a rectal biopsy detects more focal abnormalities: A prospective study of patients with inflammatory bowel disease. *Dig Dis Sci* 1982, 27:434–436.

97. Dourmashkin RR, Davies H, Wells C, *et al.*: Epithelial patchy necrosis in Crohn's disease. *Hum Pathol* 1983, 14:643–648.

98. Teague RH, Waye JD: Endoscopy in inflammatory bowel disease. In *Colonoscopy: Techniques, Clinical Practice and Colour Atlas*. Edited by Hunt RH, Waye JD. London: Chapman and Hall, 1981:343–362.

99. Samach M, Train J: Demonstration of mucosal bridging in Crohn's colitis. *Am J Gastroenterol* 1980, 74:50–54.

100. Fishman RS, Fleming CR, Stephens DH: Roentgenographic simulation of colonic cancer by benign masses in Crohn's colitis. *Mayo Clin Proc* 1978, 53:447–449.

101. Bernstein JR, Ghahremani GG, Paige ML, Rosenberg JL: Localized giant pseudopolposis of the colon in ulcerative and granulomatous colitis. *Gastrointest Radiol* 1978, 3:431–435.

102. Kuijpers TJA, Shaw MPC: Giant pseudopolyps complicating Crohn's colitis. *Fortschr Geb Rontgenstr Nuklearmed Erganzung Sbd* 1983, 139:451–453.

103. Foderaro AE, Barloon TJ, Murray JA: Giant pseudopolyposis in Crohn's disease with computed tomography correlation. *J Comput Tomogr* 1987, 11:288–290.

104. Edwards FC, Truelove FC: The course and prognosis of ulcerative colitis, III and IV. *Gut* 1964, 5:1–22.

105. Jalan KN, Sircus W, Walker RJ, *et al.*: Pseudopolyposis in ulcerative colitis. *Lancet* 1969, 2:555–559.

106. Sparberg M, Fennessy J, Kirsner JB: Ulcerative proctitis and mild ulcerative colitis: A study of 220 patients. *Medicine* 1966, 45:391–412.

107. Devroede GJ, Taylor WF, Sauer WG, *et al.*: Cancer risk and life expectancy of children with ulcerative colitis. *N Engl J Med* 1971, 285:17–21.

108. Stahl TJ, Schoetz DJ, Roberts PL, *et al.*: Crohn's disease and carcinoma: Increasing justification for surveillance? *Dis Colon Rectum* 1992, 35:850–856.

109. Schmitz-Moormann P, Pittner PM: The granuloma in Crohn's disease: Bioptical study. *Pathol Res Pract* 1984, 178:467–476.

110. Morson BC: Crohn's disease. *Proc R Soc Med* 1968, 61:79–83.

111. Schmitz-Moormann, Schag M: Histology of the lower intestinal tract in Crohn's disease of children and adolescents. Multicentric paediatric Crohn's disease study. *Pathol Res Pract* 1990, 186:479–484.

112. Markowitz J, Kahn E, Daum F: Prognostic significance of epithelioid granulomas found in rectosigmoid biopsies at the initial presentation of pediatric Crohn's disease. *J Pediatr Gastroenterol Nutr* 1989, 9:182–186.

113. Lennard-Jones JE, Melville DM, Morson BC, *et al.*: Precancer and cancer in extensive ulcerative colitis: Findings among 401 patients over 22 years. *Gut* 1990, 31:800–806.

114. Baron JH, Connell PM, Lennard-Jones JE, *et al.*: Sulphasalazine and salicylazosulphadimidine in ulcerative colitis. *Lancet* 1962, 1:1094–1096.

115. Dick AP, Grayson MJ, Carpenter RG, *et al.*: Controlled trial of sulphasalazine in the treatment of ulcerative colitis. *Gut* 1964, 5:437–442.

116. Jewell DP: Corticosteroids for the management of ulcerative colitis and Crohn's disease. *Gastroenterol Clin North Am* 1989, 18:21–34.

117. Kuritzkes R, Shanahan F: Corticosteroid therapy. In *Steroids and Inflammatory Bowel Disease: Diagnosis and Treatment*. Edited by Gitnick G. Tokyo: Igaku-Shoin, 1990:299–321.

118. Blair V, Ullman U: The influence of metronidazole and its two main metabolites on murine in vitro lymphocyte transformation. *Eur J Clin Microbiol* 1983, 2:568–570.

119. Duffy L, Daum F, Fisher SE, *et al.*: Peripheral neuropathy in Crohn's disease patients with metronidazole. *Gastroenterology* 1985, 88:681–684.

120. Gitnick G: Etiology of inflammatory bowel disease: Where have we been? Where are we going? *Scan J Gastroenterol* 1990, 25(suppl 175):93–96.

121. Podolsky DK: Inflammatory bowel disase (Part I). *N Engl J Med* 1991, 325:928–936.

122. Das KM, Eastwood MA, McManus JP, Sircus W: Adverse reactions during salicylazosulfapyridine therapy and the relation with drug metabolism and acetylator phenotype. *N Engl J Med* 1973, 289:491–495.

123. Rao SS, Cann PA, Holdsworth CD: Clinical experience of the tolerance of mesalazine and olsalazine in patients intolerant of sulphasalazine. *Scand J Gastroenterol* 1987, 22:332–336.

124. Campieri M, Lanfranchi GA, Bazzochi G, *et al.*: Treatment of ulcerative colitis with high dose 5-aminosalicylic acid enemas. *Lancet* 1981, 2:270–271.

125. Campieri M, Lanfranchi GA, Brignoa C, *et al.*: 5-Aminosalicylic acid for the treatment of inflammatory bowel disease (Letter). *Gastroenterology* 1991, 89:701–703.

126. van Hees PA, Bakher JH, van Tongeren JH: Effect of sulphapyridine, 5-aminosalicylic acid and placebo in patients with idiopathic proctitis: A study to determine the active therapeutic moiety of sulphasalazine. *Gut* 1980, 21:632–635.

127. Williams CN, Hader G, Aguino JA: Double-blind placebo-controlled evaluation of 5-ASA suppositories in active distal proctitis and measurement of extent of spread using Tc-labelled 5-ASA suppositories. *Dig Dis Sci* 1987, 32:718–755.

128. Nielsen OH, Bukhave K, Elmgreen J, Ahnfelt-Ronne I: Inhibition of 5-lipoxygenase pathway of arachidonic acid metabolism in human neutrophils by sulfasalazine and 5-aminosalicylic acid. *Dig Dis Sci* 1987, 6:577–582.

129. Craven PA, Pfanstiel J, Saito R, DeRubertis FR: Actions of sulfasalazine 5-aminosalicylic acid as reactive oxygen scavengers in the suppression of bile acid-induced increases in colonic epithelial cell loss and proliferative activity. *Gastroenterology* 1987, 92:1998–2008.

130. Daum F, Markowitz J, Rosa J, *et al.*: Does proctosigmoiditis in inflammatory bowel disease presage the imminent onset of symptoms? *J Pediatr Gastroenterol Nutr* 1989, 8:339–342.

131. Hyams J, Moore R, Leichtner A, *et al.*: Relationship of type I procollagen to corticosteroid therapy in children with inflammatory bowel disease. *J Pediatr* 1988, 112:893–898.

132. Whittington PF, Barnes HV, Bayless TM: Medical management of Crohn's disease in adolescence. *Gastroenterology* 1977, 72:1338–1344.

133. Kumana CR, Seaton T, Meghji M, *et al.* Beclomethasone dipropionate enemas for treating inflammatory bowel disease without producing Cushing's syndrome or hypothalamic-pituitary-adrenal suppression. *Lancet* 1982, 1:579–583.

134. Brattsand R: Overview of newer glucocorticosteroid preparations for inflammatory bowel diseases. *Can J Gastroenterol* 1990, 407–414.

135. Larochelle P, DuSouich P, Bolte E, *et al.*: Tixocortole pivalate, a corticosteroid with no systemic glucocorticoid effect after oral, intrarectal and intranasal application. *Clin Pharmacol Ther* 1983, 33:343–350.

136. Lofberg R, Danielsson A, Salde L: Oral budesonide ileocecal Crohn's disease: An initial experience (Abstract). *Gastroenterology* 1991, 100:A226.

137. Greenberg GR, Feagan BG, Martin F, *et al.*: Oral budesonide for active Crohn's disease: Canadian Inflammatory Bowel Disease Study Group. *N Engl J Med* 1994, 331:873–874.

138. Roth M, Ueberschaer B, Ewe K, Gross V: Scholmerich slow release budesonide includes remission in active disease with little effect on adrenal function (Abstract). *Gastroenterology* 1992, 102:A688.

139. Carpani de Kaski M, Peters AM, Lavender JP: Fluticasone propionate in Crohn's disease. *Gut* 1991, 32:657–661.

140. Present DH, Korelitz BI, Wisch N, *et al.*: Treatment of Crohn's disease with 6-mercaptopurine. *N Engl J Med* 1980, 302:981–987.

141. Markowitz J, Rosa J, Grancher K, *et al.*: Long term 6-mercaptopurine (6-MP) in adolescents with Crohn's disease. *Gastroenterology* 1991, 100:1156–1157.

142. Treem WR, Davis PM, Hyams JS: Cyclosporine treatment of severe ulcerative colitis in children. *J Pediatr* 1991, 119:994–997.

143. Benkov KF, Rosh JR, Schwersenz AH, *et al.* Cyclosporine as an alternative to surgery in children with inflammatory bowel disease. *J Ped Gastroenterol Nutr* 1994, 19:290–294.

144. Hanauer SB, Smith MB: Rapid closure of Crohn's disease fistulas with continuous intravenous cyclosporin A. *Am J Gastroenterol* 1993, 88:646–649.

145. Rohr G, Kusterer K, Schille M, *et al.*: Treatment of Crohn's disease and ulcerative colitis with 7S-immunoglobulin. *Lancet* 1987, 1:170.

146. Alperstein G, Daum F, Fisher SE, *et al.*: Linear growth following surgery in children and adolescents with Crohn's disease: Relationship to pubertal status. *J Pediatr Surg* 1985, 20:129–133.

147. Goligher JC: Ulcerative colitis. In *Surgery of the Anus, Rectum and Colon*. New York: MacMillan; 1980, 689–826.

148. Fazio VW: Toxic megacolon: Natural history and management. In *Mucosal Ulcerative Colitis*. New York: Future Publishing; 1986, 159–175.

149. Rubin CE, Haggitt RC, Burmer GC, *et al.*: *Gastroenterology* 1992, 103:1611–1620.

150. Ravitch MM, Sabiston DL, Jr: Anal ileostomy with preservation of the sphincter: A proposed operation in patients requiring total colectomy for benign lesions. *Surg Gynecol Obstet* 1947, 84:1095.

151. Ekbom A, Helmick C, Zack M, Adami HO: Ulcerative colitis and colorectal cancer. A population-based study. *N Engl J Med* 1990, 323:1228–1233.

152. Melville DM, Jass JR, Shepherd NA, *et al.*: Dysplasia and deoxyribonucleic acid aneuploidy in the assessment of precancerous changes in chronic ulcerative colitis. Observer variation and correlations. *Gastroenterology* 1988, 95:668–675.

153. Markowitz J, Grancher K, Rosa J, *et al.*: Growth failure in pediatric inflammatory bowel disease. *J Pediatr Gastroenterol Nutr* 1993, 16:373–380.

154. McIntyre PB, Powell-Tuck J, Wood SR, *et al.*: Controlled trial of bowel rest in the treatment of severe acute colitis. *Gut* 1986, 27:481–485.

155. Greenberg GR, Fleming CR, Jeejeebhoy KN, *et al.*: Controlled trial of bowel rest and nutritional support in the management of Crohn's disease. *Gut* 1988, 29:1309–1315.

156. O'Morain C, Segal AW, Levi AJ: Elemental diet as primary treatment of acute Crohn's disease: A controlled trial. *Br J Med* 1984, 288:1859–1862.

157. Saverymuttu S, Hodgson HJF, Chadwick VS: Controlled trial comparing prednisone with an elemental diet plus non-absorbable antibiotics in active Crohn's disease. *Gut* 1985, 26:994–998.

158. Motil KJ, Grand RJ, Matthews DE, *et al.*: The effect of disease, drug, and diet on whole body protein metabolism in adolescents with Crohn's disease and growth failure. *J Pediatr* 1982, 101:345–351.

159. Aiges H, Markowitz J, Daum F: Home nocturnal supplemental nasogastric feedings in growth-retarded adolescents with Crohn's disease. *Gastroenterology* 1989, 97:905–910.

160. Belli DC, Seidman E, Bouthillier L, *et al.*: Chronic intermittent elemental diet improves growth failure in children with Crohn's disease. *Gastroenterology* 1988, 94:603–610.

161. Israel DM, Hassal E: Prolonged use of gastrostomy for enteral hyperalimentation in children with Crohn's disease. *Am J Gastroenterol* 1995, 90:1084–1088.

162. Strobel CT, Byren WJ, Ament MF: Home parenteral nutrition in children with Crohn's disease: An effective management alternative. *Gastroenterology* 1979, 272–279.

163. Wood B, Watkins J, Boyle J, *et al.*: Psychological functioning in children with Crohn's disease and ulcerative colitis: Implications for models of psychobiological interaction. *J Am Acad Child Adol Psychiat* 1987, 26:774–781.

164. Gitlin K, Markowitz J, Pelcovitz D, *et al.*: Stress mediators in children with inflammatory bowel disease. In *Advances in Child Health Psychology: Proceedings of the Florida Conference*. Edited by Johnson J, Johnson S. Gainesville, Florida: University of Florida Press; 1990:54–62.

Chapter 8

Functional Bowel Disorders in Pediatrics

● ●

Functional bowel diseases are defined by a variable combination of chronic and recurrent gastrointestinal symptoms which cannot be explained by structural or biochemical abnormalities. They occur in up to 35% of the adult population. A majority of outpatient visits to pediatric gastroenterologists are for functional bowel disorders. Some functional bowel disorders are unique to children and resolve by puberty (*eg*, functional fecal retention) whereas others may be found in both age groups (*eg*, nonulcer dyspepsia, irritable bowel syndrome, intestinal pseudo-obstruction). Some disorders are common (*eg*, recurrent abdominal pain, functional fecal retention), others are rarer (*eg*, intestinal pseudo-obstruction). The pathogenesis of most functional bowel disorders is still poorly understood, but there is nearly always interaction among motor, sensory, and psychologic factors. Treatment requires establishing a supportive relationship with the child and family, reassuring that the symptom is real, and avoiding unnecessary invasive tests aimed at ruling out every "organic" disease. In extreme cases, the affected child may be totally disabled by functional pains. In such children, a multidisciplinary approach involving interested clinicians from gastroenterology, psychiatry, and pain management services is required for optimal treatment.

CARLO DI LORENZO

At the time of publication, **cisapride** was not FDA approved for use in children. Check the package insert for any change in indications and dosage and for added warnings and precautions.

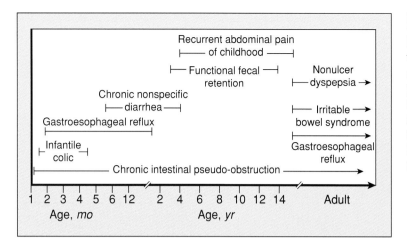

FIGURE 8-1.

Functional bowel disorders in children. There is an age-specific vulnerability to different functional bowel diseases. Sometimes different functional complaints arise at different ages in the same patient. A colicky infant may present later in life with chronic nonspecific diarrhea followed by recurrent abdominal pain and symptoms typical of irritable bowel syndrome. Other diseases, such as gastroesophageal reflux, present with different symptoms in infancy or late childhood (*see* Chapter 4 on gastroesophageal reflux in this volume).

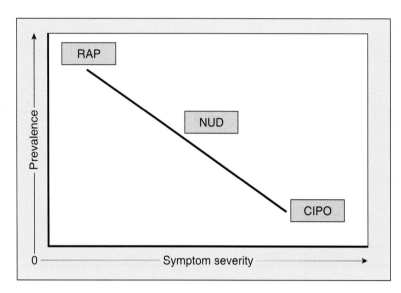

FIGURE 8-2.

Spectrum of functional bowel diseases in childhood. Recurrent abdominal pain (RAP) of childhood occurs in 10% to 15% of school-aged children [1]. Nonulcer dyspepsia (NUD) has only recently received attention as a condition affecting the pediatric patient; its incidence in children remains unknown. Chronic intestinal pseudo-obstruction (CIPO) is rare. In a membership survey of the North American Society of Pediatric Gastroenterology, CIPO was reported in only 87 children [2]. Recurrent abdominal pain may be associated with nausea, bloating, anorexia, and constipation [3], overlapping with the symptoms of NUD. In childhood NUD, eating may cause symptoms severe enough to require special means of alimentation [4], making it arduous to differentiate severe NUD from mild CIPO. It is possible to postulate that these three entities are part of an over-lapping spectrum of functional bowel diseases with RAP as the most common and benign condition at one end of the spectrum and CIPO the least common and most severe disorder at the other.

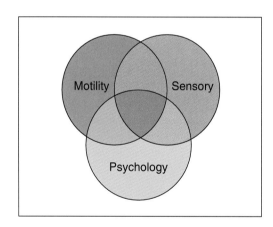

FIGURE 8-3.

Pathogenesis of functional bowel diseases. An attractive model for functional bowel diseases of childhood is one in which motility abnormalities, visceral hypersensitivity, and psychosocial vulnerability interact to generate the symptom. Motility abnormalities have been described in all functional bowel diseases. Sensory disturbances may decrease or increase the threshold for a symptom. A decreased gastric visceral threshold causes nausea or pain in response to normal or non-noxious stimuli [5]. An increased threshold for sensory response in a dilated rectum is one of the factors contributing to childhood constipation [6]. The role of psychologic factors in modulating gastrointestinal motility and sensory response is well established [7]. Decreased motility and delayed gastric emptying occur with depression, and an increased motility index is associated with anger and aggressive behavior. The variable interactions among motility, sensory, and psychologic components contribute to the heterogeneity of functional bowel diseases in children.

Manometry

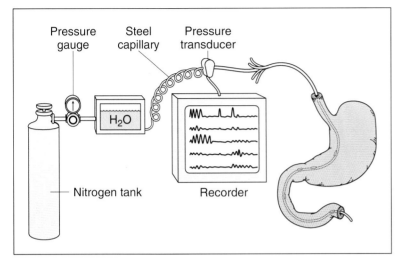

FIGURE 8-4.

FIGURE 8-4.

Perfused tube manometry. Diagram of low-compliance pneumohydraulic system of perfusion manometry. The equipment required for manometric recording consists of a low-compliance, pneumohydraulic perfusion system connected to a multilumen catheter with interposed strain gauges. The number of recording sites and their location on the catheter depends on the study design and the segment of bowel monitored. Pneumohydraulic perfusion is achieved by degassed water maintained at constant pressure (5–15 psi); the latter pressure is reduced to atmospheric levels before entering the manometry catheter by steel capillary tubing which provides a high resistance to flow. Intestinal contractions occurring at the side hole of the catheter obstruct the constant flow of water through the catheter. This resistance to water flow is determined by the amplitude and duration of the contraction; the pressure is transmitted to the strain gauge and may be recorded on a paper chart or electronic system.

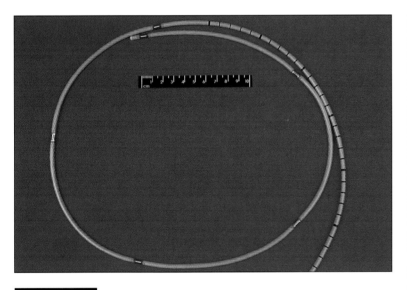

FIGURE 8-5.

Ambulatory manometry. Shown is a manometry catheter with solid-state transducers spaced 15 cm apart. The study of motility in ambulatory subjects requires that strain gauge pressure transducers be incorporated in specially designed catheters. The catheter is connected to a recorder that can be carried by the subject, as is done during prolonged intraesophageal pH monitoring. The subject is encouraged to engage in usual activities. An event marker is used to note various physiologic (sleep, meals) and pathologic (pain, vomiting) events during the recording. Data acquired during the test are subsequently downloaded to a computer that displays and analyzes the signal. Prolonged ambulatory studies allow the investigator to minimize the large inter- and intraindividual variability of gastrointestinal motility [8]. They may be used for repetitive study of variables in the same individual, such as different meals or drugs, or to investigate motor events that occur infrequently such as the high amplitude propagated colonic contractions. Another advantage of prolonged ambulatory studies is the possibility of measuring motility at night because it seems that some motor abnormalities can be better appreciated during sleep [9]. Disadvantages include the higher price and shorter half-life of the catheters and the lack of on-line display of the motility signal, which does not allow detection of catheter migration.

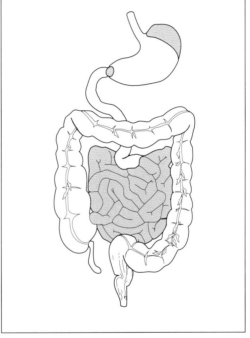

FIGURE 8-6.

Areas of the gastrointestinal tract that cause special problems for manometric recording. Some areas of the gastrointestinal tract have not been extensively studied in children by either water-perfused or solid-state manometry. Manometry is particularly suitable for the study of phasic contractions. The proximal third of the stomach, which contains the fundus, does not contract rapidly but instead exhibits slow, tonic alterations in pressure, which are poorly detected by manometric catheters. The pylorus is the most distal and narrowly tubular part of the stomach. It measures less than 1 cm in length and its function can be monitored reliably only by using several manometric ports spaced a few millimeters apart or by using a "sleeve" [10], a manometric tube appliance rarely used in children. The bowel distal to the ligament of Treitz and proximal to the ileocecal valve is difficult to access. Motility in the jejunum and ileum in children has been studied only by placing manometric catheters through jejunostomies or ileostomies.

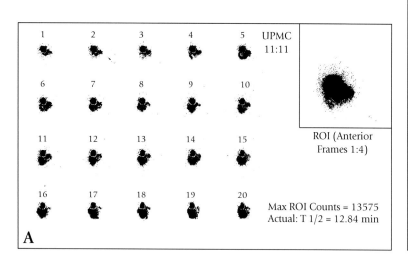

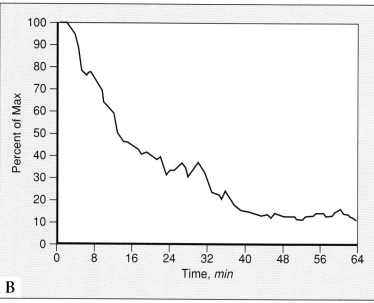

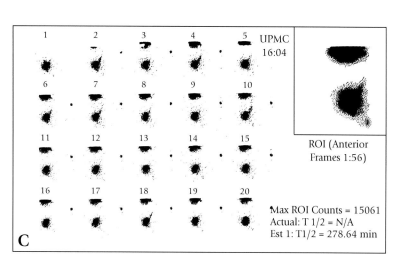

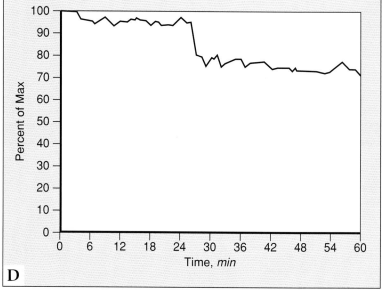

FIGURE 8-7.

Radionuclide measurement of gastric emptying (milk scan). **A–B**, Normal gastric emptying in an infant. **C–D**, Delayed gastric emptying in an infant with chronic intestinal pseudo-obstruction. The infants were given milk labeled with technetium 99m. In both figures, the images on the top left quadrant depict abdominal scintiscans taken at 1-minute intervals. Note movement of isotope from the stomach to the small intestine in *panels A* and *B*, while *panels C* and *D* show very little change in the distribution of the isotope. The reader ought also appreciate that episodes of gastroesophageal reflux with the isotope could be visualized in the esophagus by this method. The *top right corners* show the "region of interest" drawn on the gastric region. The amount of radioactivity in that region is measured and corrected for the decay of the isotope. The *bottom halves* of the two figures represent gastric emptying curves. The T1/2 (*ie,* the time it takes for the half of the meal to empty) is normal in the patient shown in *panels A* and *B* and extremely delayed in the patient viewed in *panels C* and *D*. Being noninvasive, radionuclide testing has gained wide acceptance as an indirect measure of gastric motor function. It is possible to label simultaneously the liquid and solid components of a meal with different isotopes and to obtain quantitative information on the emptying of both components. Gastric emptying is influenced by various factors, including the nature, size, consistency, and caloric content of the meal, as well as the emotional state of the patient.

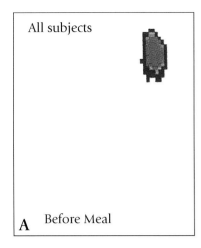 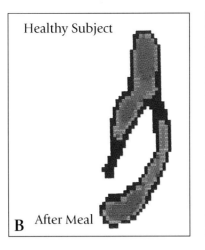 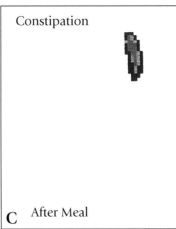 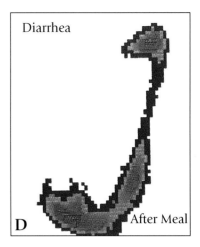

FIGURE 8-8.

Radionuclide assessment of colonic transit. A small amount of water containing technetium 99m is placed at splenic flexure (**A**) and its movement is recorded by a gamma camera. After a meal, the radioactive marker moves backward into the transverse colon and forward into the rectosigmoid region in healthy patients (**B**). In subjects with constipation secondary to colonic inertia, the marker does not move (**C**). Patients with diarrhea have an exaggerated colonic response to meals with movement of most of the marker to the rectum and passage of stools (**D**).

This technique has been used to investigate the pathophysiology of constipation in children with intestinal pseudo-obstruction [11]. It requires placement of a colonic manometry catheter with an infusion site at the splenic flexure. Scintigraphic studies in children are complicated by paucity of data in normal children and the requirement for the subject to lie motionless for an extended period under the gamma camera. (*Courtesy* of Narashima Reddy, PhD, Los Angeles, CA.)

Electrogastrography

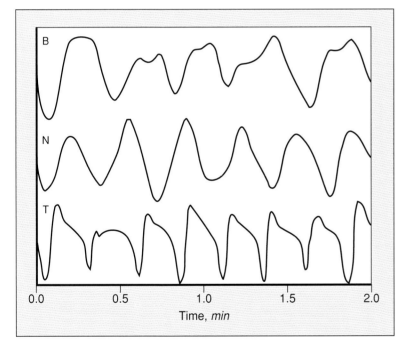

FIGURE 8-9.

Electrogastrography (EGG). Examples of EGG signals recorded from children with bradygastria (B), normal electric rhythm (N), and tachygastria (T). EGGs record gastric myoelectric activity measured from the abdominal surface with electrodes placed on the skin. The predominant rate of electrical waves recorded from the stomach of normal individuals is 3 cycles per minute (3 cpm). Amplitude of the EGG signal increases after a meal. Gastric myoelectric signals are distorted by cardiac electrical activity, respiratory movement, and body motion. Thus, the EGG requires filtration to eliminate artifacts without removing potentially useful information. The stomach can be the source of abnormally fast or slow myoelectrical signals, called *tachygastrias* (frequency > 4 cpm) or *bradygastrias* (frequency < 2.5 cpm). Abnormalities of gastric electric rhythm are found in various conditions associated with nausea and gastric dysfunction [12]. The elimination of tachygastria and bradygastria with restoration of a normal rate of 3 cpm is associated with improvement of symptoms [13]. (*Courtesy of* S. Narasimha Reddy, EngD, Los Angeles, CA.)

Ultrasonography

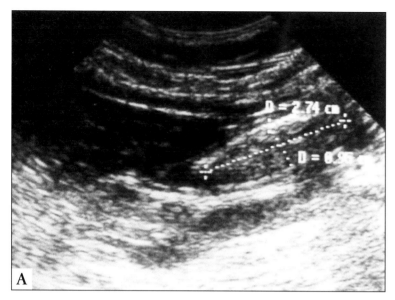 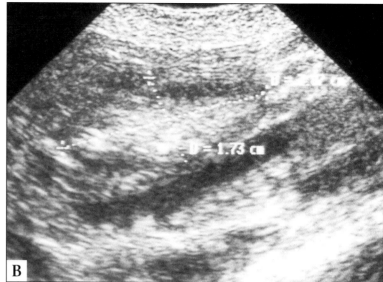

FIGURE 8-10.

Ultrasonographic measurement of gastric emptying. **A**, Ultrasonographic image of the gastric antrum after ingestion of a meal. **B**, Ultrasonographic image of the gastric antrum during fasting. Anteroposterior and longitudinal antral diameters are indicated by the letter *D*. In both images the superior mesenteric vein is shown as a hypoechogenic area below the gastric antrum. In panel A, food particles can be noticed as hyperechogenic material within the gastric antrum. Real-time ultrasonography may be used to estimate gastric volume and gastric motor activity. Comparison studies with scintigraphy and radiology have validated the ultrasonographic assessment of gastric emptying [14]. Ultrasonography is noninvasive, safe, and repeatable. The ultrasound probe is placed over the epigastrium of a supine patient. Most authors assess gastric emptying time by measuring the width of the gastric antrum at selected levels before and after the test meal. Ultrasonography has been used to evaluate the gastric emptying of infants with gastroesophageal reflux [15]. It has also been used to evaluate the transpyloric movement of gastric contents and the strength of antral contractions [16]. (**B**, *Courtesy of* Salvatore Cucchiara, MD, Naples, Italy.)

Barostat

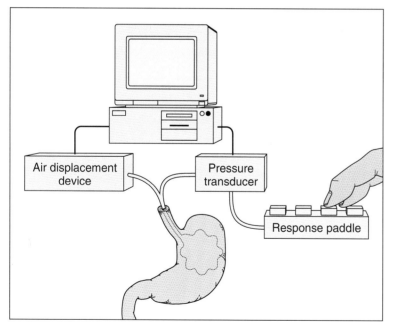

FIGURE 8-11.

Schematic diagram illustrating how the barostat operates. The barostat is a computer-driver air pump which simultaneously records pressure and volume in a balloon placed in a segment of the gastrointestinal tract. The barostat may be used to maintain a constant pressure within the balloon by changing the balloon's volume required to neutralize the organ wall contraction or relaxation. The amount of air needed to maintain a constant pressure reflects changes in tone. Compliance of the organ may be evaluated by measuring changes in pressure in response to increases in balloon volume. Visceral sensitivity is assessed by asking the patient to press buttons on a hand-held panel corresponding to different sensations. Using the barostat, it has become possible to determine that in a subgroup of patients with nonulcer dyspepsia without anatomic or motility abnormality, the threshold for symptoms is altered in response to gastric distension [17]. The barostat has been used to evaluate gastric wall compliance and gastric receptive relaxation in newborn infants [18].

RECURRENT ABDOMINAL PAIN

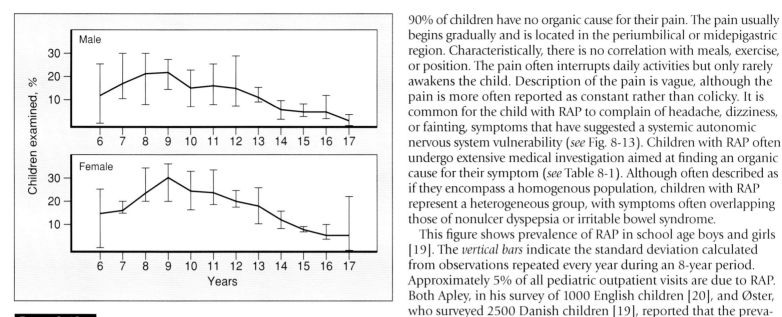

FIGURE 8-12.

Abdominal pain is one of the most common symptoms in childhood and adolescence. *Chronic* or *recurrent abdominal pain* (RAP) is defined as the presence of at least three episodes of abdominal pain occurring over a period of at least 3 months. Recurrent abdominal pain is also called *functional abdominal pain of childhood* because up to

90% of children have no organic cause for their pain. The pain usually begins gradually and is located in the periumbilical or midepigastric region. Characteristically, there is no correlation with meals, exercise, or position. The pain often interrupts daily activities but only rarely awakens the child. Description of the pain is vague, although the pain is more often reported as constant rather than colicky. It is common for the child with RAP to complain of headache, dizziness, or fainting, symptoms that have suggested a systemic autonomic nervous system vulnerability (*see* Fig. 8-13). Children with RAP often undergo extensive medical investigation aimed at finding an organic cause for their symptom (*see* Table 8-1). Although often described as if they encompass a homogenous population, children with RAP represent a heterogeneous group, with symptoms often overlapping those of nonulcer dyspepsia or irritable bowel syndrome.

This figure shows prevalence of RAP in school age boys and girls [19]. The *vertical bars* indicate the standard deviation calculated from observations repeated every year during an 8-year period. Approximately 5% of all pediatric outpatient visits are due to RAP. Both Apley, in his survey of 1000 English children [20], and Øster, who surveyed 2500 Danish children [19], reported that the prevalence of RAP seems to peak at 9 years of age. Another later peak for girls aged 13 to 14 was reported by Apley. Abdominal pain presenting before age 4 requires an in-depth evaluation to rule out organic causes. Age of onset in children older than 13 to 14 years demands a thorough evaluation of systemic inflammatory conditions and gynecologic disorders. (*Modified from* Øster [19].)

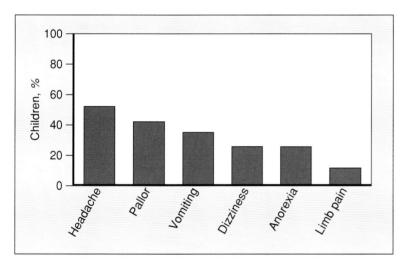

FIGURE 8-13.

Common symptoms associated with recurrent abdominal pain (RAP). Symptoms associated with RAP include headache, pallor, nausea with vomiting, and dizziness. These symptoms are upsetting to parents and physicians unfamiliar with the spectrum of RAP. Disturbances of appetite are less common; the child is usually in good health between pain attacks. Some parents report that the symptoms become more severe when the child is emotionally stressed. A thorough examination usually reveals no abnormality, although at times tenderness to deep palpation that is not localized to a particular quadrant of the abdomen may exist.

TABLE 8-1. FINDINGS SUGGESTING ORGANIC DISEASE IN CHILDREN WITH RAP

Pain away from the umbilicus
Pain that awakens patient from sleep
Radiation of pain to back, shoulder, lower extremities
Weight loss or failure to thrive
Bilious or bloody emesis
Fever
Jaundice
Dysuria
Positive family history of peptic disease, inflammatory bowel disease
Elevated sedimentation rate
Anemia
Guaiac-positive stools

TABLE 8-1.

Findings suggesting the presence of organic disease in children with recurrent abdominal pain (RAP). The presence of these features signals the need for a more extensive evaluation for organic disease. The most likely organic cause for abdominal pain is a disease involving either the genitourinary tract or the gastrointestinal tract [21]. Laboratory evaluation at the time of the first visit should include complete blood count, erythrocyte sedimentation rate, serum lipase, urinalysis and urine culture, stool examination for occult blood, ova, and parasites. When these tests yield negative results and the history and physical examination are compatible with a diagnosis of RAP, the physician should not embark in any additional invasive testing that will only reinforce in the child and the family the concept that something is seriously wrong with the child's health. The physician should instead make diagnosis of RAP and provide a thorough explanation to the patient and family of what RAP means.

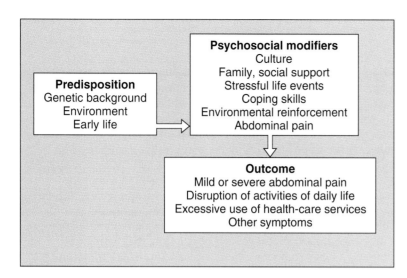

Figure 8-14.

Model for the pathogenesis of recurrent abdominal pain (RAP). Pathogenesis of RAP probably involves genetic and environmental predisposing factors with psychosocial modifiers influencing the outcome. Treatment focuses on minimizing disability and reinforcing the relative health of the child. The child must be reassured that the pain is real but that no serious organic disease is present. Reassurance is made effective by establishing a therapeutic alliance with the patient and the family. This requires the physician to be available at any time for phone consultations and to setup a schedule of return visits to monitor symptoms and for physical examinations. It is essential to reverse any reinforcement of pain behavior. Parents, schools, and physicians should support the child without directing excessive attention toward the symptom. Missing school or returning home from school because of the pain is discouraged. Self-hypnosis and relaxation techniques or low-dose tricyclic antidepressant drugs may benefit some children with RAP.

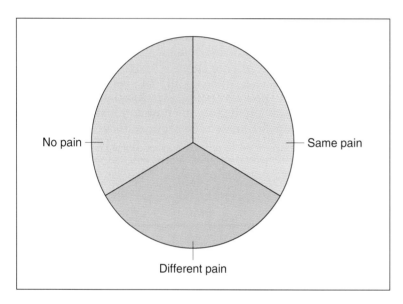

Figure 8-15.

Despite many assertions to the contrary, recurrent abdominal pain (RAP) is often not self-limited. After 5 years, approximately one third of children with RAP will have resolution of their pain, one third will continue to complain of the same symptoms, and another one third will have a different recurrent pain complaint [21]. Factors that seem to be related to worse prognosis are: (1) positive family history of abdominal symptoms; (2) male sex, in that boys suffer abdominal pain longer than girls; (3) age of onset younger than 3 years; (4) a period of more than 6 months before seeking treatment [22]; and (5) low educational level and family poverty [23].

■ NONULCER DYSPEPSIA

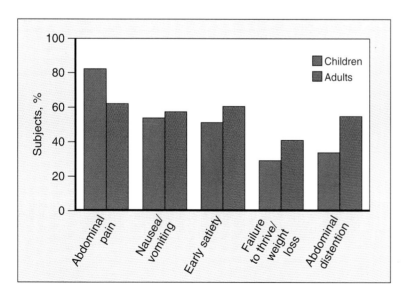

Figure 8-16.

Symptoms and signs of children and adults with nonulcer dyspepsia (NUD). NUD is a condition characterized by chronic intermittent upper abdominal symptoms without mucosal and structural abnormalities of the gastrointestinal tract. The symptoms are usually related to feedings and include epigastric pain and fullness, early satiety, nausea, belching, and vomiting. NUD is being described with increased frequency in the pediatric literature [4,24]. Children with NUD have for a long time been included under the recurrent abdominal pain (RAP) designation. They probably suffer from a particularly severe form of RAP (*see* Fig. 8-2). NUD has the same age distribution as RAP [3]. Results of physical examination and laboratory evaluation are normal. The role of gastroduodenal inflammation and *Helicobacter pylori* as a cause of NUD in children and adults is still under investigation [25,26].

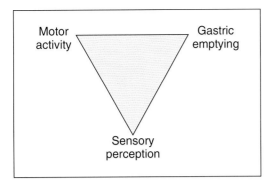

FIGURE 8-17.

Pathogenesis of symptoms in nonulcer dyspepsia (NUD). Because of the temporal relationship between symptoms and food ingestion, the stomach has been considered responsible for the abnormal interactions leading to the symptoms. Children with NUD often have antral hypomotility and either decreased frequency or decreased amplitude of phasic contractions after ingesting a solid meal [24]. Gastric emptying of a radiolabeled meal is delayed in a sizeable proportion of patients with NUD. It has been suggested that abnormal gastric electrical activity may play a pathogenic role in abnormal motility and gastric stasis in children with NUD. Normalization of gastric dysrhythmias with use of prokinetic drugs improves symptoms in children with NUD [13]. Nevertheless, up to 50% of patients with NUD have normal gastric motility and emptying. In patients with either minor or no abnormalities of gastric motor function, an abnormal gastric perception may be causing the symptoms. Increased visceral sensitivity could be secondary to decreased threshold of gastric receptors for visceral sensations, an altered modulation in the conduction of the neural signal, or an altered conscious threshold at a central level [27].

CHRONIC INTESTINAL PSEUDO-OBSTRUCTION

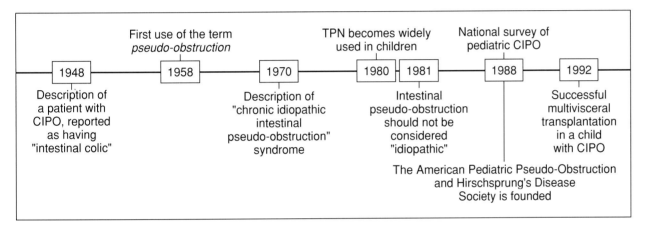

FIGURE 8-18.

Major developments in the history of chronic intestinal pseudo-obstruction (CIPO) in children. Towards the end of the 1970s interest increased in the study of gastrointestinal motility and researchers began to investigate the causes of abnormal gut motility and intestinal flow. At the same time, total parenteral nutrition (TPN) became more widely available. Children born with CIPO, who would previously have died of malnutrition and fluid and electrolyte imbalances, were able to survive. When the pathophysiology of most cases of CIPO was elucidated, it was proposed to remove "idiopathic" from the name of the syndrome [28]. During the last few years, improved nutrition, new drug regimens, and novel surgical approaches have led to an improved quality of life in most affected children and to a cure in those receiving multivisceral transplantations.

TABLE 8-2A. PRIMARY PSEUDO-OBSTRUCTION

Visceral neuropathy
  Familial
    Autosomal recessive with intranuclear inclusions
    Autosomal recessive with mental retardation and
      calcification of the basal ganglia
    Autosomal dominant with none of the above
  Sporadic
    Neuronal immaturity (preterm and term newborns)
    Aganglionosis
    Neuronal intestinal dysplasia
Visceral myopathy
  Familial
    Autosomal recessive with ptosis and external ophthalmoplegia
    Autosomal dominant
  Sporadic
    Presenting as megacystis-microcolon-hypoperistalsis syndrome

TABLE 8-2.

Causes of primary (**A**) and secondary (**B**) chronic intestinal pseudo-obstruction (CIPO) in children. Pseudo-obstruction is a clinical diagnosis based on a phenotype characterized by signs and symptoms of mechanical bowel obstruction in the absence of a physical obstruction. CIPO fits the concept of *genetic heterogeneity*, which is the common clinical presentation of several disorders different in pathophysiology, genetics, natural history, and in response to therapeutic and preventive measures.

TABLE 8-2B. SECONDARY PSEUDO-OBSTRUCTION

Disorders affecting the myenteric plexus

  Postischemic neuropathy (secondary to necrotizing
    enterocolitis, volvulus, gastroschisis)
  Postviral neuropathy (cytomegalovirus, Epstein-Barr virus,
    rotavirus)
  Generalized dysautonomia
  Diabetic autonomic neuropathy
  Chagas' disease
  Drugs (opiates, anticholinergic agents, cytotoxic agents
    used in cancer chemotherapy)
  Fetal alcohol syndrome
  Chromosomal abnormalities
  Multiple endocrine neoplasia 2B
  Radiation enteritis

Disorders affecting the intestinal smooth muscle

  Muscular dystrophies
  Scleroderma and other connective tissue diseases
  Amyloidosis
  Hypothyroidism
  Hypoparathyroidism
  Drugs (Ca2+ channel blockers)

TABLE 8-3. CHRONIC INTESTINAL PSEUDO-OBSTRUCTION

CHILDREN	ADULTS
Mostly primary	Mostly secondary
Mostly congenital	Mostly acquired
Neuropathy more common than myopathy	Myopathy more common than neuropathy
Neuropathy secondary to maturational arrest of myenteric plexus	Neuropathy secondary to degeneration of myenteric plexus
TPN frequently needed	TPN rarely needed
Absence of MMC predicts need for TPN	Absence of MMC not predictive
Presence of MMC predicts response to cisapride	Normal autonomic function predicts response to cisapride
Death likely due to complications of TPN	Death likely due to primary disease

TABLE 8-3.

Differences between chronic intestinal pseudo-obstruction (CIPO) in children and adults. Most forms of childhood CIPO are congenital and primary, whereas adults often acquire CIPO as part of systemic diseases (*eg*, diabetes, paraneoplastic syndrome, connective tissue disorder, drug-associated). Perhaps in part because of the higher energy requirement in childhood, with growth retardation reflecting caloric deprivation, more children than adults require total parenteral nutrition (TPN). The widespread use of TPN in children with CIPO has allowed them to live longer lives of better quality. The presence of the motor-migrating complex (MMC) has a much better defined prognostic role in children than in adults [29].

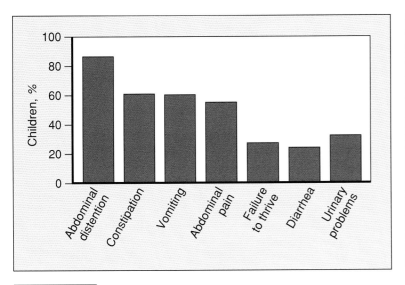

FIGURE 8-19.

Symptoms at presentation in children with chronic intestinal pseudo-obstruction (CIPO). Great variability exists in the number and intensity of symptoms in children with CIPO [30]. Typically, the child experiences nausea, emesis of possibly bile-stained vomitus, abdominal pain, and alternating constipation and diarrhea. Reduced food intake and malabsorption result in malnutrition with failure to thrive. Poor nutritional status facilitates infections and worsens motility. Abnormal motility is responsible for the constipation, but by facilitating bacterial overgrowth with steatorrhea and bile-acid malabsorption, poor motility may also lead to diarrhea. Urinary tract smooth muscle is affected in about 20% of CIPO patients. Both children with neuropathy and myopathy affecting the hollow viscera may present with a dilated and atonic bladder causing difficulty in voiding and recurrent urinary tract infections [31]. Dysphagia occurs more common in adults than in children with CIPO.

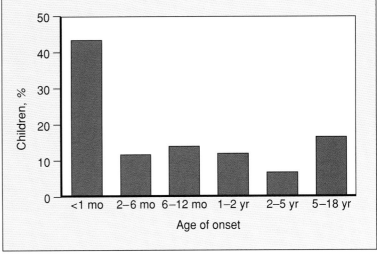

FIGURE 8-20.

Age at onset of symptoms in children with chronic intestinal pseudo-obstruction (CIPO). More than half the affected children with CIPO develop symptoms at or shortly after birth [30], and about 40% have a malrotation. In the infants with the most severe forms of the disease, the symptoms are evident within few hours of life. Children with milder forms may present during the first few months of life with vomiting, constipation, and failure to thrive. About three quarters of the children are symptomatic at the end of the first year of life and the remainder present sporadically during the first two decades. Most children experience a clinical course characterized by relative remissions and exacerbations. Factors that precipitate exacerbations include infections, general anesthesia, and psychologic and physical stress.

Diagnosis

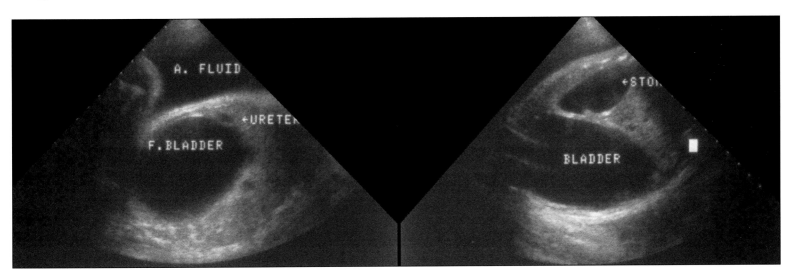

FIGURE 8-21.

Ultrasound of an infant with chronic intestinal pseudo-obstruction (CIPO) diagnosed in utero. It is possible to notice polyhydramnios and distension of the stomach and the bladder. The ultrasonographer can diagnose CIPO before birth by recognizing dilated bladder and loops of bowel with polyhydramnios. Megacystitis is one component of the *megacystis microcolon hypoperistalsis syndrome*, a diagnosis descriptive of the CIPO phenotype in some infants. Because of the severe abdominal distension, the fetuses diagnosed in utero may be stillborn, may undergo fetal surgery of the urinary tract, and often require delivery by cesarean section. At birth, they may fail to pass meconium, and thus have bilious vomiting. (*From* Hyman [32]; with permission.)

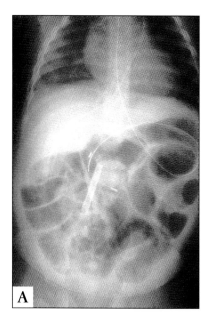

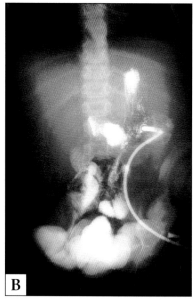

FIGURE 8-22.

Radiology in the diagnosis of chronic intestinal pseudo-obstruction (CIPO). **A**, Abdominal radiograph from a child with hollow visceral myopathy. Massive bowel dilatation and an antroduodenal manometry catheter in the stomach and duodenum are present. **B**, Barium contrast study from a child with neuropathic CIPO. Note dilated loops of distal small bowel, the tip of a central venous catheter in the chest, massive hepatomegaly (secondary to liver disease induced by total parenteral nutrition), and the presence of a gastrostomy tube.

In CIPO, radiographic studies reveal slow small-intestine transit time of contrast material with dilation of some segment of the gastrointestinal tract. Poor intestinal peristalsis leads to prolonged stasis of contrast material, so it may be prudent to use an isotonic water-soluble contrast in order to prevent barium from solidifying and forming a true physical obstruction. Air-fluid levels may be evident on abdominal radiographs. A microcolon is often recognized at birth because the colon is *unused*. In children who had previous surgery, it is difficult to differentiate between obstruction secondary to adhesions and symptoms due to pseudo-obstruction.

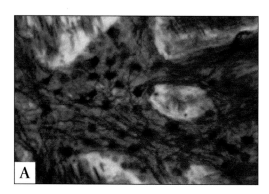

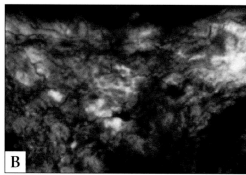

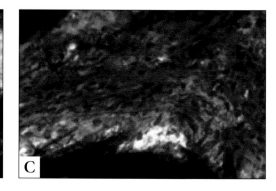

FIGURE 8-23.

Pathologic diagnosis of chronic intestinal pseudo-obstruction (CIPO). **A–C**, Silver stain of the myenteric plexus of full thickness biopsies. **A**, Biopsy specimen obtained from a normal infant. **B**, Colonic biopsy obtained from a 4-year-old with intractable constipation. The deficiency in argyrophilic neurons suggest congenital immaturity of the myenteric plexus. **C**, Jejunal biopsy obtained from a 15-year-old child with acquired pseudo-obstruction. No neurons are present in the myenteric plexus, but multiple glial-cell nuclei and few axons are present. **D**, Hematoxylin and eosin (H & E)–stained slide of a full-thickness jejunal biopsy obtained from a normal infant. Circular muscle is on the top, myenteric plexus is in the center, and longitudinal muscle is on the bottom. **E**, H & E slide of a visceral myopathy showing vacuolated muscle. **F**, In this Masson trichrome stain of a biopsy from a child with visceral myopathy, the circular muscle is vacuolated and a large amount of blue-staining collagen is present.

Surgery is performed in most cases to rule out a mechanical obstruction and confirm the diagnosis of CIPO. At surgery, a biopsy of full thickness bowel should be done to obtain a tissue diagnosis. The tissue should be processed for routine histology,

(continued on next page)

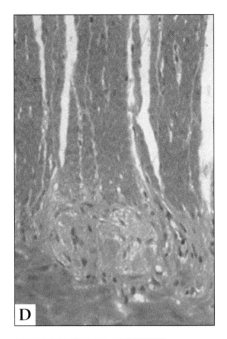
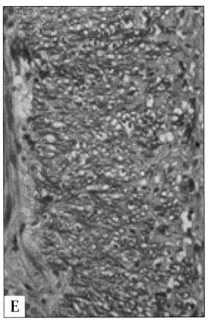
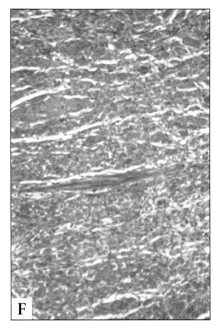

FIGURE 8-23. (*CONTINUED*)

immunohistochemistry, electron microscopy, and silver stains (Smith's technique). Using Smith's technique, tissue sections are cut parallel to the serosa. The silver staining of these sections shows the morphology of neurons, dendrites, and axons. Developmental disorders of the myenteric plexus are the most frequent causes of CIPO in childhood [31]. Maturational arrest may occur at different stages of development. Sometimes the neurons are so immature that this can be recognized on H & E stains, in other instances they may appear mature on H & E but immature on silver stains. Changes may be patchy or generalized. Compared with adults with CIPO [33], it is rare to find morphologic evidence of neural degeneration. Muscle disease may be inflammatory but is more often noninflammatory. The external longitudinal muscle is usually more involved than the internal circular muscle. The primary myopathies are characterized by muscle cell degeneration, vacuolation, and fibrosis. Fibrosis may be so massive that only few normal muscle cells are left, surrounded by a large amount of collagen. (**A–C**, **E–F**, *Courtesy of* Michael D. Schuffler, MD, Seattle, WA; **D**, *Courtesy of* Patrick Dean, MD, Memphis, TN.)

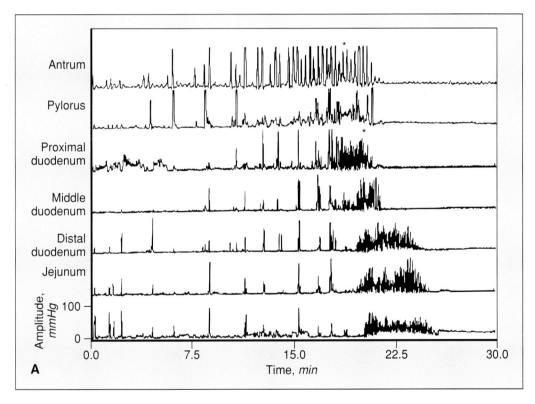

FIGURE 8-24.

Antroduodenal manometry in chronic intestinal pseudo-obstruction (CIPO). Recordings obtained using a motility catheter with recording sites spaced 5 cm apart (*A–B*) and 3 cm apart (*C*). Amplitude is reported in mmHg and time in minutes. Normal phase 3 of the motor-migrating complex (MMC) followed by phase 1 (*panel A*). The asterisks indicate antral and duodenal components of phase 3. Phase 3 of the MMC is characterized by a migrating cluster of contractions at highest possible frequency for the recording site. It is the most recognizable feature of the interdigestive motility pattern. It is followed by phase 1, during which no contractions are recognized, and phase 2, with intermittent contractions of variable amplitude.

(*continued on next page*)

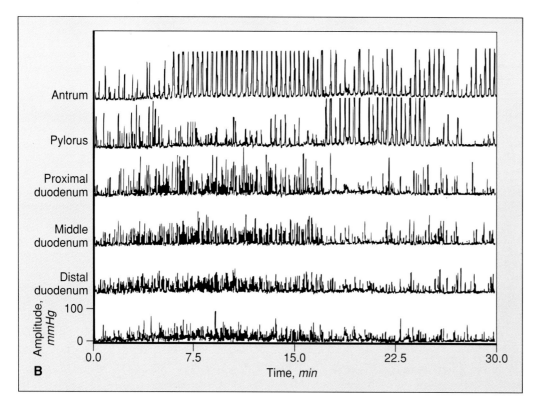

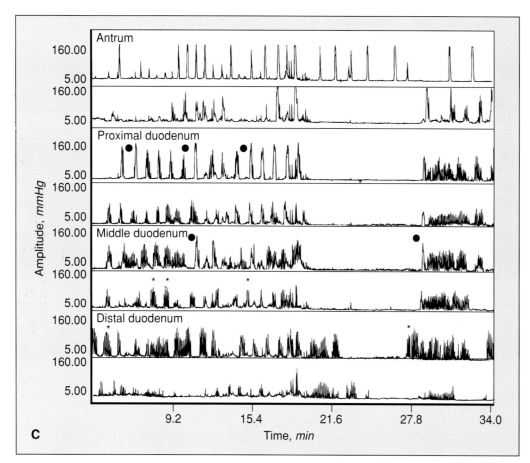

FIGURE 8-24. (*CONTINUED*)

Normal postprandial motility (*panel B*). Postprandial motility is characterized by a pattern similar to the pattern found during phase 2 of the MMC. **C,** Abnormal postprandial motility in a child with CIPO. Note the retrograde clusters of contractions (*asterisks*) propagating from the distal to the proximal duodenum, and the high-amplitude prolonged duodenal contractions (●).

Manometry is more sensitive than radiography to evaluate the strength and coordination of contractions. Diagnostic antroduodenal manometry rarely requires more than 5 hours (*ie*, 4 hours fasting and 1 hour postprandial). Antroduodenal manometry is always abnormal in children with CIPO involving the upper gastrointestinal tract [34]. A normal manometric study in a child with symptoms suggestive of CIPO should arise the suspicion of a factitious disorder [35]. Because intestinal motility is also abnormal in children with mechanical obstruction, manometry should not be used to differentiate CIPO from true bowel obstruction. After a diagnosis of CIPO has been made, antroduodenal manometry is done to determine the pathophysiologic correlates for the symptoms, to assess drug responses, and for a prognosis [29]. Increases in intraluminal pressure are inversely proportional to the gut diameter (Laplace's law). Therefore, in the presence of a dilated bowel, manometry is often uninterpretable. Care must be taken to stop all drugs with known effects on gastrointestinal motility, such as prokinetic drugs and narcotics, before performing the manometry study. (**A** and **B**, *Courtesy of* S. Narasimha Reddy, EngD, Los Angeles, CA.)

TABLE 8-4. DISCRETE MANOMETRIC ABNORMALITIES

NORMAL FEATURES
MMC during fasting

Transition from a fasting to a fed pattern
   (resembling phase 2) after a meal

ABNORMAL FEATURES DURING FASTING
Persistent low amplitude or absent contractions

Abnormal phase 3

Stationary clusters of contractions

Minute rhythm

Tonic duodenal contractions

Giant duodenal contractions

Absent phase 2 during awaking time

ABNORMAL FEATURES AFTER FEEDING
Failure to induce a fed pattern (MMC persists)

Antral hypomotility

Duodenal hypomotility

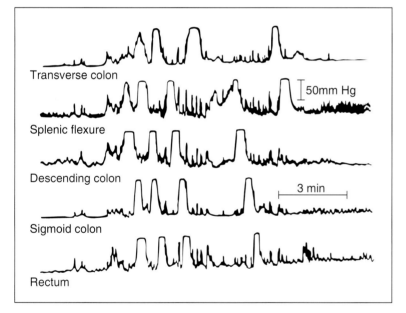

TABLE 8-4.

Discrete manometric abnormalities reported in children with chronic intestinal pseudo-obstruction (CIPO). *Low amplitude* is used when amplitude of the contractions is persistently low (< 30 mmHg in the antrum and < 15 mmHg in the duodenum). A *phase 3* is considered abnormal when it is retrograde, simultaneous, interrupted for more than 2 minutes, or fails to migrate to the most distal recording site. *Stationary cluster* is a prolonged (> 2 minutes), nonmigrating burst of contractions. *Minute rhythm* describes the presence of short (< 2 minutes) migrating clusters of contractions during more than 50% of phase 2 recording time, with no contractions in the intervals between bursts. *Tonic contractions* are considered abnormal if more than 15 mmHg amplitude and lasting longer than 30 seconds. *Giant duodenal contraction* is a contraction greater than 80 mmHg in the duodenum.

Antral and duodenal hypomotility are used when the motility index (number of contractions multiplied by mean amplitude of contractions) is less than 400 mmHg per channel in the stomach and less than 600 mmHg per channel in the duodenum in the first 30 minutes after a meal. In the absence of a dilated bowel, coordinated, persistently low-amplitude contractions suggest myopathy, whereas normal-amplitude, uncoordinated contractions correlate with histopathologic evidence of neuropathy. In children, the presence of phase 3 of the motor-migrating complex (MMC) correlates with enteral feeding [36] and a good response to cisapride. More than 80% of children without MMCs require partial or total parenteral nutrition [29].

FIGURE 8-25.

High-amplitude propagated contractions (HAPCs) in the colon. *HAPCs* are defined as colonic contractions with amplitude greater than 80 mmHg and migrating aborally over at least 30 cm. Colonic manometry differentiates causes of intractable constipation in children [37]. Three manometric features suggest normal colonic motility in children: (1) presence of HAPCs following awakening or a meal; (2) increase in motility index after a meal; and (3) absence of discrete abnormalities associated with symptoms. Colonic manometry is particularly helpful in children with chronic intestinal pseudo-obstruction limited to the colon. In the absence of generalized colonic dilatation, children whose contractions do not increase following a meal or do not produce HAPCs have a colon neuropathy. Children with no colonic contractions are more likely to have a myopathy [38]. The frequency of HAPCs in normal children is inversely proportional to the child's age.

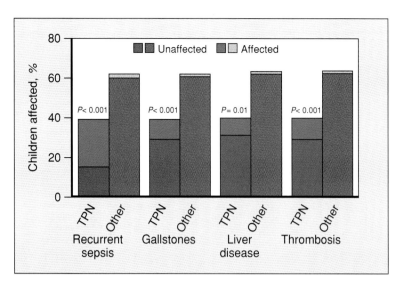

FIGURE 8-26.

Complications of total parenteral nutrition (TPN) in children with chronic intestinal pseudo-obstruction (CIPO). Approximately 40% of children with CIPO require either partial or total parenteral nutrition. In CIPO, enteral feeding is often associated with severe vomiting, abdominal distension and pain, and food refusal. In these children, home TPN becomes a life-saving treatment, allowing them to achieve normal growth and development [39]. Unfortunately, TPN is also the least desirable means of improving nutritional status because of its high rate of complications and high costs. Most morbidity and mortality in children with CIPO results from the infectious or hepatic complications of TPN. Thus, every effort should be extended to maximize enteral nutrition in children with CIPO.

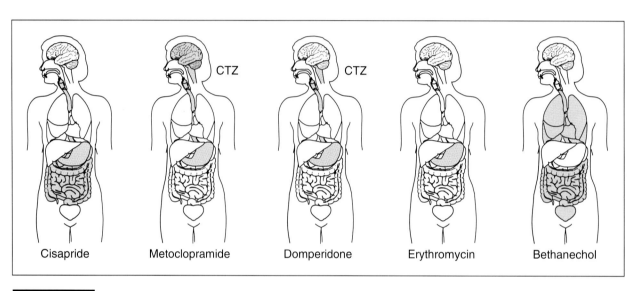

FIGURE 8-27.

Sites of action of prokinetic drugs used in children with chronic intestinal pseudo-obstruction (CIPO). Prokinetic drugs are helpful only in a minority of children with CIPO. *Cisapride* binds to serotonin receptors on nerve fibers within the myenteric plexus, facilitating the release of acetylcholine at the neuromuscular junction. Its action is relatively specific for the gastrointestinal tract. Cisapride increases lower esophageal sphincter (LES) pressure and stimulates motility from the stomach to the small intestine. Cisapride improved gastric emptying in adults with CIPO [40] and increased duodenal motility in children with CIPO [41]. The action of cisapride on the colon is less established. Diarrhea and abdominal cramping are common but transient side effects. *Metoclopramide* is a dopamine-receptor antagonist with activity both in the gastrointestinal tract and the brain. It accelerates gastric emptying and increases amplitude of esophageal peristalsis and the resting pressure of the LES in children with gastroesophageal reflux [42]. It seldom improves symptoms in children with CIPO. Metoclopramide rapidly crosses the blood-brain barrier and blocks the dopamine receptors in the brain. Side effects of metoclopramide include irritability, insomnia, drowsiness, fatigue, depression, and extrapyramidal movement disorders. Metoclopramide also inhibits the emetic effects of apomorphine and levodopa by binding to the chemoreceptor trigger zone (CTZ) of the lateral reticular formation. *Domperidone* is mainly a peripheral dopamine-receptor antagonist. It has most of the pharmacologic effects of metoclopramide on the gastrointestinal tract. Because of its relative inability to cross the blood-brain barrier, domperidone has fewer extrapyramidal and central nervous system side effects. Domperidone improves nausea and vomiting by its action on the CTZ, a structure located outside the blood-brain barrier [43]. Domperidone causes increased levels of prolactin with consequent gynecomastia, galactorrhea, and menstrual irregularities after prolonged use. *Erythromycin* is a motilin-receptor agonist which improves gastric emptying in patients with severe gastroparesis [44]. It stimulates high-amplitude, 3-per-minute antral contractions in children with neuropathic CIPO [45]. It is given at lower doses (1–3 mg/kg IV or 3–5 mg/kg po) than those required for its antibiotic effects. Erythromycin does not appear to be effective for more generalized motility disorders. *Bethanechol* is a muscarinic agonist which increases LES pressure [46]. It has never been shown to benefit children with CIPO. Because its action is not restricted to the gastrointestinal tract, bethanechol has a high frequency of undesirable side effects which limit its use, including hypotension, bronchospasm, salivation, flushing, diarrhea, and urinary urgency. (*Adapted from* Hyman [46a]; with permission.)

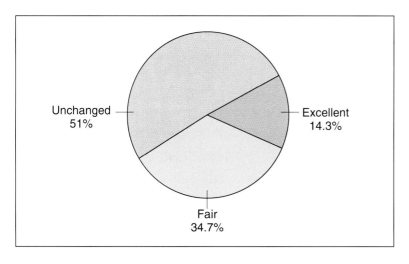

FIGURE 8-28.

Symptomatic response to cisapride in children with chronic intestinal pseudo-obstruction (CIPO). In a double-blind, placebo-controlled study of the effect of a short-term cisapride administration, cisapride increased the strength and number of duodenal contractions in a heterogeneous group of children with CIPO [41]. Gastric emptying was unchanged. Cisapride did not initiate the motor-migrating complex (MMC) in children without it nor did it inhibit discrete motility abnormalities. In an open-labeled trial involving a larger number of children with CIPO, a minority of patients had an excellent symptomatic response, about a third had fair improvement and more than half did not improve. Cisapride was more likely to help children with MMCs and no bowel dilatation. Because of its excellent safety profile, cisapride should be tried in children with CIPO. The lack of a formulation approved for parenteral administration makes the delivery of the drug challenging in children with CIPO and with delayed gastric emptying.

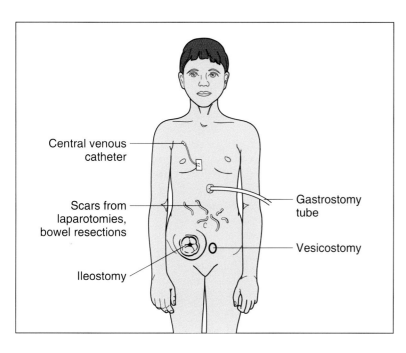

FIGURE 8-29.

Surgeries commonly performed in children with chronic intestinal pseudo-obstruction (CIPO). Many children with CIPO undergo repeated exploratory laparotomies during episodes of acute pseudo-obstruction. Unnecessary abdominal surgery should be avoided in children with CIPO because adhesions may develop, creating a diagnostic challenge each time there is a new obstructive episode and also because children with CIPO often suffer from prolonged postoperative ileus. Gastrostomy has been shown to reduce the number of hospitalizations in adults with CIPO [47]. It may be used to decompress a dilated bowel, thus relieving nausea and pain related to gastric distension, or to provide a route for continuous or bolus enteral feedings and administration of medications. Jejunostomies are sometimes successful for continuous enteral feedings when oral and gastrostomy feedings had failed [36]. Central venous catheter placement is necessary in children who fail enteral feedings. Vesicostomy may obviate the need for repeated daily urinary catheterizations in infants with urinary system involvement. Colectomy with creation of ileostomy is curative in selected children with CIPO limited to the colon. It provides symptomatic relief in children with dilated colon or those incapable of having spontaneous bowel movements. Fundoplication is rarely indicated in CIPO. Following fundoplication, symptoms may change from vomiting to repeated retching because the underlying gastroparesis is not corrected, but rather is complicated by outlet obstruction at the lower esophageal sphincter [48]. Results of pyloroplasty and Roux-en-Y gastrojejunostomy to improve gastric emptying have been disappointing.

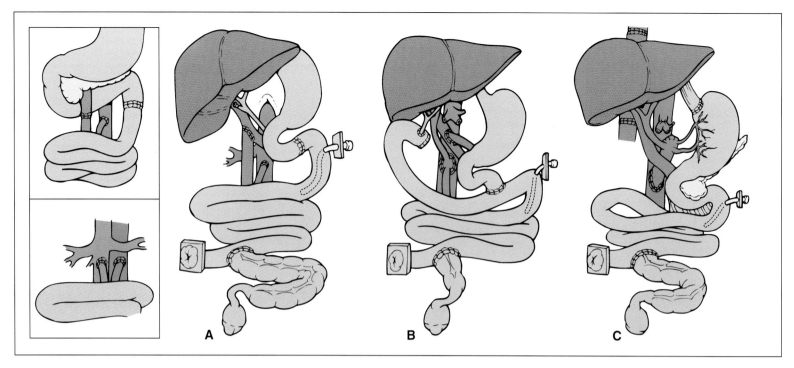

FIGURE 8-30.

Small-bowel transplant. **A**, Isolated small-bowel transplant. The arterial anastomosis is from donor superior mesenteric artery to aorta. The donor mesenteric vein is anastomosed to the recipient portal vein [49]. **B**, Small-bowel liver transplant. A patch including the celiac axis and superior mesenteric artery is directly anastomosed to the recipient aorta. Venous return is by means of hepatic vein-vena cava anastomoses [50]. **C**, Multivisceral transplant. The celiac axis and superior mesenteric artery are anastomosed to a graft of donor aorta that is anastomosed to recipient abdominal aorta. The donor hepatic vein drains into the donor vena cava that is anastomosed to the recipient vena cava [49].

Since the introduction of FK506, a more potent immunosuppressant than cyclosporine, several centers perform small-bowel transplantation, alone or in combination with liver, and other viscera in patients with chronic intestinal pseudo-obstruction

(CIPO). Current experience is that although surgical techniques have been successful, postoperative management is complex. Complications include infection, rejection, and post-transplant lymphoproliferative disease. Because of the high rates of morbidity and mortality associated with the procedure, children with CIPO must suffer from end-stage liver disease to be considered candidates for combined liver-intestine transplantation. Isolated liver transplantation in children with gut failure is likely to subject the transplanted liver to the same insults that damaged the native liver. At the time of transplantation a gastrostomy is also performed to permit continuous enteral alimentation; an ileostomy is placed to allow frequent endoscopic and histologic monitoring. After 1 or 2 months, the child is allowed ad libitum oral intake and the gastrostomy may be closed. (**A**, *Adapted from* Todo *et al.* [48]; **B–C**, *Adapted from* Starzl *et al.* [51].)

CONSTIPATION

Background and epidemiology

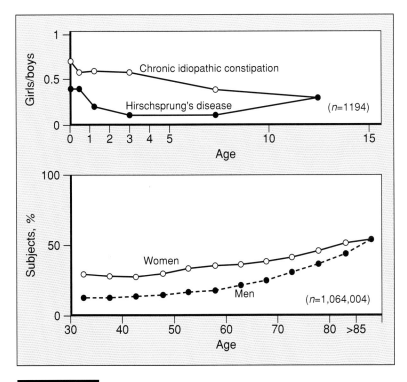

FIGURE 8-31.

In childhood, constipation is more common among boys than girls. In adulthood, it is more common among women [51]. Constipation is the chief complaint in 3% of all pediatric outpatient visits and up to 25% of children referred to pediatric gastroenterologists have a disorder of defecation [52,53]. As illustrated in the figure, the ratio of females to males varies along the life span. Childhood constipation is equally distributed among different social classes with no relation to family size, ethnic background, or age of the parents [54]. The incidence of childhood constipation increases when a parent, a sibling, or a twin is constipated. (*Adapted from* Devroede [50].)

TABLE 8-5. CONSTIPATION

CHILDREN	ADULTS
More common in boys	More common in women
Resolves at puberty	Begins at puberty
Withholding behavior	Straining behavior
Fecal incontinence very common	Fecal incontinence less common
High-fiber diet rarely helpful	High-fiber diet helpful
Surgery never indicated in functional constipation	Surgery successful in selected patients
Better prognosis	Worse prognosis

TABLE 8-5.

Comparison between childhood and adulthood constipation. Constipation in children differs significantly from constipation in adults. Diagnostic and therapeutic approaches need to be adjusted to patient's age.

Etiology and pathogenesis

TABLE 8-6. CAUSES OF CONSTIPATION IN CHILDREN

Functional
Anatomic
  Anorectal malformations
  Strictures
  Tumors
Neurogenic conditions
  Hirschsprung's disease
  Cerebral palsy and
    developmental retardation
  Myelodysplasia
  Spinal cord trauma
  Neurofibromatosis
  Intestinal neuronal dysplasia and
    other visceral neuropathies
  Botulism

Systemic and metabolic disorders
  Electrolyte abnormalities (hypokalemia,
    hypercalcemia)
  Hypothyroidism
  Cystic fibrosis
  Diabetes mellitus
  Malabsorption
  Multiple endocrine neoplasia type 2B
Drugs
  Opiates, anticholinergics, anticonvulsants,
    tryciclic antidepressants, antacids, sucralfate,
    iron, vitamin D intoxication, and lead ingestion
Diet

TABLE 8-6.

Causes of constipation in children. Many organic disorders can cause constipation, but only a minority of children have organic or anatomic causes for the condition. In neurologically devastated children, constipation is common and the cause may be multifactorial. The absence of normal skeletal muscle tone and coordination may result in a poor defecatory effort. When tube feedings are used, the absence of dietary fiber may be constipating. Sensory or motor abnormalities may exist due to affected enteric neurons, just as there are abnormalities in the central nervous system. Anticonvulsant drugs often cause constipation. In children with spinal cord injury or dysraphism, the external anal sphincter and levator ani muscles, which depend on sacral nerves 2, 3, and 4, may be impaired. Children with myelomeningocele have both constipation and fecal incontinence [54].

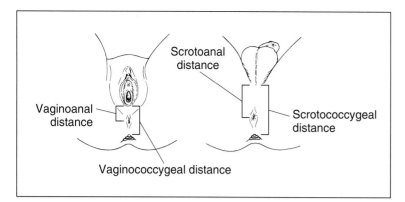

Figure 8-32.

Normal position of anus [56]. Anatomic abnormalities of the anus and rectum are frequently associated with constipation. Anterior displacement of the anus is more common in females and is associated with a posterior rectal shelf and an abnormal angle of descent for the fecal mass so that constipation occurs [57]. Anterior displacement of the anus should be suspected when the anus is located less than one half the distance from the scrotum to the coccyx, or less than one third the vagina-coccyx distance in girls [56]. Anal stenosis presents with thin ribbons of stool and fecal accumulations. Anal membranes and imperforate anus with or without fistulas are recognized during the examination of the newborn. (*Adapted from* Bar-Maor *et al.* [56].)

TABLE 8-7. CONSTIPATION AND HIRSCHSPRUNG'S DISEASE

FEATURE	FUNCTIONAL CONSTIPATION	HIRSCHSPRUNG'S DISEASE
Delayed passage of meconium	Rare	Common
Symptoms from birth	Rare	Common
Soiling	Common	Rare
Obstructive symptoms	Rare	Common
Withholding behavior	Common	Rare
Large caliber stools	Common	Rare
Enterocolitis	Never	Possible
Rectal ampulla	Enlarged	Narrowed
Stool in ampulla	Common	Rare
Male predominance	Yes	Yes

Table 8-7.

Differentiating features between functional constipation and Hirschsprung's disease. The incidence of Hirschsprung's disease is 1 in 5000 live births and is found in fewer than 1% of children presenting for the first time with constipation. There are sufficient differences between these two entities so that in most cases rectal biopsy, anorectal manometry, and radiologic tests are unnecessary. When the clinical presentation is consistent with functional constipation, it is wise to treat the child before embarking on a series of tests to "rule out Hirschsprung's disease" or other colonic neuromuscular diseases.

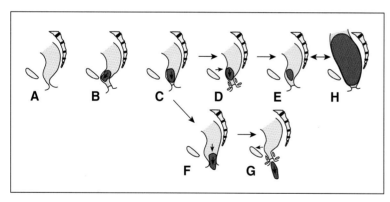

Figure 8-33.

Pathophysiology of functional fecal retention. Most children with constipation have functional or behavioral problems that cause their symptom. The most common nonorganic cause of constipation and encopresis in children is *functional fecal retention* [52]. Functional fecal retention has been called psychogenic megacolon, and idiopathic or retentive constipation. It is often caused by fear of defecation and the voluntary withholding of stool. This figure is a schematic representation of normal defecatory function and chronic stool withholding. **A**, The rectum is empty; there is no urge to stool. The internal anal sphincter is closed. The resting tone of the pelvic floor muscles holds the sides of the anal canal in apposition, keeping it closed. **B**, Stool enters the rectum and presses on the rectal wall, causing a sense of fullness. **C**, Distention of the rectal wall causes reflex relaxation of the internal anal sphincter, allowing the stool to descend into contact with the upper end of the anal canal. This causes conscious awareness that passage of stool is imminent. **D**, The pelvic floor muscles contract to maintain continence, moving the stool upwards. **E**, If the stool remains in this higher location after the pelvic floor returns to its resting tone, stool will no longer be in contact with the anoderm. Accommodation by the smooth muscle lessens rectal wall tension and the urge to defecate abates. **F**, Defecation occurs when the pelvic floor relaxes below the level of resting tone; this opens the anal canal to intrarectal pressure. The accompanying Valsalva maneuver propels the stool down the short, wide anal canal. **G**, *Automatic* contraction of the pelvic floor occurs when the stool is no longer in contact with the upper end of the anal canal, and this propulsive force expels the stool completely. **H**, If a child repeatedly responds to the defecatory urge by withholding (*panels C and D*), a fecal mass accumulates. It becomes more difficult to pass, especially if it is too firm to be extruded without painfully stretching the anal opening. As the pelvic floor muscles fatigue, anal closure becomes less competent and retentive fecal soiling with soft or liquid stool occurs. (*Adapted from* Hyman *et al.* [52].)

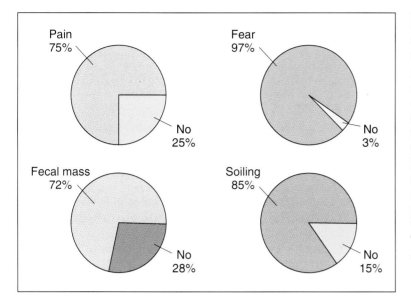

FIGURE 8-34.

Clinical features of childhood functional constipation [58]. Children who suffer from functional fecal retention display retentive posturing. Children develop this condition when defecatory activities are associated with pain and fear. Instead of relaxing the pelvic floor during the Valsalva maneuver so that stool might pass, they recruit the gluteal muscles in an attempt to avoid defecation. They consistently make a conscious decision to postpone defecation. When a child decides not to have a bowel movement, stool accumulates in the rectum and soiling may occur. The soiling may be misinterpreted as diarrhea and the child receives antidiarrheal agents which worsen the constipation. The parents may become angry and punish the child who they believe is consciously responsible for soiling underwear. There is risk that with increasing duration of this problem, the child will develop an increasingly negative self-image.

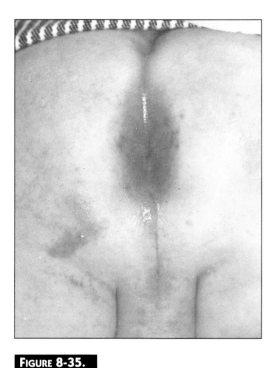

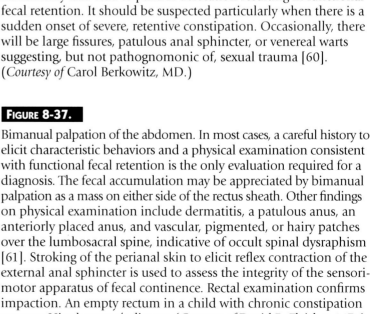

FIGURE 8-35.

Streptococcal perianal disease. The fear of pain associated with defecation may originate from past experience with the passage of hard stools, an anal fissure, or from less common sources, such as group A β-hemolytic streptococcal perianal infection [59]. Signs and symptoms of this condition include perianal dermatitis, itching, rectal pain, and blood-streaked stools. Penicillin is used for treatment. Relapses occur in 30% to 40% of patients.

FIGURE 8-36.

Sexual abuse with anal penetration. Sexual abuse with anal penetration may also lead to painful defecation resulting in functional fecal retention. It should be suspected particularly when there is a sudden onset of severe, retentive constipation. Occasionally, there will be large fissures, patulous anal sphincter, or venereal warts suggesting, but not pathognomonic of, sexual trauma [60]. (*Courtesy of* Carol Berkowitz, MD.)

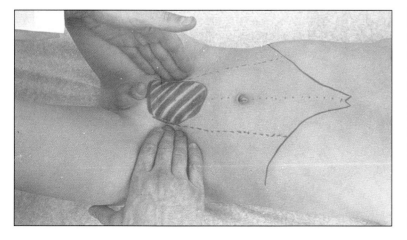

FIGURE 8-37.

Bimanual palpation of the abdomen. In most cases, a careful history to elicit characteristic behaviors and a physical examination consistent with functional fecal retention is the only evaluation required for a diagnosis. The fecal accumulation may be appreciated by bimanual palpation as a mass on either side of the rectus sheath. Other findings on physical examination include dermatitis, a patulous anus, an anteriorly placed anus, and vascular, pigmented, or hairy patches over the lumbosacral spine, indicative of occult spinal dysraphism [61]. Stroking of the perianal skin to elicit reflex contraction of the external anal sphincter is used to assess the integrity of the sensori-motor apparatus of fecal continence. Rectal examination confirms impaction. An empty rectum in a child with chronic constipation suggests Hirschsprung's disease. (*Courtesy of* David R. Fleisher, MD.)

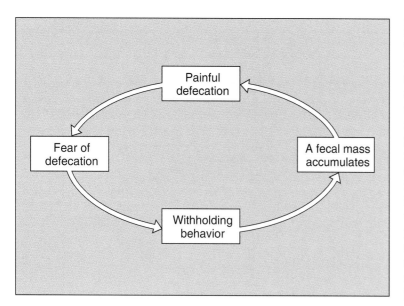

FIGURE 8-38.

Treatment of childhood functional constipation. In functional fecal retention the physician needs to provide reassurance that the condition will most likely resolve and must prescribe stool softeners to ensure painless defecation. The child needs to understand that responding to the defecatory urge and not holding back is key for the success of the treatment. There are two phases to treatment: passage of the rectal mass and maintenance. Almost every fecal mass can be softened and liquefied with sufficient quantity and duration of cathartics. Enemas are avoided because they are often interpreted by the child as a punishment [62]. After elimination of the rectal mass, treatment should be continued for several months with lower doses of cathartics. Agents commonly used in this phase include lubricants such as mineral oil, osmotic agents such as lactulose or milk of magnesia, and stimulants such as senna derivatives. The dosage of the drug is titrated to obtain the desired response. After a few months of painless and soil-free defecation, the patient is slowly weaned from the medication.

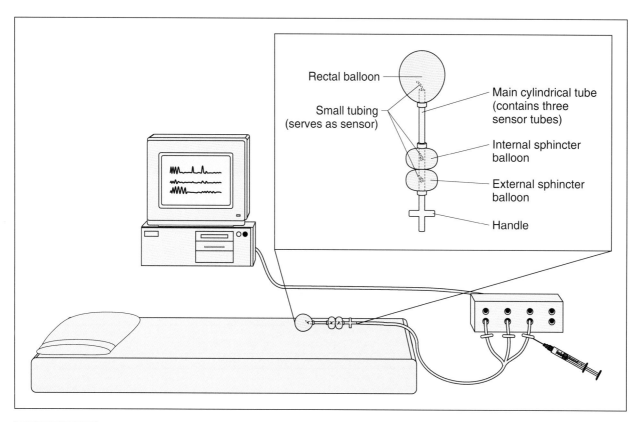

FIGURE 8-39.

Anorectal device for biofeedback training. For cooperative children older than 6 years of age, biofeedback can be used with success for treatment of both constipation and encopresis. During biofeedback training, the child is instantly provided with auditory and visual information about the external anal sphincter function. Children can learn how to relax or to contract the external anal sphincter to produce evacuation or continence. For biofeedback to be successful there must be (1) a cooperative, motivated child, (2) a sphincter able to respond (a completely denervated sphincter does not respond to biofeedback), (3) a perceptible signal (distension of the rectum) alerting the child to initiate control, and (4) a readily measurable response (sphincter contraction or relaxation) [63].

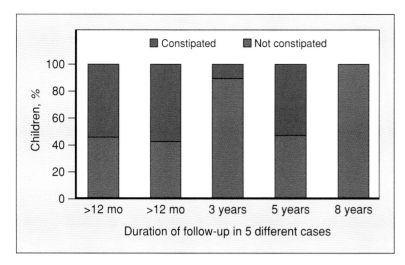

FIGURE 8-40.

Follow-up therapy of children with functional constipation and encopresis. Results from five studies [64–68]. Treatment fails in a minority of children with functional fecal retention regardless of the treatment. Subjects likely to fail are children who have suffered from functional fecal retention for several years or with early onset of constipation, children who have developed a negative self image, and children who find a secondary gain from the condition (such as attention from a parent or avoiding sexual abuse). Children with attention deficit disorder also may be difficult to treat due to their inability to focus on and respond to the urge to defecate.

REFERENCES

1. Apley J: *The Child with Abdominal Pains.* London: Blackwell Scientific Publications; 1975.

2. Vargas JH, Sachs P, Ament ME: Chronic intestinal pseudo-obstruction in pediatrics. *J Pediatr Gastroenterol Nutr* 1988, 7:323–332.

3. Boyle JT: Chronic abdominal pain. In *Pediatric Gastrointestinal Disease.* Edited by Walker WA, Durie PR, Hamilton JR, *et al.* Philadelphia: BC Decker; 1994:45–54.

4. Di Lorenzo C, Hyman PE, Flores AF, *et al.*: Antroduodenal manometry in children and adults with severe nonulcer dyspepsia. *Scand J Gastroenterol* 1994, 29:799–806.

5. Mearin F, Cucala M, Malagelada JR: The origin of symptoms on the brain-gut axis in functional dyspepsia. *Gastroenterology* 1991, 101:999–1006.

6. Loening-Baucke V: Sensitivity of the sigmoid colon and rectum in children with chronic constipation. *J Pediatr Gastroenterol Nutr* 1984, 3:454–459.

7. Almy TP: Experimental studies on the "irritable colon". *Am J Med* 1951, 10:60–67.

8. Dooley CP, Di Lorenzo C, Valenzuela JE: Variability of motor migrating complex in humans. *Dig Dis Sci* 1992, 73:723–728.

9. David D, Mertz H, Fefer L, *et al.*: Sleep and duodenal motor activity in patients with severe non-ulcer dyspepsia. *Gut* 1994, 35:916–925.

10. Dent J: A new technique for continuous sphincter pressure measurement. *Gastroenterology* 1976, 71:263–267.

11. Di Lorenzo C, Reddy SN, Villanueva Meyer-J, *et al.*: Simultaneous colonic manometry and transit in children. *Gastroenterology* 1990, 98:345.

12. Cucchiara S, Riezzo G, Minella R, *et al.*: Electrogastrography in nonulcer dyspepsia. *Arch Dis Child* 1992, 67:613–617.

13. Cucchiara S, Minella R, Riezzo G, Auricchio S: Reversal of gastric electrical dysrhythmias by cisapride in children with nonulcer dyspepsia. *Dig Dis Sci* 1992, 37:1136–1140.

14. Marzio L, Giacobbe A, Conoscitore P, *et al.*: Evaluation for the use of ultrasonography in the study of liquid gastric emptying. *Am J Gastroenterol* 1989, 84:496–500.

15. LiVoti G, Tulone V, Bruno R, *et al.*: Ultrasonography and gastric emptying: evaluation in infants with gastroesophageal reflux. *J Pediatr Gastroenterol Nutr* 1992, 14:397–399.

16. King PM, Adam RD, Pryde A, *et al.*: Relationship of human antroduodenal motility and transpyloric fluid movement: Noninvasive observations with real-time ultrasound. *Gut* 1984, 25:1384–1391.

17. Mayer EA, Gebhart GF: Basic and clinical aspects of visceral hyperalgesia. *Gastroenterology* 1994, 107:271–293.

18. Di Lorenzo C, Mertz H, Rehm D, *et al.*: Gastric sensory response in newborn infants. *Gastroenterology* 1994, 106:A488.

19. Øster J: Recurrent abdominal pain, headache and limb pains in children and adolescents. *Pediatrics* 1972, 50:165–170.

20. Apley J, Naish N: Recurrent abdominal pain: A field survey of 1000 school children. *Arch Dis Child* 1958, 33:165–170.

21. Rappaport L: Recurrent abdominal pain: Theories and pragmatics. *Pediatrician* 1989, 16:78–84.

22. Apley J, Hale B: Children with recurrent abdominal pain: How do they grow up? *Br Med J* 1973, 3:7–9.

23. Magni G, Pierri M, Donzelli F: Recurrent abdominal pain in children: A long term follow up. *Eur J Pediatr* 1987, 146:72–74.

24. Cucchiara S, Bortolotti M, Colombo C, *et al.*: Abnormalities of gastrointestinal motility in children with nonulcer dyspepsia and in children with gastroesophageal reflux disease. *Dig Dis Sci* 1991, 36:1066–1073.

25. Tytgat GNJ, Noach LA, Rauws EAJ: Is gastroduodenitis a cause of chronic dyspepsia? *Scan J Gastroenterol* 1991, 26(suppl 182):33–36.

26. Glassman MS, Schwartz SM, Medow MS, *et al.*: Campylobacter pylori related gastrointestinal disease in children: Incidence and clinical findings. *Dig Dis Sci* 1989, 34:1501–1504.

27. Mayer EA: Functional bowel disorders and the visceral hyperalgesia hypothesis. In *Basic and Clinical Aspects of Chronic Abdominal Pain.* Edited by Mayer EA, Raybould HE. New York: Elsevier; 1993:3–28.

28. Snape WJ Jr: Taking the "idiopathic" out of intestinal pseudo-obstruction. *Ann Int Med* 1981, 95:646–647.

29. Hyman PE, Di Lorenzo C, McAdams L, *et al.*: Predicting the clinical response to cisapride in children with chronic intestinal pseudo-obstruction. *Am J Gastroenterol* 1993, 88:832–836.

30. Vargas JH, Sachs P, Ament ME: Chronic intestinal pseudo-obstruction syndrome in pediatrics. Results of a national survey by members of the North American Society of Pediatric Gastroenterology and Nutrition. *J Pediatr Gastroenterol Nutr* 1988, 7:323–332.

31. Krishnamurthy S, Heng Y, Schuffler M: Chronic intestinal pseudo-obstruction in infants and children caused by diverse abnormalities of the myenteric plexus. *Gastroenterology* 1993, 104:1398–1408.

32. Hyman PE, DiLorenzo C: Chronic intestinal pseudo-obstruction. In *Pediatric Gastrointestinal Disease.* Edited by Wylie R and Hyams JS. Philadelphia: WB Saunders; 1993.

33. Krishnamurthy S, Schuffler MD: Pathology of neuromuscular disorders of the small intestine and colon. *Gastroenterology* 1987, 93:610–639.

34. Hyman PE, McDiarmid SV, Napolitano J, *et al.*: Antroduodenal motility in children with chronic intestinal pseudo-obstruction. *J Pediatr* 1988, 112:899–905.

35. Hyman PE: Chronic intestinal pseudo-obstruction. In *Pediatric Gastrointestinal Motility Disorders. Edited by Hyman PE, Di Lorenzo C. New York: Academy Professional Information Services; 1994:115–128.*

36. Di Lorenzo C, Flores AF, Buie T, Hyman PE: Intestinal motility and jejunal feedings in children with chronic intestinal pseudo-obstruction. *Gastroenterology.* 1995, 108:1379–1385.

37. Di Lorenzo C, Flores AF, Reddy SN, Hyman PE: Colonic manometry differentiates causes of intractable constipation in children. *J Pediatr* 1992, 120:690–695.

38. Di Lorenzo C, Flores AF, Reddy SN, *et al.*: Colonic manometry in children with chronic intestinal pseudo-obstruction. *Gut* 1993, 34:803–807.

39. Mughal MM, Irving MH: Treatment of end stage chronic intestinal pseudo-obstruction by subtotal enterectomy and home parenteral nutrition. *Gut* 1988, 29:1613–1617.

40. Camilleri M, Brown ML, Malagelada JR: Impaired transit of chyme in chronic intestinal pseudo-obstruction: correction by cisapride. *Gastroenterology* 1986, 91:610–626.

41. Di Lorenzo C, Reddy SN, Villanueva-Meyer J, *et al.*: Cisapride in children with chronic intestinal pseudo-obstruction. *Gastroenterology* 1991, 101:1564–1570.

42. Spino M: Pharmacologic treatment of gastrointestinal motility. In *Pediatric Gastrointestinal Disease. Edited by Walker WA, Durie PR, Hamilton JR, et al. Philadelphia, PA: BC Decker Inc; 1994:1735–1746.*

43. Niemegeers CJE, Schellekens KHL, Janssen PAJ: The antiemetic effects of domperidone a novel potent gastrokinetic. *Arch Int Pharmacodyn* 1980, 244:130–140.

44. Richards RD, Davenport K, McCallum RW: The treatment of idiopathic and diabetic gastroparesis with acute intravenous and chronic oral erythromycin. *Am J Gastroenterol* 1993, 88:203–207.

45. Di Lorenzo C, Flores AF, Tomomasa T, Hyman PE: Effect of erythromycin on antroduodenal motility in children with chronic functional gastrointestinal symptoms. *Dig Dis Sci* 1994, 39:1399–1405.

46. Orenstein SR, Lofton SW, Orenstein DM: Bethanechol for pediatric gastroesophageal reflux: A prospective, blind, controlled study. *J Pediatr Gastroenterol Nutr* 1986, 5:549–555.

46a. Hyman PE: Gastroesophageal Reflux: One reason why baby won't eat. *J Pediatr* 1994, 125(suppl):S103–S109.

47. Pitt HA, Mann LL, Berquist WE, *et al.*: Chronic intestinal pseudo-obstruction: Management with total parenteral nutrition and a venting enterostomy. *Arch Surg* 1985, 120:614–618.

48. Di Lorenzo C, Flores AF, Hyman PE: Intestinal motility in symptomatic children after fundoplication. *J Pediatr Gastroenterol Nutr* 1991, 12:169–173.

49. Todo S, Tzakis AG, Abus-Elmagd K, *et al.*: Intestinal transplantation in composite visceral grafts or alone. *Ann Surg* 1992, 216:223–234.

50. Starzl TE, Todo S, Tzakis AG, *et al.*: The many faces of multivisceral transplantation. *Surg Gynecol Obstet* 1991, 172:335–344.

51. Devroede G: Constipation. In *Gastrointestinal Disease: Pathophysiology, Diagnosis, Management. Edited by Sleisinger MH, Fordran JS. Philadelphia: WB Saunders; 1989:331–368.*

52. Hyman PE, Fleisher D: Functional fecal retention. *Practical Gastroenterology* 1992, 16:29–37.

53. Loening-Baucke VA, Younoszai MK: Abnormal anal sphincter response in chronically constipated children. *J Pediatr* 1982, 100:213–218.

54. Anthony EJ: An experimental approach to the psychopathology of childhood: Encopresis. *Br J Med Psychol* 1957, 30:146.

55. Younoszai MK: Stooling problems in patients with myelomeningocele. *South Med J* 1992, 85:718–723.

56. Bar-Maor JA, Eitan A: Determination of the normal position of the anus. *J Pediatr Gastroenterol Nutr* 1987, 6:559–561.

57. Leape LL, Ramenofsky ML: Anterior ectopic anus: A common cause of constipation in children. *J Pediatr Surg* 1978, 13:627–629.

58. Partin JC, Hamill SK, Fischel JE, Partin JS: Painful defecation and fecal soiling in children. *Pediatrics* 1992, 89:1007–1009.

59. Kokx NP, Comstock JA, Facklam RR: Streptococcal perianal disease in children. *Pediatrics* 1987, 80:659–663.

60. Agnarsson U, Warde C, McCarthy G, Evans N: Perianal appearances associated with constipation. *Arch Dis Child* 1990, 65:1231–1234.

61. Anderson F: Occult spinal dysraphism: A series of 73 cases. *Pediatrics* 1975, 55:826–835.

62. Gleghorn EE, Heyman MB, Rudolph CD: No-enema therapy for idiopathic constipation and encopresis. *Clin Pediatr* 1991, 30:669–672.

63. Loening-Baucke VA: Anorectal manometry and biofeedback training. In *Pediatric Gastrointestinal Motility Disorders. Edited by Hyman PE, DiLorenzo C. New York: Academy Professional Information Services; 1994:231–252.*

64. Abrahamian FR, Lloyd-Still JD: Chronic constipation in children: A longitudinal study of 186 patients. *J Pediatr Gastroenterol Nutr* 1984, 3:460–467.

65. Loening-Baucke V: Factors determining outcome in children with chronic constipation and fecal soiling. *Gut* 1989, 30:999–1006.

66. Davidson M, Kugler MM, Bauer CH: Diagnosis and management in children with severe and protracted constipation and obstipation. *J Pediatr* 1963, 62:261–275.

67. Staiano AM, Andreotti MR, Greco L, *et al.*: Long term follow-up of children with chronic idiopathic constipation. *Dig Dis Sci* 1994, 39:561–564.

68. Bellman M: Studies on encopresis. *Acta Pediatr Scand* 1966, 170(suppl):1–150.

Chapter 9

Cystic Fibrosis

PETER R. DURIE

Cystic fibrosis (CF) is the most common lethal autosomal recessive disorder among whites. It is a generalized disease that affects various secreting epithelial tissues, but clinical evidence is provided by pulmonary and gastrointestinal manifestations. Heterozygotes with one normal CF allele and one mutant allele are entirely asymptomatic. A child born to two CF carriers has a one-in-four chance of being affected with CF by acquiring a mutation from each parent. Disease frequency varies considerably among ethnic groups; it is highest among people of Northern European origin, among whom approximately 1 in 2500 births is affected. It is extremely rare in people of Asian or African origin.

Despite considerable advances in clinical ability to identify specific CF mutations, the diagnosis of CF is still established by quantitative sweat iontophoresis. This test is based on the observation by di Sant'Agnese and colleagues that the concentration of salt in the sweat of CF patients is greatly elevated [1]. In the 1930s, it was separated from other celiac syndromes by identifying the dual involvement of the pancreas and the lungs in affected patients [2,3]. At that time, the demonstration of pancreatic insufficiency was the key to the clinical diagnosis. In the 1950s, Gibbs, Bostick, and Smith [4] showed that steatorrhea was not seen in all patients. Since then, it has become increasingly apparent that the clinical expression of the disease is extremely variable.

In the years before the CF gene was identified, research into the etiopathogenesis of this disorder was hampered by the inability to differentiate the basic defect from secondary effects of the disease. Most research strategies were based on identifying differences between heterozygotes and affected individuals in cells and bodily fluids. Over a period of more than 4 decades of research, no protein or biochemical abnormality was identified that could be convincingly viewed as the primary defect. In contrast, electrophysiologic studies were quite helpful. Quinton initially showed that chloride permeation was defective in the sweat duct [5]; this work was quickly followed by evidence of a similar defect in the respiratory tract epithelium. Subsequent work in the isolated secretory coil of the sweat gland, respiratory epithelium [6], and isolated secretory cells in culture demonstrated that affected epithelia had unresponsive cyclic AMP (cAMP)–mediated chloride channels within the apical membrane [7]. These observations were confirmed after the CF gene was cloned [8]. Patch clamp techniques have been used to show that specific chloride channels that open in the presence of cAMP–dependent protein kinase and ATP in normal cells do not do so in cells cultured from CF patients [9].

The predominant clinical feature of CF is respiratory tract involvement, in which obstruction of airways by sticky mucus gives rise to infection, especially with *pseudomonas* species. Most patients experience gastrointestinal difficulties; 85% show pancreatic insufficiency caused by obstruction of small pancreatic ducts. Among neonates, over 10% of affected patients present with bowel obstruction resulting from meconium ileus. Up to 5% of patients develop overt liver disease, frequently in adolescence or adulthood [10]. Subclinical liver disease is much more common, however. Infertility among affected males is virtually universal. Undernutrition is a cause of morbidity in affected children, adolescents, and young adults [11].

In most patients, the prognosis depends entirely on the pulmonary complications. Symptoms of airway disease usually begin insidiously as chronic pulmonary infection caused by the plugging of small airways by thick viscid secretion, which in turn leads to widespread destruction of the bronchioles, bronchiectasis, atelectasis, and emphysema with progressive respiratory failure and death. Over the past 2 to 3 decades, however, considerable improvement has been made in survival rates throughout the world. Median survival for patients in Canada is 32 years for males and 28 years for females. The great discrepancy in survival between sexes remains unexplained. Females appear to do almost as well as males until the early teens, but in late adolescence and adulthood deteriorate at a much faster rate [12]. Both males and females who do not have sufficient pancreatic disease to produce steatorrhea have better pulmonary function than their more common counterparts with pancreatic insufficiency [13].

GENETIC AND ELECTROPHYSIOLOGIC BASIS OF CYSTIC FIBROSIS

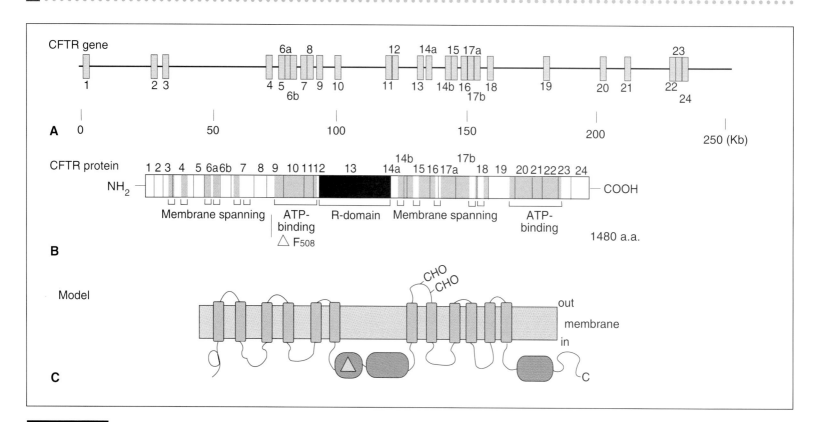

FIGURE 9-1.

A–C, Identification of the cystic fibrosis (CF) gene. In 1989, following concerted efforts by various investigators throughout the world, the CF gene was identified by Lap-Chee Tsui and J. Riordan of the University of Toronto, in collaboration with Francis Collins of the University of Michigan [8]. The CF gene, which is on the long arm of chromosome 7, comprises 27 exons spanning 230 kb of DNA. The gene product (initially thought to be comprised of 24 exons), named the *cystic fibrosis transmembrane conductance regulator* (CFTR), is a protein of 1480 amino acids. The predominant mutation, which accounts for approximately 70% of all the CFTR gene mutations worldwide, is a three base-pair deletion in exon 10 of the CFTR gene, which results in the loss of a single amino acid, phenylalanine, at codon 508 (ΔF508). (*Adapted from* Tsui [14].)

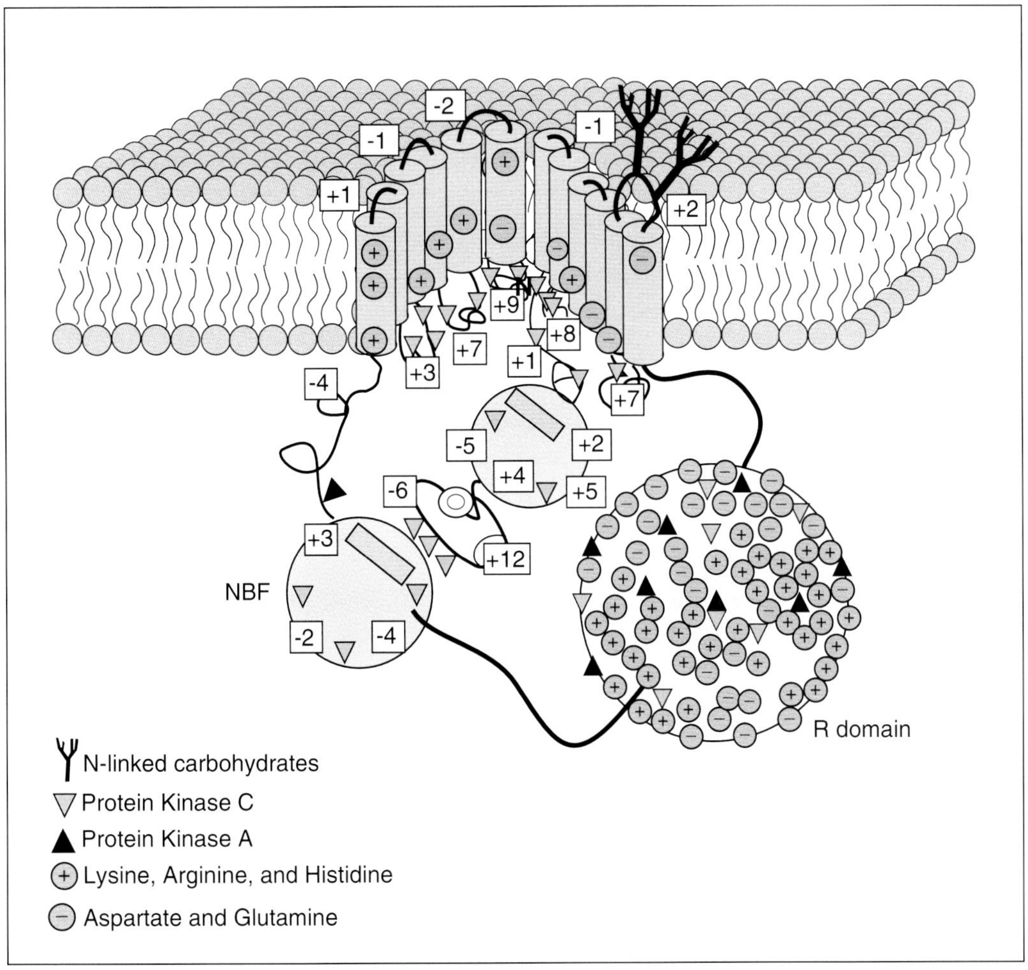

-2
-1
-1
+1
+2
+9
+8
-4
+3
+7
+1
+7
-5
+2
+4
+5
-6
+3
+12
NBF
-2
-4
R domain
N-linked carbohydrates
Protein Kinase C
Protein Kinase A
Lysine, Arginine, and Histidine
Aspartate and Glutamine

FIGURE 9-2.

The deduced primary amino acid sequence of the cystic fibrosis transmembrane conductance regulator (CFTR) immediately suggested that the gene product was a membrane channel. This schematic model of the CFTR protein, which is situated within the cell membrane, shows membrane-spanning helices on each half of the molecule, which is shown as cylinders. The green spheres show two nucleotide binding folds (NBF); the light blue sphere shows large polar regulatory domain (R domain). Individual charged amino acids within the R domain are shown. Potential phosphorylation sites and N-glycosylation linkages are as shown. The predicted amino acid sequence of CFTR showed striking homology to a superfamily of membrane-associated proteins involved in active transport known as the ATP-binding cassette (ABC) superfamily. Members of this superfamily have several features in common, notably the presence of transmembrane domains and nucleotide binding folds. (*Adapted from* Riordan [8].)

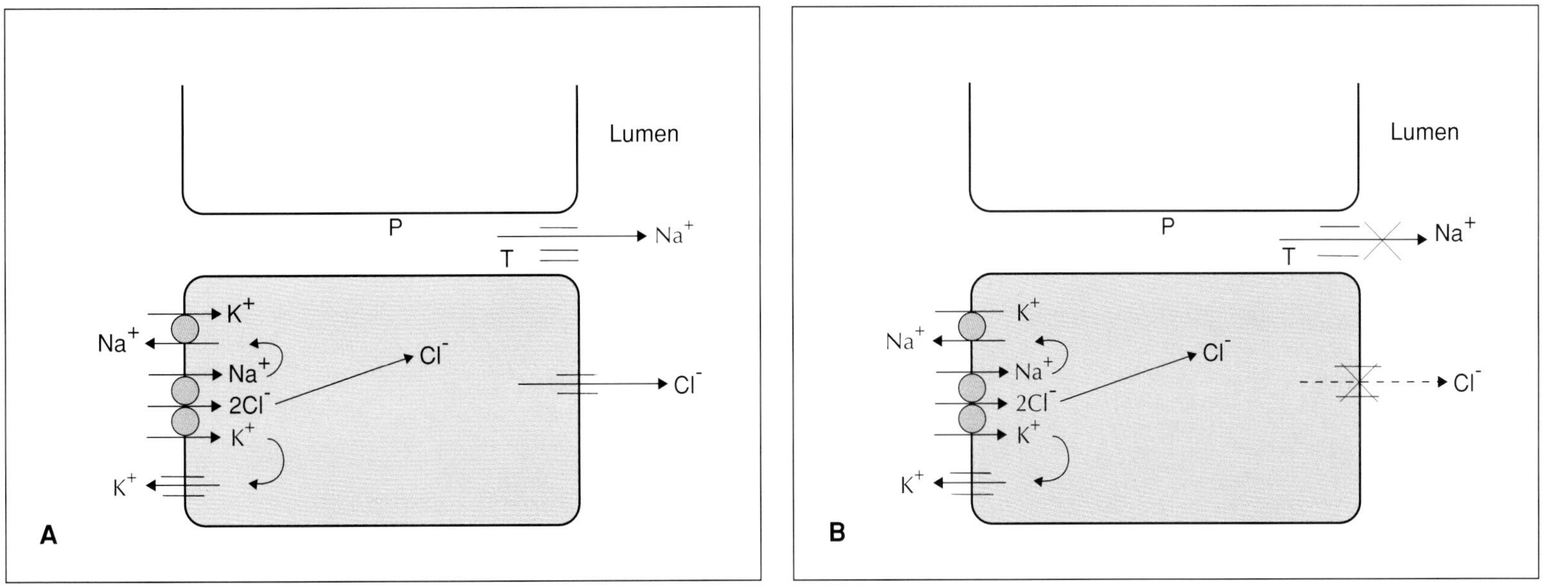

Lumen
P
T
Na+
Na+
K+
Na+
2Cl-
K+
Cl-
Cl-
K+
A
Lumen
P
T
Na+
Na+
K+
Na+
2Cl-
K+
Cl-
Cl-
K+
B

FIGURE 9-3.

Epithelial cell transport. **A**, Apical chloride channels are important elements in the secretion of sodium chloride by epithelial cells. In a typical epithelial cell, basolateral membrane transport processes give rise to accumulation of chloride intracellularly to levels that exceed the electrochemical potential in the cell exterior. When the apical chloride channel opens, the electrochemical gradient allows chloride to exit through the apical membrane. This generates a lumen-negative voltage that stimulates exit of sodium through paracellular-tight junctions. Secretion of water follows the movement of sodium and chloride. **B**, In cystic fibrosis, the cystic fibrosis transmembrane conductance regulator chloride channel is absent or defective. Consequently, chloride efflux from the apical membrane is impaired, which in turn prevents the movements of sodium paracellularly. The net *effect* of defective apical chloride channels would lead to diminished secretory volume. Na^+—sodium; Cl^-—chloride; K^+—potassium; P—paracellular route; T—tight junction. The *circles* in the basolateral membrane denote coupled ion transporters. (*Adapted from* Forstner and Durie [15].)

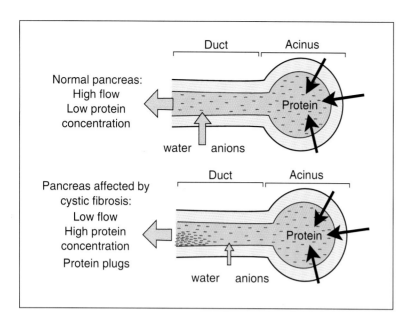

FIGURE 9-4.

The pancreas affected by cystic fibrosis is most vulnerable to lumenal concentration defects caused by the high protein content of acinar secretions and dependence on ductal cystic fibrosis transmembrane conductance regulator for anion (chloride and bicarbonate) and fluid secretion. When ductal water flow is reduced owing to defective anion secretion, protein concentration in the duct rises. High protein concentration causes precipitation of protein and plugging of duct lumina [16,17]. In contrast, the sweat duct is unaffected pathologically because of low protein load and high flow rate. (*Adapted from* Forstner and Durie [15].)

PATHOLOGY

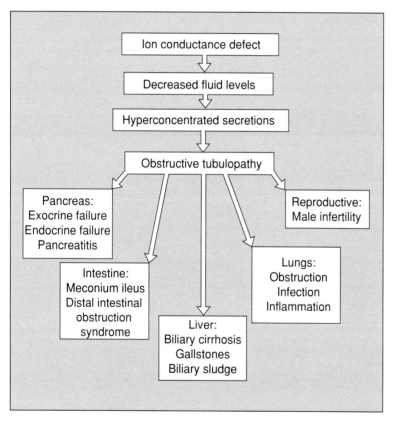

FIGURE 9-5.

Pathophysiology of cystic fibrosis. The ion conductance defect in epithelial tissues almost always results in reduced fluid flow within epithelia of organs normally possessing cystic fibrosis transmembrane conductance regulator (CFTR) expression. Absent or dysfunctional CFTR would be expected to lead to functional consequences in organs with a high concentration of macromolecules in the lumen of the ducts. A variety of organs listed in this figure are affected pathologically when proteins or other macromolecules precipitate, form plugs, slow ductal flow, and lead to blockage. (*Adapted from* Forstner and Durie [15].)

TABLE 9-1. THE PATHOLOGY OF CYSTIC FIBROSIS

Organ	Physiologic Changes	Pathology
Lung	Distal airway obstruction, glandular hyperplasia, mucous hypersecretion	Early—terminal bronchiolar plugging, peribronchiolar inflammation Late—mucus casts, atelectasis, bronchiectasis, emphysema, cor pulmonale
Pancreas	Decreased volume and increased concentration of secretions	Early—duct plugging, dilatation, acinar atrophy Late—fibrous and fatty replacement, and loss of islets
Intestine	Concentrated secretions, mucus altered—hyperglycosylated and hypersulfated	Meconium plug, distal ileum; crypt dilatation; meconium peritonitis; distal intestinal obstruction syndrome; constipation
Liver	Reduced bile salt secretion, increased circulating bile salt concentration	Early—bile ductular hyperplasia, eosinophilic plugging of intrahepatic bile duct, focal biliary cirrhosis Late—multilobular cirrhosis
Gallbladder	Reduced bile salt pool, lithogenic bile	Cystic duct occlusion, hypoplastic gallbladder, gallstones
Salivary glands	High calcium concentration	Inspissated mucus in intercalated ducts, mild inflammation
Epididymis and vas deferens	Reduced secretions	Absent—fibrous replacement

TABLE 9-1.

Pathology of cystic fibrosis (CF). Nearly all lesions in the disease have an obstructive element whereby a duct or air passage is blocked by mucus and/or other proteins. The airway and pancreatic lesions have the most adverse effects on health, but hepatic, intestinal, and reproductive tissues are also significantly affected pathologically. The pathologic changes closely mirror CF transmembrane conductance regulator (CFTR) expression on the epithelial cell surface of the respective organs.

The lung is not affected until after birth. Mucous plugging of small bronchioles and local inflammation are the earliest features. There is impaired clearance of airway secretions, which allows chronic infections to develop in the small airways, giving rise to chronic inflammation and progressive damage.

In contrast to the lung, the pancreas is affected in utero. At birth, intralobar ducts are plugged with proteinaceous material. Acinar cells show progressive atrophy. In time, both acini and proximal ducts atrophy and are replaced by fibrous tissue and fat. In the early stages, endocrine elements are relatively preserved, but islets also begin to disappear during adolescence. CF-associated diabetes mellitus is a common problem among adolescents and adults.

The intestine may also be affected in utero because of the low flow rate of intestinal contents. Rubbery masses of meconium may accumulate and obstruct the terminal ileum, giving rise to meconium ileus. After birth, predominantly in adolescence and adulthood, intermittent subacute intestinal obstruction with inspissated mucofeculent material is common.

CF-associated liver disease is characterized by small biliary ducts obstructed by eosinophilic material. This produces a patchy form of liver disease, focal biliary cirrhosis. In a small percentage of affected individuals, more extensive multilobular cirrhosis develops. The gallbladder is frequently atrophic and filled with mucus. The cystic duct and the intrahepatic and extrahepatic ducts may be filled with mucus and sludge.

The vas deferens is occluded in almost all males with CF. Thus, virtually all males with CF are sterile. In females, increased viscosity of cervical mucus has been described. Pathology is minimal, however. Healthy females with CF successfully conceive and are capable of carrying pregnancies to term. (*From* Forstner and Durie [15]; with permission.)

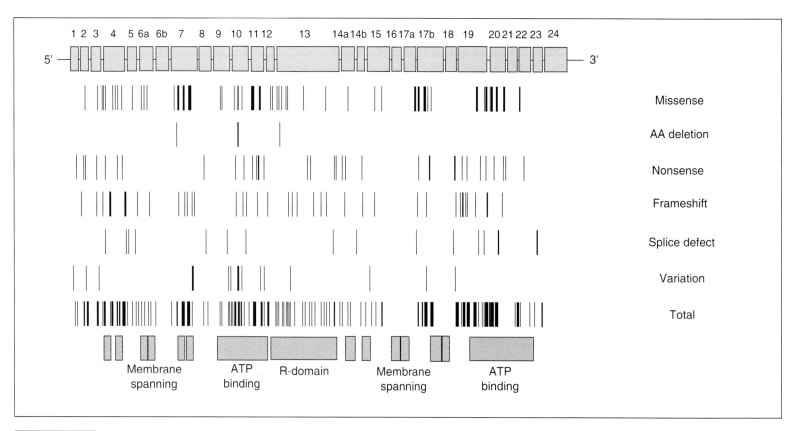

FIGURE 9-6.

Distribution of cystic fibrosis transmembrane conductance regulator (CFTR) gene mutations. The predominant mutation that causes cystic fibrosis (ΔF508) accounts for approximately 70% of mutant chromosomes screened [18]. Under the leadership of Dr. L.-C. Tsui, the Cystic Fibrosis Genetic Analysis Consortium was formed in 1989 to pool knowledge and information concerning CFTR gene mutations. To date the Consortium has identified more than 500 sequence alterations. Most of these mutations are almost certainly associated with the disease. The distribution and nature of the mutations in the CFTR gene are shown. The boxes at the top represent exons; the functional domains of the CFTR protein are shown at the bottom. Each vertical bar shows the location of a mutation reported to the CF Genetic Analysis Consortium (as of May 1992). A variation suggests a benign amino acid substitution. (*From* Tsui [19]; with permission.)

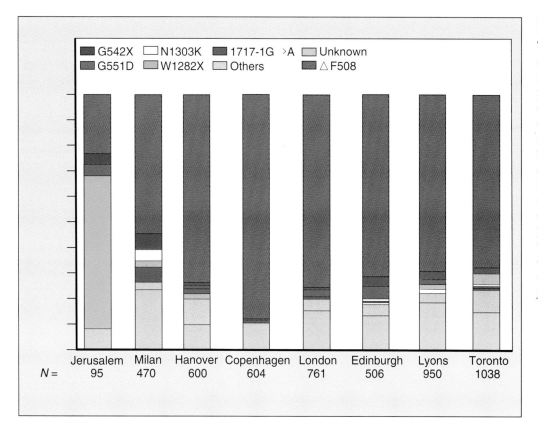

FIGURE 9-7.

The relative frequencies of the common cystic fibrosis transmembrane conductance regulator (CFTR) gene mutations in selected population centers are shown. A founder effect is apparent for some of the more common mutations. For example, ΔF508 accounts for almost 90% of CFTR mutations detected in the Danish population, suggesting that this mutation originated in Northeastern Europe. In contrast, ΔF508 accounts for only 22% of the cystic fibrosis chromosomes in the Ashkenazi Jewish population living in Israel. In that population, the nonsense mutation W1282X is common. It should be noted that a number of mutations remain unknown. (*Adapted from* Tsui [19]; with permission.)

TABLE 9-2. CLINICAL CHARACTERISTICS OF 293 PATIENTS ACCORDING TO GENOTYPE AND PANCREATIC-FUNCTION STATUS*

CHARACTERISTIC	ΔF508/ΔF508		ΔF508/OTHER		OTHER/OTHER	
	PI	PS	PI	PS	PI	PS
Patients, no	149	2	84	33	9	16
Patients with meconium ileus, %	22 (15)	0	10 (12)	0	4 (44)	0
Age at diagnosis, yr[†]	1.8±3.3	0.6±0.1	2.8±4.1[‡]	8.4±7.6	4.2±10.2[‡]	11±6
Sweat chloride level at diagnosis, mmol/L[†]	106±16	112±15	108±18[‡]	94±18	115±15[‡]	89±15
Current age, yr[†]	17±10	10±6	18±11[‡]	26±9	11±11[‡]	23±9
Current weight percentile[†]	39±30	32±2	42±31[‡]	64±29	31±31[‡]	73±19
Current height percentile	40±28	73±12	45±28	50±26	44±35	55±21
Current weight for height, %[†]	100±12	86±2	98±14[‡]	108±15	95±8[‡]	110±15

*PI denotes pancreatic insufficiency, and PS pancreatic sufficiency. Plus-minus values are means ±SD.
[†]P<0.001 by analysis of variance of five means (group in which n = 2 was not included in analysis).
[‡]Significantly different from the value for patients with pancreatic sufficiency within each genotype group (P<0.05, with Bonferroni's correction).

TABLE 9-2.

Clinical characteristics. Coincident with the accumulation of knowledge of cystic fibrosis transmembrane conductance regulator (CFTR) gene mutations, clinicians have gained considerable insight into genotype-phenotype relationships. Among the various clinical findings, the most striking association is with the presence or absence of pancreatic insufficiency. Of patients with cystic fibrosis, 293 were evaluated for the presence of the most common CFTR gene mutation (ΔF508); the results were compared with the clinical manifestations of the disease [20]. Of the patients, 52% were homozygous for the mutation, 40% were heterozygous, and 8% had other undefined mutations. The patients who are homozygous for the mutation had been diagnosed as having cystic fibrosis at an early age; in 99% of these patients pancreatic insufficiency was present. In contrast, only 72% of the heterozygous patients and 36% of the patients with other genotypes had pancreatic insufficiency. Patients with pancreatic insufficiency in all three genotype groups had similar clinical characteristics, reflected by an earlier diagnosis, similar sweat chloride values at diagnosis, similar severity of pulmonary disease, and similar percentile for weight. By comparison, the heterozygous-genotype and other genotype groups that did not have pancreatic insufficiency were older and had milder disease. They had lower sweat chloride values at diagnosis, normal nutritional status, and as a group, pulmonary function was better after adjustment for age. (*Adapted from* Kerem *et al.* [20]; with permission.)

PANCREATIC INSUFFICIENCY

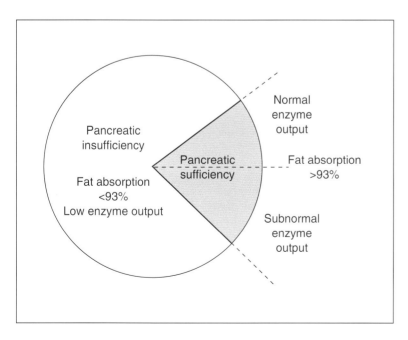

FIGURE 9-8.

The term *pancreatic insufficiency* describes patients who have evidence of maldigestion due to pancreatic failure. Those who absorb fat normally are often said to have normal pancreatic function, but when evaluated by quantitative measure of pancreatic function, they frequently have exocrine function that is below the normal level. It seems appropriate to use the term *pancreatic sufficiency* to define a patient who lacks steatorrhea and does not require pancreatic enzymes with meals. Overall prognosis and management of the patients with pancreatic sufficiency are somewhat different from that of patients with pancreatic insufficiency. Pancreatic sufficiency is an operational term and does not imply that the ability to secrete anions, fluid, and zymogens is normal. (*Adapted from* Forstner and Durie [15].)

TABLE 9-3. CLASSIFICATION OF CF GENE MUTATIONS AS SEVERE OR MILD WITH RESPECT TO PANCREATIC FUNCTION

Type of mutation	Severe (location)	Mild (location)
Missense (point mutation)	I148T (exon 4)	R117H (exon 4)
	G480C (exon 9)	R334W (exon 7)
	V520F (exon 10)	
	G551D (exon 11)	R347P (exon 7)
	R560T (exon 11)	A455E (exon 9)
	N1303K (exon 21)	P574H (exon 12)
Single amino acid deletion	ΔF508 (exon 10)	
	ΔI507 (exon 10)	
Stop codon (nonsense)	Q493X (exon 10)	
	G542X (exon 11)	
	R553X (exon 11)	
	W1282X (exon 20)	
Splice junction	621 + 1G → T (intron 4)	
	1717-1G → T (intron 10)	
Frameshift	556delA (exon 4)	
	3659delC (exon 19)	

TABLE 9-3.

Investigations of families with more than one affected member showed that the presence of pancreatic sufficiency or pancreatic insufficiency is highly concordant within families [21]. To evaluate the genetic basis of this observation, complete genotypes were determined in 394 patients in whom pancreatic status was well documented. The data showed that, with very few exceptions, each genotype was associated with pancreatic insufficiency only or with pancreatic sufficiency only. This finding is consistent with the hypothesis that the pancreatic function phenotype is determined by the genotype at the cystic fibrosis transmembrane conductance regulator (CFTR) gene locus. More specifically, the pancreatic sufficiency phenotype occurs in patients carrying one or two "mild" CFTR gene mutations, whereas the pancreatic insufficiency phenotype occurs in patients with two "severe" alleles. All the nonsense (stop codon), splice junction, and frameshift mutations were "severe" with respect to pancreatic function status. ΔF508 and ΔI507, which are single amino acid deletions, are also severe with respect to the pancreas. Interestingly, the study showed that missense mutations (amino acid substitutions) could be either severe or mild. (*Adapted from Kristidis et al.* [22]; *with permission.*)

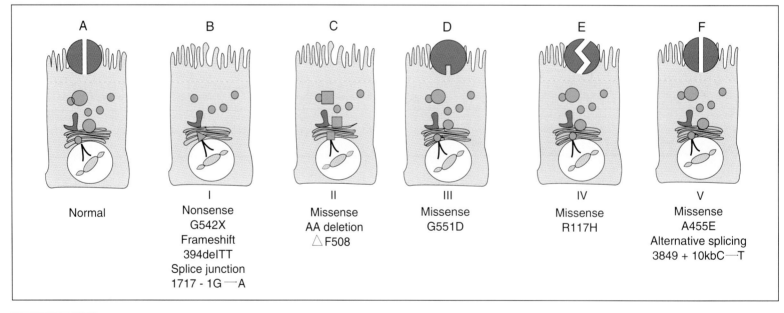

A — Normal

B — I
Nonsense
G542X
Frameshift
394delTT
Splice junction
1717 - 1G ⎯ A

C — II
Missense
AA deletion
△F508

D — III
Missense
G551D

E — IV
Missense
R117H

F — V
Missense
A455E
Alternative splicing
3849 + 10kbC ⎯ T

FIGURE 9-9.

Attempts have been made to define the different mutations into classes according to the functional properties of the gene product with respect to chloride regulation. A modified classification system, originally proposed by Tsui [19], is shown. **A,** Normal mutations. **B,** Class I represents gene mutations for which the intact cystic fibrosis transmembrane conductance regulator (CFTR) protein product is not formed. Most nonsense mutations fit into this category. **C,** Class II represents the forms of mutation CFTR that fail to traffic to the apical membrane under physiologic conditions. ΔF508 is the most striking example of this class of mutations. **D,** Class III mutant CFTR proteins include those that are inserted into the apical membrane but fail to respond to stimulation with cyclic adenosine monophosphate (cAMP). The relatively common missense mutation G551D is an example of a class III mutation. **E,** Class IV mutants produce protein that reach the apical membrane, generate cAMP-regulated apical membrane chloride current, but have altered channel properties, resulting in a reduction in the amount of current. Most mutations in this class are represented by the "mild" pancreatic sufficient CFTR gene mutations outlined in Table 9-3. **F,** Class V mutations are extremely rare. They result in reduced synthesis of normal functioning CFTR because of defective processing or aberrant splicing at alternative sites. Class IV and class V mutations have a strong association with the pancreatic sufficient phenotype. (*From Wilchanski et al.* [23]; *with permission.*)

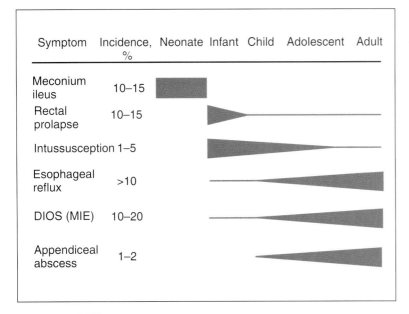

Symptom	Incidence, %	Neonate	Infant	Child	Adolescent	Adult
Meconium ileus	10–15					
Rectal prolapse	10–15					
Intussusception	1–5					
Esophageal reflux	>10					
DIOS (MIE)	10–20					
Appendiceal abscess	1–2					

FIGURE 9-10.

Gastrointestinal manifestations vary with age and disease progression. Approximately 10% to 15% of cystic fibrosis (CF) patients present at birth with signs and symptoms of intestinal obstruction. The cause is a plug of meconium in the terminal ileum that is acquired in utero. Half the cases are complicated by volvulus and atresia with or without attendant meconium peritonitis. Rectal prolapse occurs in almost 20% of patients, usually between 1 and 2.5 years of age [25]. In almost half these cases, episodes of prolapse precede diagnosis. Rectal prolapse has a tendency to resolve spontaneously.

Gastroesophageal reflux that may cause severe esophagitis and esophageal stricture increases in frequency with age, being more common in older children or adults with chronic pulmonary disease [26]. Distal intestinal obstruction syndrome (DIOS) or meconium ileus equivalent (MIE) occurs mainly in patients with pancreatic insufficiency [27]. It results from inspissated fecal masses that adhere tightly to the intestinal mucosa, particularly in the ileocecal area. An abdominal mass can be palpated in the abdomen. Complete bowel obstruction is rare; more often it causes partial bowel obstruction with intermittent abdominal pain that may result in loss of appetite and weight loss. Classical symptoms of acute appendicitis seem to be relatively rare in CF. More frequently, patients develop an appendicial abscess that is frequently misdiagnosed as DIOS.

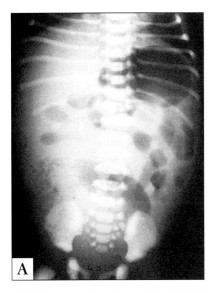

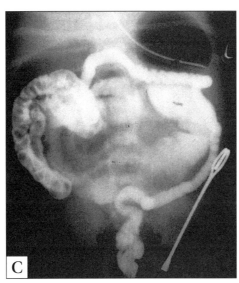

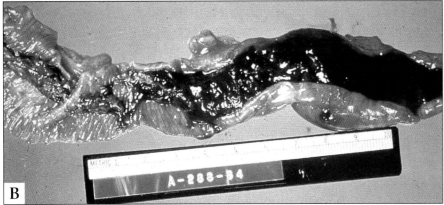

FIGURE 9-11.

Meconium ileus. **A,** A plain radiograph of the abdomen shows numerous gas-filled loops, displaced by meconium in the right lower quadrant. Small, multiple bubbles of gas are obvious within the meconium. No air is present in the rectum. **B,** Resected surgical specimen of the ileum from a patient with cystic fibrosis (CF) with meconium ileus. Rubbery, inspissated meconium is adherent to the intestinal mucosa (ileum is dissected open longitudinally). **C,** Water-soluble air contrast enema of a newborn with CF and complicated meconium ileas. A microcolon is demonstrated. Meconium plugs are shown in the ileum, which is opacified with contrast material. (**A,** *From* Forstner and Durie [15]; with permission.)

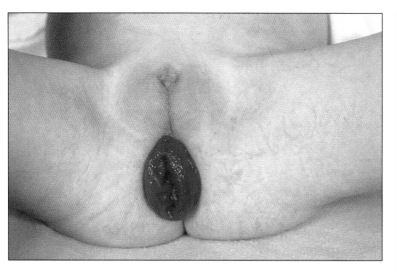

FIGURE 9-12.

Rectal prolapse, which usually occurs during passage of a large bowel motion, can be a frightening condition for parents of young children. It is hardly ever associated with major medical complications and is easily reduced manually. This condition usually resolves spontaneously by 3 to 4 years of age. Surgical intervention is not advocated, unless the condition is persistent.

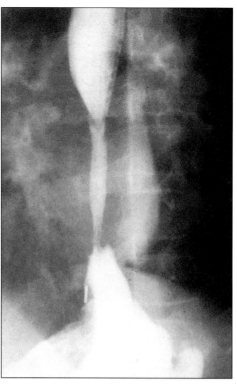

FIGURE 9-13.

A barium esophagogram in a 7-year-old girl with cystic fibrosis and advanced pulmonary disease. A severe distal esophageal stricture resulting from reflux esophagitis is demonstrated.

DISTAL INTESTINAL OBSTRUCTION SYNDROME

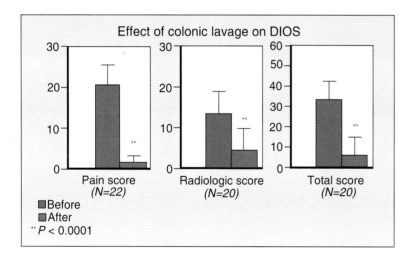

FIGURE 9-14.

Effect of colonic lavage on distal intestinal obstruction syndrome (DIOS). Episodes of DIOS are usually chronic and recurrent in the susceptible patient. Symptoms may be relieved by intestinal lavage with a balanced isotonic, polyethylene glycol-salt solution delivered orally or through a nasogastric tube. In patients with cystic fibrosis who sought medical attention for DIOS, treatment was initiated with the lavage solution. Although 14 patients chose to drink the solution, the 8 remaining patients elected to use a nasogastric tube. The solution was administered at the average rate of 1 liter per hour with an average volume of 5.6 liters. All but one patient reported impressive improvement when assessed by a semi-quantitative scoring system designed to assess the severity of pain and the degree of fecal impaction on plain abdominal radiograph [27]. (*Adapted from* Koletzko *et al.* [27]; with permission.)

HEPATOBILIARY DISEASE

TABLE 9-4. HEPATOBILIARY COMPLICATIONS OF CYSTIC FIBROSIS

HEPATIC COMPLICATIONS	REPORTED FREQUENCY, %
Neonatal cholestasis	Uncommon
Fatty liver	15–30
Focal biliary cirrhosis	11–70
Multilobular cirrhosis	2–5
Liver failure	Rare
BILIARY COMPLICATIONS	
Microgallbladder	5–20
Cholelithiasis	10
Intrahepatic biliary disease	Unknown
Extrahepatic biliary disease	Unknown
Common bile duct obstruction	Unknown

TABLE 9-4.

Liver disease, characterized by prolonged cholestatic jaundice, may be the presenting feature of cystic fibrosis (CF) in the neonate. The onset may be delayed several weeks with manifestations suggestive of biliary atresia, but jaundice usually resolves spontaneously. Investigations usually focus on other causes of neonatal jaundice. Isolated hepatomegaly without cholestasis may also be seen in infancy and early childhood. This may result from steatosis when the liver is smooth, soft, and only moderately enlarged. The etiology and significance of hepatic steatosis in CF remain an enigma. Focal biliary cirrhosis is, by far, the most common hepatic complication; incidence as high as 70% is reported on postmortem examination. A small number of patients develop advanced multilobular cirrhosis with portal hypertension and hypersplenism. Hyperbilirubinemia is rare. Overt liver failure is an unusual complication in CF.

Abnormalities of the biliary tract are quite common. Patients frequently have nonfunctioning microgallbladders whereas others have distended gallbladders as if obstructed. Gallstones are common. Cholangiographic studies reveal abnormalities of both the intrahepatic and extrahepatic ducts in a large percentage of older patients. Common bile duct obstruction due to fibrosis of the head of the pancreas has been postulated as a major cause of CF-associated liver disease. Other studies have questioned the high prevalence of this abnormality. Intrahepatic and extrahepatic ductal filling defects appear to be present in a large percentage of patients. Some of these changes, which resemble sclerosing cholangitis, are probably due to intraluminal accumulation of sludge or protein and mucus. (*Adapted from* Forstner and Durie [15].)

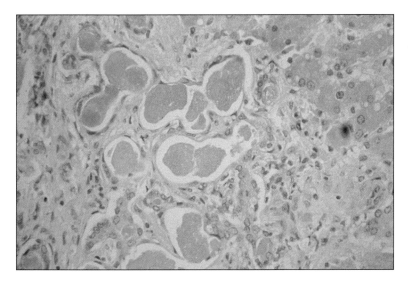

FIGURE 9-15.

A portal area from the liver biopsy of a patient with cystic fibrosis who also has focal biliary cirrhosis. Marked eosinophilic plugging of bile ductules is present. Bile ductules are increased in number and their cells are flattened. Periductal cell infiltration, bile duct proliferation, and increased fibrosis are common in scattered portal tracts. The patchy, focal nature of these lesions makes interpretation using needle liver biopsy to determine the severity of liver disease problematic. (*From* Forstner and Durie [15]; with permission.)

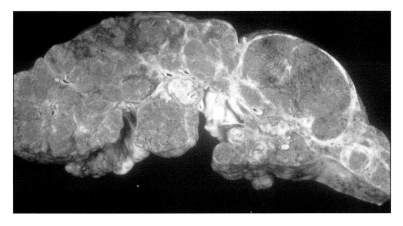

FIGURE 9-16.

Cut section of a postmortem liver from a patient with cystic fibrosis (CF) and multilobular cirrhosis. This patient had portal hypertension and hypersplenism. Gross cholestasis and nodular cirrhosis are present. Patients with advanced multilobular cirrhosis rarely die of hepatic failure. As life expectancy increases, however, clinical problems associated with CF liver disease, such as recurrent refractory variceal bleeding, hypersplenism, intractable ascites, and portosystemic encephalopathy will no doubt become more common. Some of these patients may be aided by hepatic transplantation.

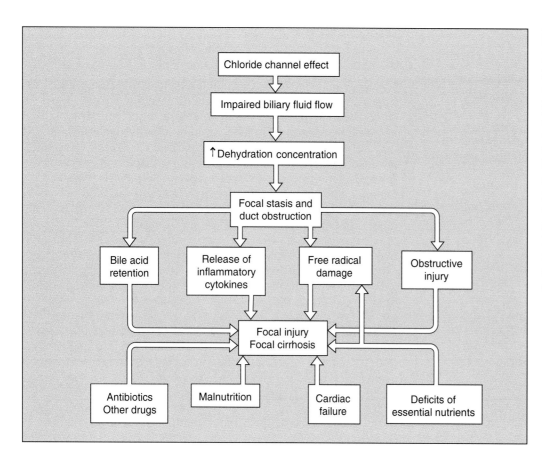

FIGURE 9-17.

Pathogenesis of hepatic injury. A variety of factors could contribute to hepatic injury and cystic fibrosis. The basic defect could result in reduced flow within small intrahepatic ducts. Mechanical obstruction caused by mucus plugs, intra- or extrahepatic lithiasis, distal stenosis of the common bile duct, or right cardiac failure could contribute to liver injury. Hepatotoxic factors include toxic bile acids together with various antibiotics and other pharmacotherapy. Free radical injury (with vitamin E deficiency), the presence of chronic malnutrition, or deficits of essential nutrients (fatty acids and taurine) might be expected to mediate hepatic injury as well.

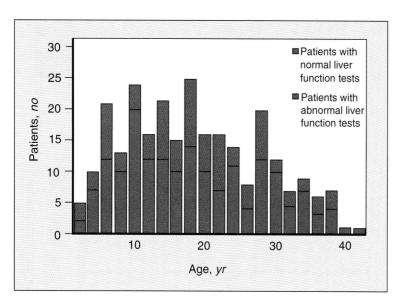

FIGURE 9-18.

No completely satisfactory methods exist for evaluating patients with cystic fibrosis (CF) for the presence or severity of liver disease [10]. Routine liver enzyme tests such as alkaline phosphatase and aspartate transaminase are mildly elevated in about 40% of CF patients. Liver enzyme test abnormalities are usually 150% to 200% higher than normal. The precise cause and significance of these abnormalities are unknown. Some patients with advanced multilobular cirrhosis can have normal results of routine liver tests. This figure shows the frequency of abnormal alkaline phosphatase with or without aspartate transaminase activities with age in patients who are homozygous for ΔF508.

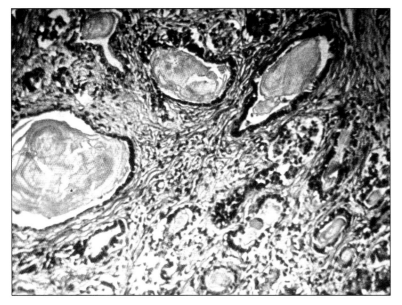

FIGURE 9-19.

Histologic section of a pancreas from a patient with cystic fibrosis. Pancreatic damage begins in utero with accumulation of protein-aceous secretory material within small pancreatic ducts [28]. The obstructive process causes dilatation of the duct lumina, which is followed by progressive degradation and atrophy of the acini. In patients with pancreatic insufficiency, advanced acinar destruction is present by the first few years of life and exocrine glands become replaced by fibrous tissue and fat. Initially, endocrine tissue is relatively preserved but as patients grow older islet cells are lost and the glands become completely replaced with fibrous tissue. Pancreatic calcification and cystic changes are occasionally seen in older patients.

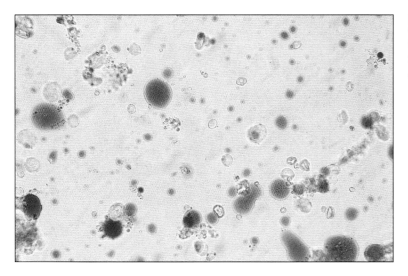

TABLE 9-5. TESTS OF PANCREATIC FUNCTION

DIRECT	INDIRECT	BLOOD
Intubation tests	Stool microscopy	Pancreatic enzymes
Hormone stimulants	72-hr fecal fat	Pancreatic polypeptide
	Stool enzymes	
Natural stimulants	Bentiromide	
	Fluorescein dilaurate	
	Breath tests	

TABLE 9-5.

Diagnosis of pancreatic function status. Several indirect and direct tests of pancreatic function are available for defining pancreatic status. Simple methods such as microscopic examination of a stool smear for neutral fat droplets are helpful, but more quantitative methods, such as determining 72-hour fecal fat losses while the patient's fat intake is measured, can be used to define the presence or absence of pancreatic insufficiency. Deficient secretion of pancreatic enzymes in stool can be ascertained by analysis of stool chymotrypsin activity. Alternative, indirect tests of pancreatic function, such as bentiromide or fluorescein dilaurate, can be helpful for distinguishing pancreatic insufficient and pancreatic sufficient patients and for monitoring pancreatic function in those with pancreatic sufficiency. More complex direct intubation studies are of value for defining the residual pancreatic capacity of patients with pancreatic sufficiency.

FIGURE 9-20.

Sudan red stain for fecal fat in cystic fibrosis (CF). Stool smear of a patient with CF stained with sudan-red. Numerous stained fat droplets are seen.

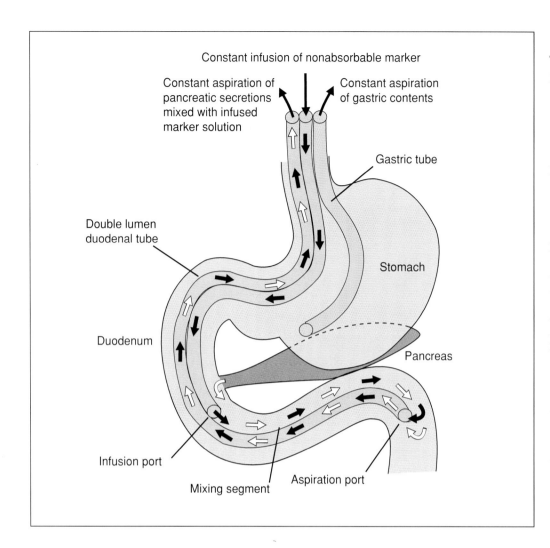

FIGURE 9-21.

The complex, direct method for assessing pancreatic function is represented diagrammatically. A double lumen tube is inserted into the duodenum. The tube is constructed so that one lumen opens proximally at the ampulla of Vater and the second lumen, which has several distal ports, is positioned distally at the ligament of Treitz. A nonabsorbable marker solution is infused into a proximal port at a constant rate. Pancreatic juice mixed with infused marker solution is aspirated distally by low-pressure suction. Following equilibration of marker solution with pancreatic juice, duodenal juice mixed with marker is collected while continuously and simultaneously infusing secretin and cholecystokinin at doses known to achieve maximal pancreatic stimulation. A separate nasogastric tube facilitates aspiration of gastric juice and minimizes contamination of duodenal contents with acid and pepsin. Use of a nonabsorbable marker permits correction for distal losses of fluid and enzyme by assuming that, after equilibration has been attained, the degree of distal loss of marker equals pancreatic enzyme and fluid loss. (*Adapted from* Couper *et al.* [29].)

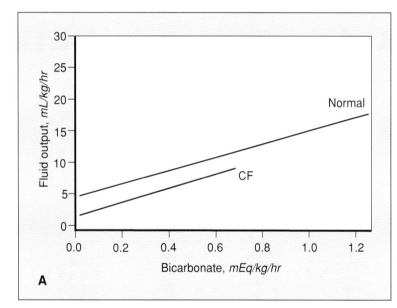

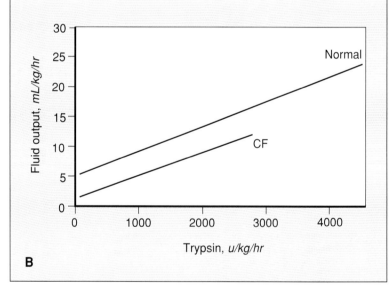

FIGURE 9-22.

A–B, The invasive, complex nature of the direct pancreatic function test tends to discourage its routine use. It is particularly helpful, however, for diagnosing cystic fibrosis (CF) or excluding the diagnosis in difficult cases. Deficits in anion levels (chloride and bicarbonate) and fluid secretion in CF compared with normal controls provide evidence of the underlying defect within epithelial cells of the pancreatic duct. (*Adapted from* Kopelman *et al.* [17].)

FIGURE 9-23.

The direct pancreatic function test is helpful in delineating the pancreatic reserve in patients who are pancreatically sufficient. More than 98% of exocrine pancreatic capacity must be lost before signs and symptoms of steatorrhea develop.

Range of pancreatic function

100% ⟷ 1% ⟷ 0%

Pancreatic sufficiency — Pancreatic insufficiency

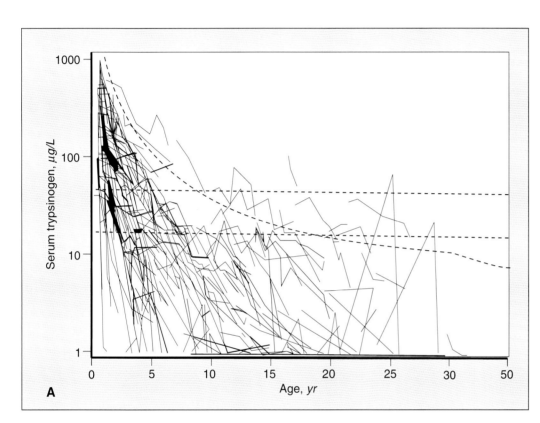

A

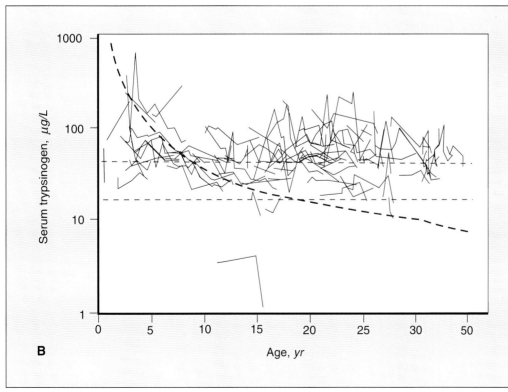

B

FIGURE 9-24.

Pancreatic enzymes, such as trypsinogen, can be detected in sera by immunologic techniques. This technique can be used to define pancreatic disease in cystic fibrosis (CF). Serum trypsinogen levels are greatly elevated in the blood of newborn infants with CF, presumably because of an obstruction of the small pancreatic ducts and regurgitation of pancreatic enzymes into the circulation. This test is used for screening neonates for CF. Longitudinal monitoring of serum trypsinogen can also be useful for predicting loss of pancreatic function. **A**, Serial measurements of serum trypsinogen in 233 patients with CF and pancreatic insufficiency. *Parallel dotted lines* indicate the normal range of values. The *curved dotted line* indicates the upper limits (95% confidence limits) for pancreatically insufficient measurements. As the pancreas atrophies, serum trypsinogen values drop, reaching subnormal values in patients by 7 to 8 years of age. **B**, Serial measurements of serum trypsinogen in 78 patients with CF and pancreatic sufficiency. The *parallel dotted lines* indicate the normal range of values. The *curved dotted line* indicates the upper limits (95% confidence limits) for the patients with pancreatic insufficiency. Most patients show widely fluctuating values within or above the normal range. One patient with unusually low results of a serum trypsinogen test died of gastrointestinal lymphoma.

TABLE 9-6. CLINICAL SIGNS OF MALNUTRITION IN CYSTIC FIBROSIS

IN INFANCY AND CHILDHOOD	IN LATE CHILDHOOD AND ADOLESCENCE
Growth retardation	Growth retardation
Delayed bone age	Weight deficit
Weight deficit	Muscle wasting
Muscle wasting	Delayed puberty
Pot belly	Hepatomegaly
Rectal prolapse	Hypoalbuminemia
Hypoalbuminemia	Osteopenia
Edema	Ataxia
Anemia	Ophthalmoplegia
Bruising	
Bleeding	
Skin rash	
Hepatomegaly	
Developmental delay	

TABLE 9-6.

Clinical features of malnutrition. Signs and symptoms of malnutrition vary according to the patient's age, but most are related to a protein-calorie deficit or malabsorption of essential nutrients [15]. Most patients with cystic fibrosis (CF) and pancreatic insufficiency present in infancy with some manifestations of maldigestion and are often malnourished. The abdomen is distended and muscles appear wasted, particularly in the buttocks and thighs. Growth failure is an early sign. The appearance of edema, hypoalbuminemia, and anemia herald severe protein-calorie malnutrition; this generally occurs in infants under the age of 6 months. Growth retardation is a variable feature during childhood. In general, patients improve rapidly with adequate attention to caloric requirements, vitamin needs, and pancreatic enzyme supplementation. In most CF centers, nutritional support is now viewed as an integral part of the multidisciplinary care of patients with CF. Aggressive programs have been instituted to prevent malnutrition. It is now generally accepted that the primary objective of nutritional management is to achieve normal nutrition and growth for children of all ages.

TABLE 9-7. DISORDERS CAUSED BY DEFICITS OF ESSENTIAL NUTRIENTS

Fat-soluble vitamin deficiency	
A	Raised intracranial pressure
	Conjunctival xerosis
	Night blindness
D	Rickets
	Osteomalacia
E	Hemolytic anemia (infants)
	Neuropathy
	Ophthalmoplegia
	Ataxia
	Diminished vibration sense and proprioception
K	Coagulopathy
Water-soluble vitamin deficiency	B_{12} deficiency in PI patients not receiving or non-compliant to enzyme therapy
Salt depletion	Lethargy
	Weakness
	Dehydration
	Metabolic alkalosis
Essential fatty acid deficiency	Desquamation
	Thrombocytopenia
	Poor wound healing

TABLE 9-7.

Deficits of essential nutrients. Fat-soluble vitamin deficiencies caused by malabsorption are common in untreated pancreatically insufficient (PI) patients. These include night blindness, ataxia, and neuropathy. Deficiencies of water-soluble vitamins are rare. Vitamin deficiencies are preventable with appropriate therapy (pancreatic enzymes and supplemental fat-soluble vitamins). Salt depletion, because of excessive sweating, particularly in hotter climates, may cause symptoms of hyponatremia. Signs and symptoms of essential fatty acid deficiency may be present before diagnosis but are rare in nourished, appropriately treated, patients. Biochemical evidence of essential fatty acid deficiency may persist following therapy, however.

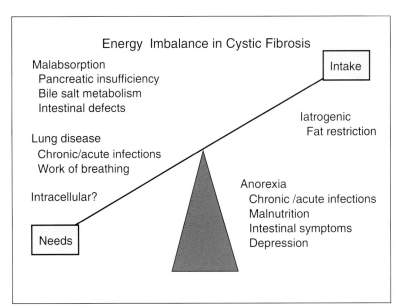

Energy Imbalance in Cystic Fibrosis

Malabsorption
  Pancreatic insufficiency
  Bile salt metabolism
  Intestinal defects

Lung disease
  Chronic/acute infections
  Work of breathing

Intracellular?

Needs

Intake

Iatrogenic
  Fat restriction

Anorexia
  Chronic /acute infections
  Malnutrition
  Intestinal symptoms
  Depression

FIGURE 9-25.

Pathogenesis of energy imbalance in cystic fibrosis (CF). Various complex-related and unrelated factors may give rise to energy imbalance in patients with CF [11]. The net effect on growth potential varies from patient to patient, according to differences in disease expression and with disease progression. Expressed in simple terms, an energy deficit results from an imbalance between energy needs and intake, which in turn is determined by three factors: energy losses, energy expenditure, and energy intake.

TABLE 9-8. ENERGY IMBALANCE CAUSED BY CYSTIC FIBROSIS

INCREASED NEEDS	REDUCED INTAKE
Increased intestinal losses	Reduced intake
Pancreatic insufficiency	Iatrogenic fat
Bile salt metabolism	Anorexia
Hepatobiliary disease	Feeding disorders
Regurgitation from	Depression
gastroesophageal reflux	Esophagitis
Increased urinary losses	
Diabetes mellitus	
Increased energy expenditure	
Pulmonary disease	
Primary defect?	

TABLE 9-8.

Causes of energy imbalance in cystic fibrosis (CF). Fecal nutrient losses from maldigestion and malabsorption are known to contribute to energy imbalance. Despite improvements in the enzymatic potency and intestinal delivery of ingested pancreatic enzyme supplements, many patients continue to have severe maldigestion even when treated with adequate amounts of enzymes. Calorie restriction, especially with reduced dietary fat to relieve symptoms, may cause energy imbalance and adversely affect growth. It is suggested that energy intakes in cystic fibrosis exceed normal requirements, but in reality energy needs are extremely variable. Some patients with CF do have a higher energy expenditure than normal. Some studies have hinted at the possibility that the CF gene might have a direct effect on basal metabolism. Conversely, chest infections with or without inflammatory mediators or the energy expended in breathing may also raise energy expenditure. Patients with CF are prone to psychologic and gastrointestinal complications that might limit oral intake.

TABLE 9-9. GENETIC DEFECTS AND RESTING ENERGY EXPENDITURE IN CYSTIC FIBROSIS

	ΔF508/ ΔF508	ΔF508/ OTHER	OTHER/ OTHER
n	31	29	18
REE, *% predicted*	121	109	104
FEV$_1$	56	63	97

TABLE 9-9.

To evaluate the possibility that the genetic defect in cystic fibrosis (CF) has a direct effect on basal metabolism, O'Rawe and colleagues [30] demonstrated evidence of increased resting energy expenditure (REE) in patients homozygous for the most common CF transmembrane conductance regulator gene mutation (ΔF508). In contrast, energy expenditure was only moderately increased in those with ΔF508/other and other/other genotypes. These investigators did not control for lung function or nutritional status, both of which could affect energy expenditure. Lung disease or lung infection increases REE; undernutrition may result in a decreased REE. (*Adapted from* O'Rawe *et al.* [30].) FEV$_1$—forced expiratory volume in 1 second.

TABLE 9-10. ENERGY EXPENDITURE AND LUNG DISEASE IN CYSTIC FIBROSIS

	ΔF508/ ΔF508 PI	ΔF508/ OTHER PI	F508/ OTHER PS
n	14	9	9
WFH, %	103	106	116
Body Fat, %	16	14	16
FEV₁	94	98	90
REE, % predicted	104	105	101

TABLE 9-10.

In a separate study the two confounding variables (malnutrition and lung disease) were accounted for by study males with normal nutritional status and good lung function—forced expiratory volume in 1 second (FEV_1>75% predicted). Little, if any, increase in resting energy expenditure (REE) was seen in normally nourished males with cystic fibrosis (CF) with good lung function [31]. Furthermore, we were unable to demonstrate any difference in REE in patient groups with different genotypes. Thus, if there is a genetic basis for increased REE in patients with CF, its effects must be minimal. PI—pancreatic insufficiency; PS—pancreatic sufficiency; WFH—weight as a percentage of ideal weight for height. (*Adapted from* Fried *et al.* [31].)

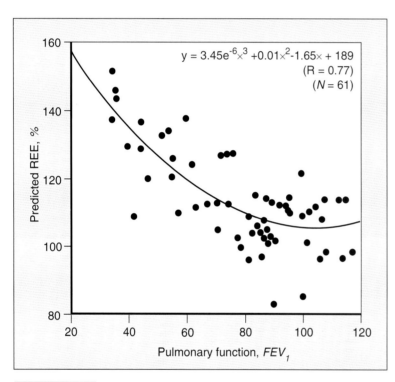

$$y = 3.45e^{-6}x^3 + 0.01x^2 - 1.65x + 189$$
$$(R = 0.77)$$
$$(N = 61)$$

FIGURE 9-26.

Resting energy expenditure (REE) (as a percentage of predicted) versus pulmonary function in normally nourished males with cystic fibrosis. Lung function appears to be a major determinant of increased REE. As forced expiratory volume in 1 second (FEV_1) falls below 75% of predicted levels, REE rises in a curvilinear (quadratic) fashion, reaching values as high as 150% above predicted levels. At least two factors appear to affect REE. The first is a normal response to negative energy balance with a reduction in energy expenditure. The second, an increase in energy expenditure, appears to be related to the severity of lung function. The precise cause of increased resting energy expenditure remains to be elucidated. (*Adapted from* Fried *et al.* [31]; with permission.)

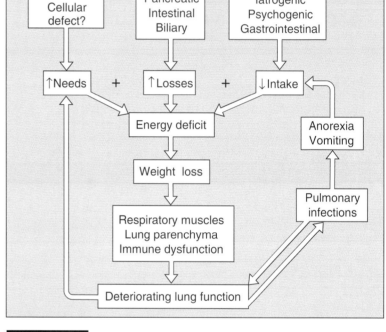

FIGURE 9-27.

Pathogenesis of an energy deficit. A proposed model to explain the cause of the energy deficit in patients with cystic fibrosis, which defines the web of independent and interdependent variables that may give rise to chronic malnutrition and growth failure. Most patients are able to maintain normal growth velocity and nutritional status by adherence to a good dietary routine, particularly when lung function is relatively unimpaired. Decline in pulmonary function and the development of malnutrition are closely interrelated, however. As lung function worsens, most commonly in adolescents and young adults, several factors may contribute to an energy deficit. More frequent and severe infections, coupled with the systemic effects of inflammatory mediators, may induce anorexia. Clinical depression, as a reaction to a chronic illness, may cause reduced intake. Weight loss causes loss of fat tissue and then muscle wasting. Respiratory muscle wasting could adversely affect respiratory motion, prevent effective coughing, and contribute to increasing lung disease. Malnutrition may impair immune function and lung elasticity. A vicious cycle is established wherein lowering lung function contributes to the nutritional deficit, which inevitably leads to endstage pulmonary failure and death. (*From* Durie and Pencharz [32]; with permission.)

REFERENCES

1. di Sant'Agnese P, Darling R, Perera G, Shea E: Abnormal electrolyte composition of sweat in cystic fibrosis of the pancreas. *Pediatrics* 1953, 12:549–563.

2. Fanconi G, Uehlinger E, Knauer C: Das Coelioksyndrom bei angeborener zystisher Pankreas Fibromatose and Bronchicktasis. *Wein Med Wochnenschr* 1936, 86:753–756.

3. Anderson D: Cystic fibrosis of the pancreas and its relation to celiac disease. *Am J Dis Child* 1938, 56:344–399.

4. Gibbs GE, Bostick WL, Smith PM: Incomplete pancreatic deficiency in cystic fibrosis of the pancreas. *J Pediatr* 1950, 37:320–325.

5. Quinton PM: Chloride impermeability in cystic fibrosis. *Nature* 1983, 301:421–422.

6. Knowles MR, Gatzy JT, Boucher RC: Relative ion permeability of normal and cystic fibrosis nasal epithelium. *J Clin Invest* 1983, 71:1410–1417.

7. Sato K, Sato F: Defective beta adrenergic response of cystic fibrosis sweat glands in vivo and in vitro. *J Clin Invest* 1984, 73:1763–1771.

8. Riordan JR, Rommens JM, Kerem BS, *et al.*: Identification of the cystic fibrosis gene: Cloning and characterization of complementary DNA. *Science* 1989, 245:1066–1073.

9. Bear CE, Li C, Kartner N, *et al.*: Purification and functional reconstitution of the cystic fibrosis transmembrane conductance regulator (CFTR). *Cell* 1992, 68:809–818.

10. Durie PR: Cystic fibrosis: Gastrointestinal and hepatic complications and their management. *Semin Pediatr Gastroenterol Nutr* 1993, 4:3.

11. Pencharz PB, Durie PR: Nutritional management of cystic fibrosis. *Annu Rev Nutr* 1993, 13:111–136.

12. Corey ML: Longitudinal studies in cystic fibrosis. In *Perspectives in Cystic Fibrosis*. Edited by Sturgess J. Proceedings of the Eighth International Congress in Cystic Fibrosis. Mississauga, Ontario, Canada: Imperial Press; 1980:246.

13. Gaskin K, Gurwitz D, Durie PR, *et al.*: Improved respiratory prognosis in patients with cystic fibrosis with normal fat absorption. *J Pediatr* 1982, 100:857–862.

14. Tsui L-C: The cystic fibrosis transmembrane conductance regulator gene. *Am J Respir Crit Care Med* 1995, 151:547–553.

15. Forstner G, Durie PR: Cystic fibrosis. In *Pediatric Gastrointestinal Disease. Pathophysiology, Diagnosis, Management*. Edited by Walker WA, Durie PR, Hamilton JR, et al. Philadelphia: BC Decker; 1991: 1179–1197.

16. Kopelman H, Durie PR, Gaskin K, *et al.*: Pancreatic fluid secretion and protein hyperconcentration in cystic fibrosis. *N Engl J Med* 1985, 312:329–334.

17. Kopelman H, Corey M, Gaskin K, *et al*: Impaired chloride secretion as well as bicarbonate secretion underlies the fluid secretory defect in the cystic fibrosis pancreas. *Gastroenterol* 1988, 95:349–355.

18. Kerem BS, Rommens JM, Buchanan JA, *et al.*: Identification of the cystic fibrosis gene: Genetic analysis. *Science* 1989, 245:1073–1080.

19. Tsui L-C: The spectrum of cystic fibrosis mutations. *Trends Genet* 1992, 8:392–398.

20. Kerem E, Corey M, Kerem B-S, *et al.*: The relation between genotype and phenotype in cystic fibrosis—analysis of the most common mutation (ΔF508). *N Engl J Med* 1990, 323:1517–1522.

21. Corey M, Durie PR, Moore D, *et al.*: Familial concordance of pancreatic function in cystic fibrosis. *J Pediatr* 1989, 115:274–277.

22. Kristidis P, Bozon D, Corey M, *et al.*: Genetic determination of exocrine pancreatic function in cystic fibrosis. *Am J Hum Genet* 1992, 50:1178–1184.

23. Wilchanski M, Zielenski J, Markiewicz D, *et al.*: Correlation of sweat chloride concentration classes of the cystic fibrosis transmembrane conductance regulator gene mutations. *J Pediatr* 1995, 127:705–710.

24. Kerem E, Corey M, Kerem B, *et al.*: Clinical and genetic comparisons of patients with cystic fibrosis, with or without meconium ileus. *J Pediatr* 1989, 114:767–773.

25. Stern R, Izant RJ, Boat TF, *et al.*: Treatment and prognosis of rectal prolapse in cystic fibrosis. *Gastroenterology* 1986, 82:707–710.

26. Scott RB, O'Laughlin EV, Gall DG: Gastroesophageal reflux in patients with cystic fibrosis. *J Pediatr* 1985, 106:223–227.

27. Koletzko S, Stringer DA, Cleghorn GJ, Durie PR: Lavage treatment of distal intestinal obstruction syndrome in children with cystic fibrosis. *Pediatrics* 1989, 83:727–733.

28. Oppenheimer E, Esterly J: Cystic fibrosis of the pancreas. *Arch Pathol Lab Med* 1973, 96:149–154.

29. Couper R, Durie P: Pancreatic function tests. In *Pediatric Gastrointestinal Disease. Pathophysiology, Diagnosis, Management*. Edited by Walter WA, Durie PR, Hamilton JR, *et al.* Philadelphia: BC Decker; 1991; 1341–1353.

30. O'Rawe A, McIntosh I, Dodge J, *et al*: Increased energy expenditure in cystic fibrosis is associated with specific mutations. *Clin Sci* 1992, 82:71–76.

31. Fried MD, Durie PR, Tsui L-C, *et al.*: The cystic fibrosis gene and resting energy expenditure. *J Pediatr* 1991, 119:913–916.

32. Durie PR, Pencharz PB: A rational approach to the nutritional care of patients with cystic fibrosis. *J R Soc Med* 1989, 82(Suppl 16):11–20.

Chapter 10

Anorectal Malformations

ALBERTO PEÑA

Anorectal malformations represent a spectrum of defects, ranging from the benign and noncomplex with good functional prognosis to more severe cases involving malformations in the genitourinary and sexual structures, with poor prognosis for bowel and urinary function. Generally, children with complex malformations present with poor anal sphincter tone, flat perineum, and no clear midline intergluteal groove. As a result, these children need a three-staged surgical repair—colostomy, main repair (pull-through), and colostomy closure. The most frequent surgical approach for the main repair is termed *posterior sagittal anorectoplasty*. Those children with relatively benign malformations, that is, "low" defects, do not need such extensive surgical repair; they simply receive an anoplasty without a colostomy.

Many patients achieve very satisfactory bowel and urinary control whereas others either remain fecally incontinent or suffer from important functional disorders. These last two groups require a great deal of medical care and long-term follow-up.

An early accurate diagnosis and an effective and efficient therapeutic approach during the newborn period in a baby born with an anorectal malformation are essential to achieving optimal results in all states of surgical repair. The natural history of these defects, diagnostic methods, and medical and surgical therapy are reviewed here with special emphasis on the most practical aspects.

INCIDENCE

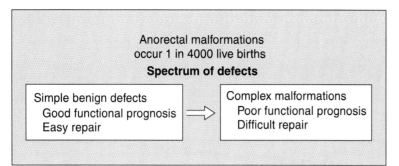

Anorectal malformations
occur 1 in 4000 live births
Spectrum of defects

| Simple benign defects
Good functional prognosis
Easy repair | ⟹ | Complex malformations
Poor functional prognosis
Difficult repair |

FIGURE 10-1.

Anorectal malformations occur in 1 of 4000 live births [1–3]. The term *anorectal malformation* encompasses multiple congenital defects of the rectum as well as urinary or sexual structures with various degrees of complexity that require different types of treatment with different prognosis for bowel and urinary control as well as sexual function. Most children with anorectal malformations have an abnormal communication between the rectum, the genitourinary tract, or the perineum; this communication is called a *fistula*. The chances of a couple having a second child with an anorectal malformation is approximately 1% [4].

TABLE 10-1. CLASSIFICATION OF ANORECTAL ANOMALIES

MALES		FEMALES	
Low defects (perineal fistula)	No colostomy required	Perineal fistula	No colostomy required
Rectourethral bulbar fistula Rectourethral prostatic fistula Rectobladder neck fistula Imperforate anus without fistula Rectal atresia and stenosis	Colostomy required	Vestibular fistula Imperforate anus without fistula Rectal atresia and stenosis Persistent cloaca	Colostomy required

TABLE 10-1.

Classification of anorectal anomalies. Only the very low and simple defects (perineal fistula) can be repaired without a protective colostomy.

NEONATAL APPROACH

TABLE 10-2. NEONATAL APPROACH

QUESTIONS TO BE ANSWERED

Does the patient need a colostomy?

Does the patient have an associated defect requiring emergency treatment?

Do not make decisions before 24 hrs

TABLE 10-2.

The diagnosis of an anorectal malformation is rarely missed, even by a nonmedical person. The physical examination of the newborn must always include the perineum, the genitalia, and the patency of the anus. There is, however, one specific type of imperforate anus in which the external appearance of the anus is normal and the obstruction is located approximately 2 cm above the anal opening; this defect is called *rectal atresia*. It is frequently diagnosed late because of a lack of suspicion, and sometimes the diagnosis is made when the nurse tries to take the rectal temperature. At other times, in cases of mild defects, the diagnosis is missed owing to a deficient initial examination, (*eg*, one performed in a hurry).

Once the diagnosis of imperforate anus (anorectal malformation) has been established, the efforts of the medical team, including nurses, neonatologists, and pediatric surgeons, are centered on the following goals: (1) to provide general medical support; (2) to determine whether or not the baby suffers from other associated defects that require immediate attention; (3) to determine whether the baby needs a temporary colostomy (high defects) or whether the defect can be treated by a minor operation called *anoplasty*; and (4) to give moral and psychologic support to the parents, providing relevant information concerning the diagnosis, tests, treatment, and prognosis.

Besides the routine evaluation, vital signs, and observation, the surgeon must specifically request the following relevant information, which will help to achieve the previously-mentioned goals: (1) abdominal distention, (2) vomiting, (3) presence of meconium in the perineum of a male baby or in the genitalia of a female baby, (4) voiding pattern, and (5) presence of meconium in the urine of a male baby as detected by filtering the urine through a gauze placed at the tip of the penis or by urinalysis. This information, plus a meticulous examination of the perineum and genitalia, as well as some special tests, will help the surgeon decide about the next therapeutic action.

Associated defects

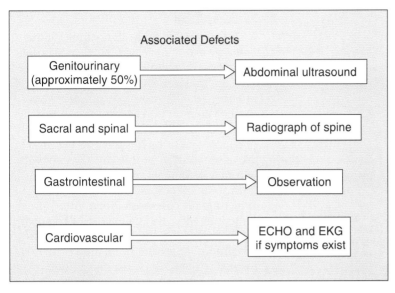

FIGURE 10-2.

The most frequently associated defects that may require immediate attention are those of the urinary tract. Approximately 50% of all cases of anorectal malformations have an associated urologic defect. This frequency varies depending on the type of defect [5,6]. Therefore, every baby with an anorectal malformation requires an ultrasound examination of the abdomen to detect a urinary obstruction. This test is the most valuable initial test of the urinary tract. If results of this test are abnormal, a more specialized urologic evaluation will be indicated. This evaluation is particularly important in cases of high malformations. Patients with a persistent cloaca and patients with a rectobladder neck fistula have almost a 90% chance of suffering from a urologic defect [5,6]; those cases, therefore, represent a urologic emergency. The urologic diagnosis must be established before the colostomy is opened. In this way the surgeon must be prepared to perform a urinary diversion at the same time of the colostomy opening (when indicated).

A radiologic evaluation of the spine and sacrum is always indicated because of the high frequency of associated sacrospinal defects. Other associated defects may affect the gastrointestinal tract, including esophageal atresia, duodenal atresia, or atresia in other locations. Cardiovascular anomalies are also frequently associated. Cardiac evaluation with electrocardiography (EKG) and echocardiography (ECHO) will be performed only if the baby shows any cardiovascular symptoms.

Colostomy opening versus anoplasty

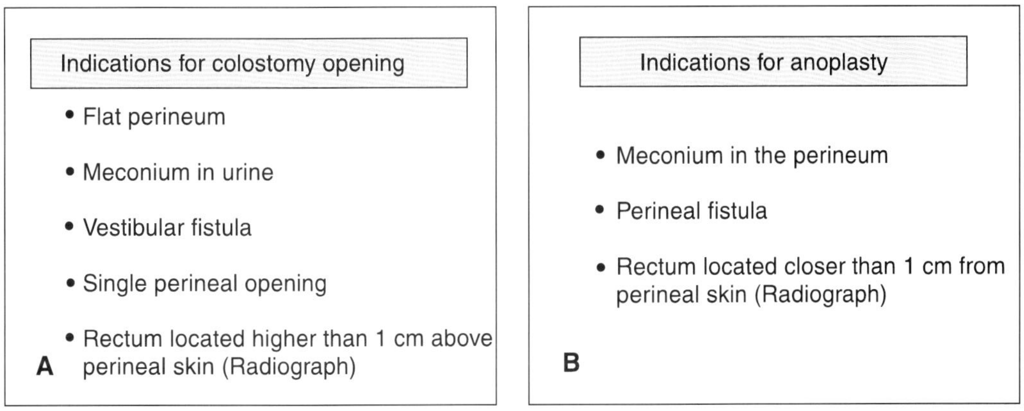

Indications for colostomy opening

- Flat perineum

- Meconium in urine

- Vestibular fistula

- Single perineal opening

- Rectum located higher than 1 cm above
A perineal skin (Radiograph)

Indications for anoplasty

- Meconium in the perineum

- Perineal fistula

- Rectum located closer than 1 cm from perineal skin (Radiograph)

B

FIGURE 10-3.

The opening of an intestinal diversion, called *colostomy*, is considered necessary to decompress the bowel, save the baby's life, and eventually, to avoid infection during the postoperative period of the main repair of the defect. This operation is indicated in most of the malformations mentioned in Table 10-1. The decision is made based on the clinical information in 80% to 90% of the cases, and requires a radiologic evaluation in the remaining 10% to 20%. This decision is taken after 24 hours of observation. General indications for a colostomy versus an anoplasty are shown in **A** and **B**.

Radiologic evaluation to determine the height of the defect

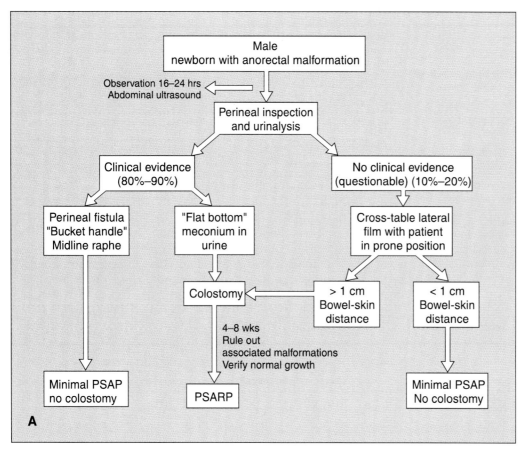

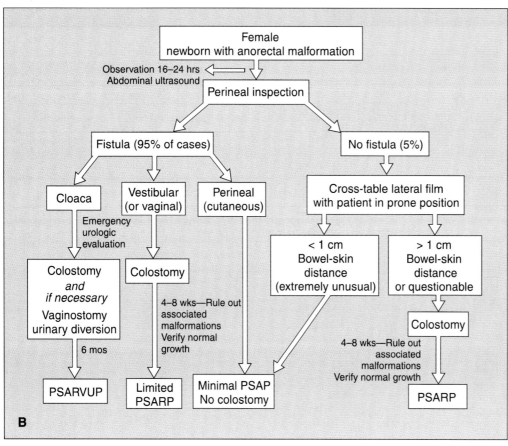

FIGURE 10-4.

A–B, Decision-making algorithms for the management of male and female newborns. As previously mentioned, in 80% to 90% of cases, the decision concerning the opening of a colostomy versus anoplasty can be taken on purely clinical grounds. However, there are babies in whom the previously mentioned signs (*see* Fig. 10-3) are not present or prominent enough, with whom a specific radiographic study is indicated. Traditionally, this study is an "invertogram" or upside-down film [7]. This study must be taken after 24 hours of life in order for the baby to have enough intraluminal pressure in the bowel to distend with gas the most distal blind portion of the rectum. A lead (radiopaque) marker is placed in the perineum, the baby is then turned upside down for 2 to 3 minutes, and a strictly lateral film of the pelvis is taken. The gas inside the distended blind rectum gives a radiolucent image; the distance between the radiopaque marker (skin) and the blind rectum is measured, providing valuable information concerning the height of the defect. During the study, the nurse must remain close to the baby to prevent hypothermia and to assist the baby in cases of vomiting or cyanosis. Recently, a view taken with the baby in prone position (face down) with the pelvis elevated, called *cross-table lateral film* [8], has proved to be equally informative while avoiding the risks of vomiting, aspiration, and respiratory distress that have been seen during the traditional invertogram. PSAP—posterior sagittal anoplasty; PSARP—posterior sagittal anorectoplasty; PSARVUP—posterior sagittal anorectovagino-urethroplasty.

Normal anorectal anatomy

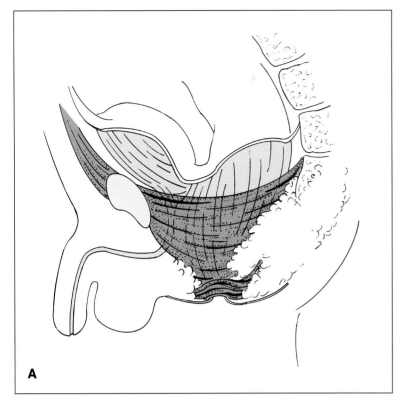

A

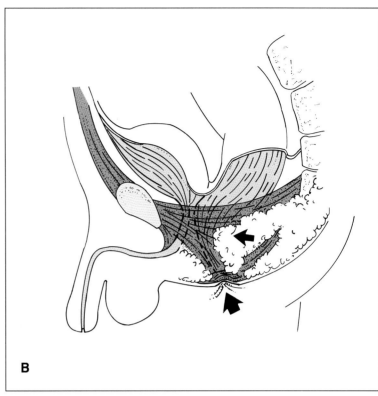

B

C

FIGURE 10-5.

Sagittal view of the normal sphincteric anatomy in a normal male during sphincter relaxation (**A**) and contraction (**B**); **C** shows the same view in a normal female. The voluntary sphincteric mechanism in both patients is represented by a funnel-like muscle structure extending from the middle of the pelvis down to the skin of the perineum.

Perineal fistula

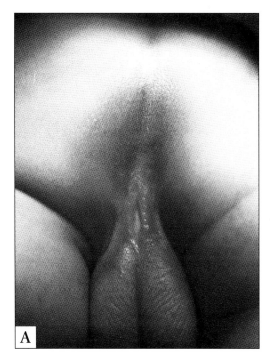

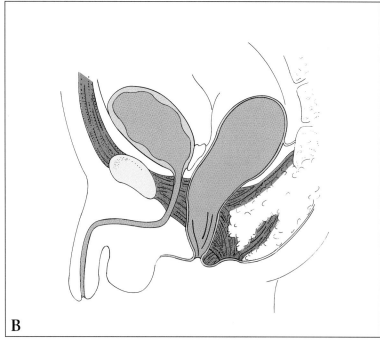

FIGURE 10-6.

When the rectum opens into the perineum, it is a low malformation called *perineal fistula*. This is a benign condition, does not require a protective colostomy, and has an excellent prognosis for future bowel function (**A** and **B**). It is best treated with a small operation called *posterior sagittal anoplasty* (PSAP), which is usually performed in newborns. Babies with perineal fistula rarely have associated malformations. Their perineum looks almost normal and they have a prominent intergluteal groove. During the first 24 hours of life, they usually pass meconium through a small fistula orifice located somewhere in the midline, anterior to the anal dimple, in the perineum, at the base of the scrotum, or sometimes at the base of the penis. Sometimes they show a midline "black-ribbon-like" subepithelial meconium fistula, and at other times they have a prominent midline skin tag located in the anal dimple, below which one can pass an instrument. This last defect is called *bucket-handle malformation.*

Rectourethral bulbar fistula

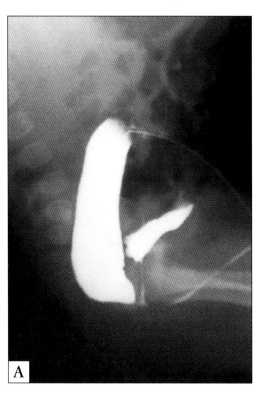

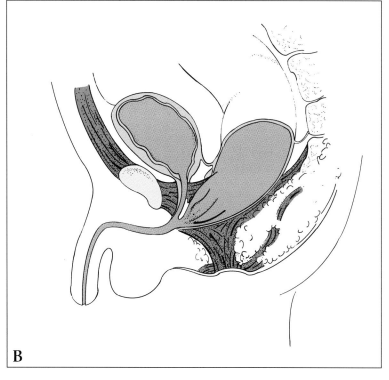

FIGURE 10-7.

Most male patients with anorectal malformations have an abnormal communication between the rectum and the urinary tract called *rectourinary fistula*. The specific location of the fistula has important therapeutic and prognostic implications.

A–B, In cases of rectourethral bulbar fistula, the rectum communicates with the lower posterior portion of the urethra called *bulbar*. The sacrum is usually

(*continued on next page*)

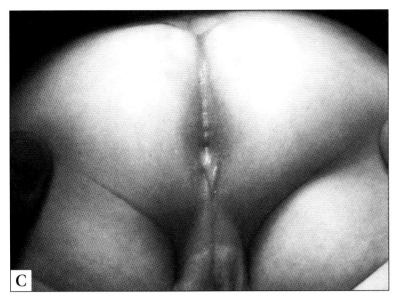

FIGURE 10-7. (CONTINUED)

normal, indicating in general a good prognosis for bowel and urinary function. Most of the time, meconium can be detected by filtering the urine through a gauze placed at the tip of the penis or can be confirmed by urinalysis. The passing of meconium through urine usually occurs after 16 to 24 hours of life, when enough intraluminal bowel pressure has been developed to force the meconium through the fistula. **C,** The perineum is usually almost normal; babies with recto-urethral-bulbar fistulae have a prominent midline groove and a noticeable anal dimple, indicating the presence of a good sphincteric muscle mechanism. A colostomy is indicated followed by a final repair called *posterior sagittal anorectoplasty* done on an elective basis later in life. Incidence of associated urologic defects is about 20% to 30% [5,6].

Rectourethral prostatic fistula

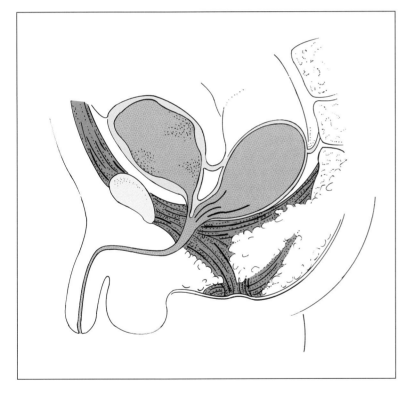

FIGURE 10-8.

In cases of rectourethral prostatic fistula, the rectum communicates with the upper portion of the posterior urethra, passing through prostatic tissue. The sacrum is frequently abnormal, indicating that these patients have different degrees of nerve deficiency in the pelvis, which means that the prognosis for bowel control in the future life of these babies is not as good as with the previous two defects. The passing of meconium through the urethra follows the same pattern described for rectourethral bulbar fistula cases. The perineum shows a tendency to be slightly flat with a small prominent midline groove and a rather inconspicuous anal dimple, indicating the sphincteric muscle mechanism is not well developed. The therapeutic approach is the same as described for cases of bulbar-urethral fistula, and the chances of having an associated urologic malformation are slightly higher than in cases of bulbar fistula [5,6].

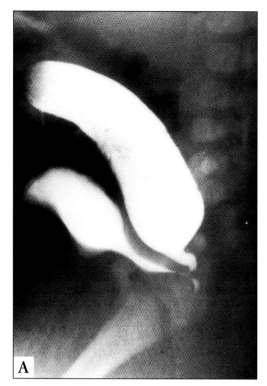

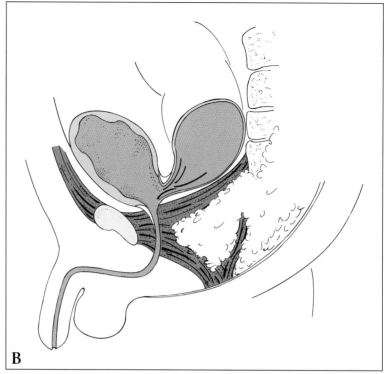

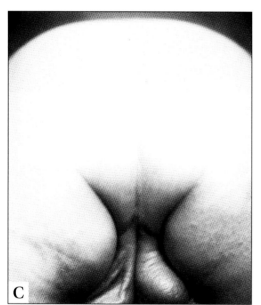

FIGURE 10-9.

Rectobladder neck fistula is the most uncommon defect with a recto-urinary fistula seen in male patients. **A–B,** The rectum communicates with the bladder neck and the sacrum is usually very abnormal, indicating the existence of a serious nerve deficiency, which will translate into a poor prognosis for future bowel control. Sometimes the patient also suffers from urinary incontinence. The passing of meconium through the urinary tract may occur earlier than in the previously described cases owing to the fact that the fistula is bigger. **C,** The perineum is most likely flat, with little or no midline groove and an absent anal dimple, indicating that these babies have very poorly developed sphincters. The chances of having an associated urinary defect is higher than 80% [5,6], and therefore an ultrasound study of the abdomen is mandatory, followed by a urologic evaluation, if indicated, prior to the opening of the colostomy. The main repair in these cases is performed later in life on an elective basis and includes a posterior sagittal anorectoplasty plus a laparotomy to mobilize a rectum that cannot be mobilized from below. Fortunately, this defect occurs in approximately 10% of all the male cases [9].

Female defects

Perineal fistula

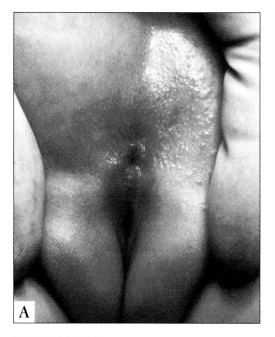

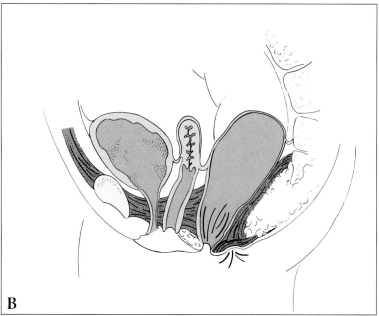

FIGURE 10-10.

Clinical diagnosis of the specific type of defect and deciding whether to open a colostomy in cases of female patients are usually easier than in male patients because approximately 90% of female patients have a fistula to the genitalia or to the perineum [9].

A–B, Perineal fistula is the most benign defect seen in female patients. The rectum opens through an abnormal orifice (fistula) located in the perineum, (ie, between the genitalia and the anal dimple). Characteristics of the sacrum, associated defects, prognosis for bowel function, and treatment are the same as mentioned for this defect in male patients (see Fig. 10-6).

Vestibular fistula

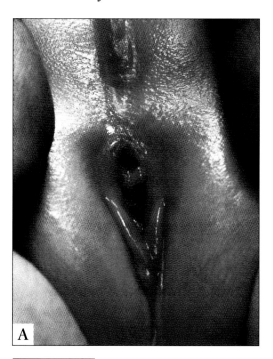

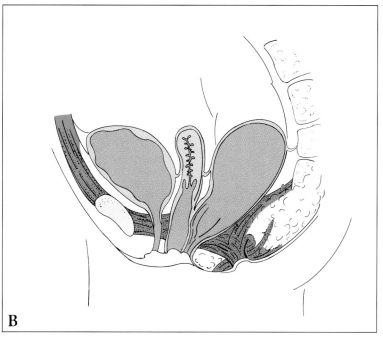

FIGURE 10-11.

A–B, Vestibular fistula is by far the most frequent defect seen in females [9]. The rectum opens through an abnormally narrow orifice located in the vestibule of the genitalia, (ie, immediately outside the hymen). The sacrum is usually normal and the perineum is consistent with the presence of good sphincteric mechanisms. More than 90% of patients with vestibular fistula achieve bowel control when adequately managed. The incidence of associated urinary malformations is lower than 20% [5,6]. A colostomy is indicated during the first few days of life, but it does not have to be opened on an emergency basis because the fistula usually allows the decompression of the bowel. The colostomy is still indicated, however, to avoid dilatation of the bowel and to protect the final repair (posterior sagittal anorectoplasty), which must be done later in life on an elective basis. Even when these patients have a fistula, one must not expect to see meconium coming out through the genitalia before 20 hours of life.

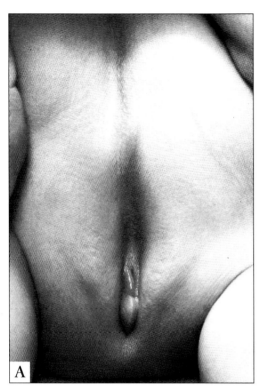

A

FIGURE 10-12.

A–C, Persistent cloaca, a complex malformation, is defined as a defect in which the rectum, vagina, and urinary tract are fused together into a common channel that communicates exteriorly through a single perineal orifice located at the normal urethral site. These defects represent a spectrum because one can expect an enormous variety of anatomic forms, characteristics of the sacrum, quality of sphincters, and associated defects. The diagnosis of a persistent cloaca is easily established purely on clinical grounds; the patient's genitalia appear to be smaller than normal, and a meticulous inspection and the separation of the labia disclose a single perineal orifice, which is characteristic of this defect. These patients may have a full spectrum of sphincter development, showing anything from a completely "flat bottom" with minimal or no sphincters to an almost normal midline groove with a prominent anal dimple, indicating the presence of a good sphincteric mechanism. Likewise, the sacrum may show different degrees of development, which accounts for the great variation of prognosis for bowel and urinary control. A patient suffering from a cloaca has about a 90% chance of having an associated urologic defect [5,6]; therefore, as in the cases of bladder neck fistulas in males, these patients represent a potential urologic emergency, and thus, an abdominal ultrasound examination must always be performed prior to the opening of a colostomy followed by a urologic workup when necessary. These babies need a diverting colostomy, and many times during the same procedure, some sort of urinary diversion (vesicotomy, ureterostomy) or vaginal diversion (vaginostomy) in cases of obstructed, distended vaginas. When the baby is older than 6 months, the entire malformation is repaired with an operation called *posterior sagittal anorectovaginourethroplasty.* This procedure is a long, complex, meticulous operation done in a few specialized centers. About 40% of the time it is necessary to open the abdomen simultaneously with the posterior approach to reach and mobilize a very highly located rectum or vagina.

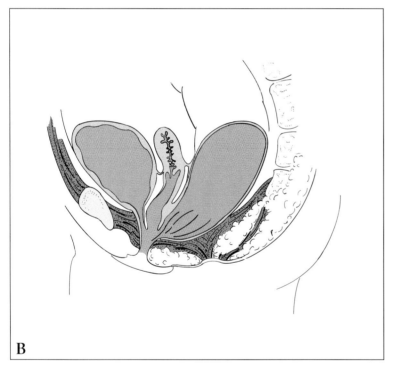

B

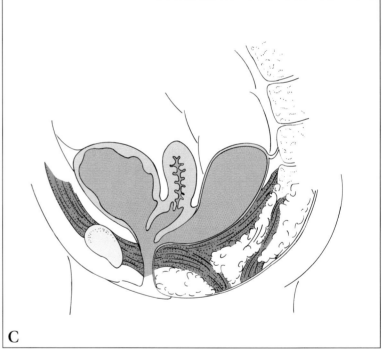

C

COLOSTOMY CREATION

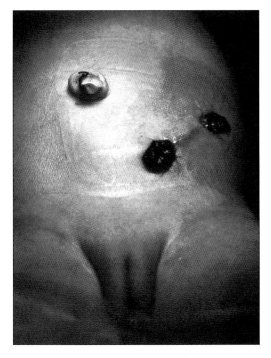

FIGURE 10-13.

The formation of a colostomy prior to the repair of an anorectal malformation is indicated in cases except those considered very low, such as cases of perineal fistulas. The best type of colostomy is a descending type with stomas separated enough to allow the use of a stoma bag in the functional site [10].

In cases of female babies with cloacas, the surgeon must establish a urologic diagnosis prior to the opening of the colostomy. More than 90% of these children are born with defects, such as vesicoureteral reflux, hydronephrosis, absent kidney, ureteropelvic obstruction, or megacystogenic or neurogenic bladder, to name a few. During the newborn period, it is sometimes necessary to decompress the urinary tract on a temporary basis, (eg, by forming a ureterostomy or suprapubic cystostomy). Later in life, the entire urologic defect will be corrected. Over 50% of these patients suffer from overdistended hemivaginas with a septum in between. These dilated structures compress the trigone interfering with the drainage of the ureters. These patients, therefore, need a vaginostomy to be created at the same time as the colostomy. After patients recover from the colostomy opening (and the vaginal or urinary diversion when necessary), they are discharged and followed up by the pediatrician.

Preposterior sagittal anorectoplasty

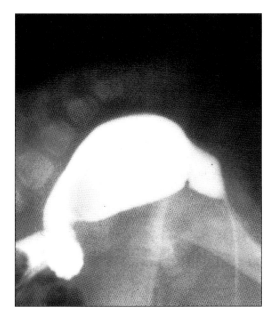

FIGURE 10-14.

A distal colostogram is the most important radiologic study to determine the location of the most distal part of the bowel and to document the presence and location of a fistula between the bowel and the urogenital tract. This test is generally done on an outpatient basis [11].

The posterior sagittal anorectoplasty is a complex detailed operation. Generally, this second stage of the surgical repair is performed in patients older than 1 month of age, provided the baby is growing and developing normally. It entails a midline posterior sagittal incision. The rectum is then meticulously separated from the genitourinary tract, dissected, and freed enough to reach its normal site without tension. The fistula site is then closed. With the use of an electrical muscle stimulator, the limits of the sphincteric mechanism are determined, and the rectum is placed in its optimal location to achieve the best functional results. Two weeks after the main repair, a program of anal dilatations is started. The dilatations prevent the anal stricture from scar tissue formation around the anus. Eventually, after about 6 to 8 weeks, the parent will reach the "desired size" predetermined by the surgeon. Once the desired size of dilatation has been reached, the colostomy can be closed (*see* Table 10-3A for the desired size of dilators for different ages). The operation entails taking down both stomas and performing a bowel anastomosis to re-establish colon continuity.

POSTOPERATIVE BOWEL FUNCTION

TABLE 10-3A. DESIRED SIZE OF DILATORS FOR DIFFERENT AGES

1–4 months old	#12 Hegar
4–8 months old	#13 Hegar
8–12 months old	#14 Hegar
1–4 years old	#15 Hegar
Older than 4 years	#16 Hegar

TABLE 10-3B. PROTOCOL FOR TAPERING ANAL DILATATIONS

Once a day for 1 month
Every other day for 1 month
Twice a week for 1 month
Once a week for 1 month
Once a month for 3 months

TABLE 10-3.

A, Desired size of of dilators for different ages. B, Protocol for tapering the frequency of anal dilatations.

TABLE 10-4. INDICATORS FOR BOWEL CONTROL

INDICATORS OF GOOD PROGNOSIS FOR BOWEL CONTROL	INDICATORS OF POOR PROGNOSIS FOR BOWEL CONTROL
Normal sacrum	Abnormal sacrum (more than two vertebrae missing)
Prominent midline groove (good muscles)	Flat perineum (poor muscles)
Rectal atresia	Rectobladder neck fistula
Vestibular fistula	Some rectoprostatic fistulas
Most patients with imperforate anus without a fistula	Some rectovaginal fistulas
Low cloaca	
Most patients with urethral bulbar fistula	
Some patients with rectoprostatic fistula	
Exceptional cases of rectobladder fistulas	
Low defects (perineal fistulas)	

TABLE 10-4.

Patients who have surgical procedures for anorectal malformations may achieve bowel control or may suffer from different degrees of fecal incontinence. The surgeon can say in advance which patients have good functional prognosis and which patients have poor prognosis.

TABLE 10-5. PROGNOSTIC SIGNS

GOOD PROGNOSTIC SIGNS	BAD PROGNOSTIC SIGNS
Good bowel movement pattern (1–3 bowel movements per day and no soiling between bowel movements)	Urinary incontinence (dribbling of urine)
Urinary control	Constant soiling and passing stool
Evidence of sensation when passing stool (pushing, making faces)	No sensation (no pushing)

TABLE 10-5.

We do not expect children born with anorectal malformations to become toilet trained for stool before 2.5 to 3 years of age. Before that age, however, there are some signs that have a prognostic value concerning the possibility for these patients becoming toilet trained.

Patients born with poor prognostic malformations or showing bad prognostic signs are offered a *Bowel Management Program*, which keeps them clean and thus more socially accepted because it is unlikely they will become toilet trained.

BOWEL MANAGEMENT PROGRAM

TABLE 10-6A. TYPES OF FECAL INCONTINENCE

INCONTINENCE WITH CONSTIPATION	INCONTINENCE WITH DIARRHEA
Rectum preserved	Absent rectosigmoid
Megasigmoid	Status post-abdominoperineal procedures with endorectal dissection
Status post-anoplasty, sacral approach, posterior sagittal anorectoplasty	Status post-colectomies

TABLE 10-6B. BOWEL MANAGEMENT FOR PATIENTS SUFFERING FROM FECAL INCONTINENCE

GOALS

To clean the colon once a day
To keep the colon quiet in between enemas or irrigations

TABLE 10-6.

Three specific factors must be present for the child to be fecally continent. First, the child needs to have sensation within the rectum. Children born with anorectal malformations lack the intrinsic sensation to differentiate between stool or gas passing through the rectum. Therefore, many times the child may unknowingly soil. Second, the child needs to have good motility of the colon. High-amplitude peristaltic waves that traverse to the colon occur many times each day in infants and are associated with movement of luminal contents into the rectum. Children with anorectal malformations most frequently suffer from hypomotility of the rectosigmoid, the stool remaining stagnant, causing constipation, and encopresis (overflow incontinence). Also, the rectum does not empty in discrete episodes, but rather keeps passing stool constantly, which may significantly interfere with bowel continence. Third, the child needs to possess good voluntary muscles or sphincteric mechanism. These muscles allow for good control and retention of stool. Children with anorectal malformations lack different degrees of development of their sphincteric mechanism.

A, Patients suffering from fecal incontinence consecutive to the treatment of imperforate anus can be divided into two well-defined groups. Patients suffering from fecal incontinence with constipation were mainly subjected to operations in which the rectum is preserved (anoplasties, posterior sagittal anorectoplasty, and sacroperineal pull-throughs). Patients suffering from fecal incontinence with diarrhea were mainly subjected to operations in which the rectum and sometimes the sigmoid colon were resected (abdominoperineal procedures, endorectal resections), or the patient loses a portion of the colon for some other reason or suffers from some sort of condition that produces diarrhea. Each of these groups of patients must be treated in a different way.

B, The basis of the *Bowel Management Program* consists in teaching the parents or patient (when more than 12 years old) to clean the colon everyday by the use of enemas or colonic irrigations, followed by finding a mechanism to keep the colon quiet for the following 24 hours to avoid soiling episodes and involuntary bowel movements. This last goal is achieved by the use of specific diets and medications, such as loperamide. The goal is usually achieved within 1 week through a process of trial and error.

TABLE 10-7. BOWEL MANAGEMENT ACCORDING TO TYPE OF INCONTINENCE

WITH CONSTIPATION	WITH DIARRHEA
Emphasis in large enemas or irrigations (large volume)	Low-volume enemas
No diet	Constipating diet
No medications	Loperamide or diphenoxylate

TABLE 10-7.

Bowel management in patients with constipation is geared toward the cleaning of the colon and, therefore, emphasizes large enemas or colonic irrigations. There is no need to use any special diet or medication.

We use Fleet's (phosphate) enemas (C.B. Fleet Co., Lynchburg, VA) mostly because of their convenience. However, pure saline enemas are often just as effective and, of course, cheaper. Children over 8 years of age may receive one adult Fleet enema daily; children between 3 to 8 may receive only one pediatric Fleet a day. Patients should never receive more than one Fleet enema per day; more than that exposes the child to phosphate intoxication and hypocalcemia. The Fleet enema administered in a routine way is expected to provoke a bowel movement followed by a period of 24 hours of complete cleanliness, in which case there is no more treatment required. If one enema is not enough to clean the colon, however, the patient requires a more aggressive treatment. High colonic washings are indicated with a Foley catheter attached to the tip of the bottle of the Fleet enema.

If the child soils at any point during the following 24 hours, it means that the bowel was not washed enough and, therefore, a more aggressive technique must be conducted that may include increasing the volume of the enema or administering a second saline enema 30 minutes later. The program is very individualized and the parents (and the child if they are old enough) learn to look at the consistency and amount of stool obtained after the enema. After a time, the parents will know when the enema was not effective and when they need to repeat it with saline solution.

Patients with constipation

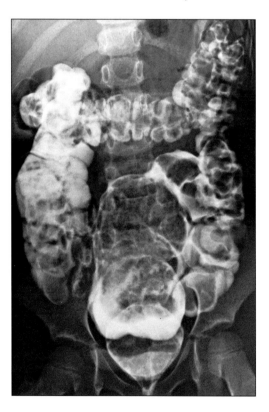

FIGURE 10-15.

There is one specific group of patients who are subjected to a surgical repair of an anorectal malformation for which a good prognosis has been assigned based on the quality of the sacrum and type of sphincters. The operation is performed in a technically correct manner and the rectosigmoid is preserved. This patient is expected to be toilet trained for stool and to suffer from some degree of constipation. Yet, some patients have severe constipation associated with a megasigmoid [12]. They may sometimes go a week without bowel movements. They are referred to the doctor with the diagnosis of "fecal incontinence." A contrast enema demonstrates the presence of a giant megasigmoid. They require a very aggressive program of enemas to be kept clean. An alternative is to offer them an operation consisting of resection of the most dilated portion of their megasigmoid. This operation may not only make them more manageable but may also make them fecally continent, which demonstrates that they were not really fecally incontinent but rather suffered from severe constipation, encopresis, or overflow pseudoincontinence [12]. When the constipation is not so severe, administration of laxatives can have the same effect as the operation.

Patients with diarrhea

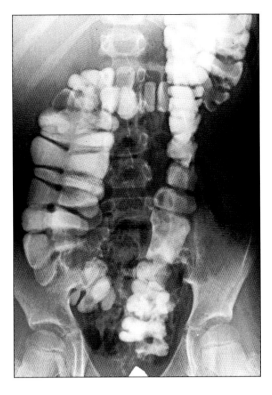

FIGURE 10-16.

Patients with diarrhea, by definition, have a short colonic transit time. Most of these patients do not have a rectosigmoid because it was resected during the repair of their defect. In other words, they do not have a reservoir. As a consequence, even when an enema may clean their colon, they pass stool fairly soon after the application of the enema because the stool travels relatively quickly from the cecum to the descending colon and the anus. To prevent this, we recommend a constipating diet or medications to slow down the colon, such as loperamide (*see* Table 10-6). A list of constipating meals is given to the parents to be promoted as part of the regular diet of the patient as well as a list of laxative meals to be avoided, which must be part of their "blacklist." Most sensitive parents know which meals provoke diarrhea and which constipate their child. Patients with diarrhea are the more difficult to manage. Sometimes, despite all of their efforts, the patients may have a very active or a very short colon. In this case, we must accept that the patient is not manageable. In this last circumstance, we offer the patient a permanent colostomy. Fortunately, however, such a situation is exceptional.

In patients subjected to a successful *Bowel Management Program* [13,14] using enemas, the parents frequently ask if this program will be needed for life. The answer is "yes" for patients born with a defect with a poor prognosis (very high defect, poor sacrum, and poor sphincters). However, because we are dealing with a spectrum of defects, there are patients with some degree of bowel control. We subject them to the *Bowel Management Program* because we do not want to expose them to occasional embarrassing accidents of uncontrolled bowel movements at school. However, as time goes by, the patients become more cooperative, more interested, and more concerned about the problem. It is conceivable that later in life a patient may stop using enemas and remain clean by following a specific regimen of a disciplined diet with regular meals to provoke bowel movements at a predictable time. Thus, every summer patients with some potential for bowel control can experiment on how well they can control their bowel movements without the help of enemas.

Lately, we have been performing a special operation for patients with fecal incontinence reluctant to accept enemas. This operation is an appendicostomy, which is also called the *Malone procedure* [15]. The cecal appendix is connected to the umbilicus in a rather inconspicuous manner. Once a day while sitting on the toilet the patient passes a feeding tube through the umbilicus into the cecum, and by gravity the saline solution runs through the colon and comes out with stool through the anus. My experience with this procedure is limited to six patients, but all of them expressed their satisfaction with this procedure.

This description does not, by any means, exhaust our *Bowel Management Program*. There are many variations depending on patient need. We have found that it takes dedication, determination, consistency, and love for everyone involved. Children who have completed the *Bowel Management Program* and remain clean for 24 hours experience a new sense of confidence based on an improved quality of life.

■ REFERENCES

1. Brenner EC: Congenital defects of the anus and rectum. *Surg Gynecol Obstet* 1915, 20:579–588.

2. Santulli TV: Treatment of imperforate anus and associate fistulas. *Surg Gynecol Obstet* 1952, 95:601–614.

3. Truffler GA, Wilkinson RH: Imperforate anus: A review of 147 cases. *Can J Surg* 1962, 5:169–177.

4. Murken JD, Albert A: Genetic counseling cases of anal and rectal atresia. *Prog Pediatr Surg* 1976, 9:115–118.

5. Rich MA, Brock WA, Peña A: Spectrum of genitourinary malformations in patients with imperforate anus. *Pediatr Surg Int* 1988, 3:110–113.

6. Parrot TS: Urologic implications of anorectal malformations. *Urol Clin North Am* 1985, 12:13–21.

7. Wangensteen OH, Rice CO: Imperforate anus: A method of determining the surgical approach. *Ann Surg* 1930, 92:77–81.

8. Narasimharao KA, Prassad GR, Katariya S: Prone cross-table lateral view: An alternative to the invertogram in imperforate anus. *AJR Am J Roentgenol* 1983, 140:227–229.

9. Peña A: Posterior sagittal anorectoplasty: Results in the management of 332 cases of anorectal malformations. *Pediatr Surg Int* 1988, 3:94–104.

10. Wilkins S, Peña A: The role of colostomy in the management of anorectal malformations. *Pediatr Surg Int* 1988, 3:105–109.

11. Gross GW, Wolfson PJ, Peña A: Augmented-pressure colostogram in imperforate anus with fistula. *Pediatr Radiol* 1991, 21:560–562.

12. Peña A, El Behery M: Megasigmoid: A source of pseudo incontinence in children with repaired anorectal malformations. *J Ped Surg* 1993, 28:1–5.

13. Peña A: Advances in the management of fecal incontinence secondary to anorectal malformations. In *Surgery Annual*. Edited by Nyhus LM. Connecticut: Appleton & Lange; 1990:143–167.

14. Peña A: Current management of anorectal anomalies. *Surg Clin North Am* 1992, 72:1393–1416.

15. Malone PS, Ransley PG, Kiely EM: Preliminary report: The antegrade continence enema. *Lancet* 1990, 336:1217–1218.

Chapter 11

Pediatric Liver Disease

PHILIP ROSENTHAL

Pediatric hepatology has been transformed from a mainly descriptive discipline of the liver disorders of infancy and childhood to a discipline more like its adult counterpart in that it has undergone an explosion in acquisition of understanding of the genetic, biochemical, and virologic bases of hepatic diseases. Pediatric liver transplantation has become highly successful and has been instrumental in expanding clinical knowledge of various pediatric hepatic disorders. Many hereditary disorders that affect the liver now have new and novel therapies as a result of this research. Major advances in molecular biologic techniques have allowed localization of many hepatic hereditary disorders to specific genes; the dawn of selective gene therapy to correct inborn errors of metabolism is quickly approaching.

This chapter is devoted to liver disorders in infancy and childhood. I have attempted wherever possible to describe the fetal and neonatal development of the liver and contrast this with adult function in an attempt to highlight the unique aspects of hepatic disorders presenting in childhood. Thus, I attempt to discuss specifically pediatric aspects of diseases knowing that other chapters deal with the complications of many of these same disorders that occur in adulthood. This chapter is a compilation of both the common and more unusual hepatic disorders associated with childhood. Because so many of the metabolic disorders present during infancy, a significant portion of this chapter is devoted to such disorders.

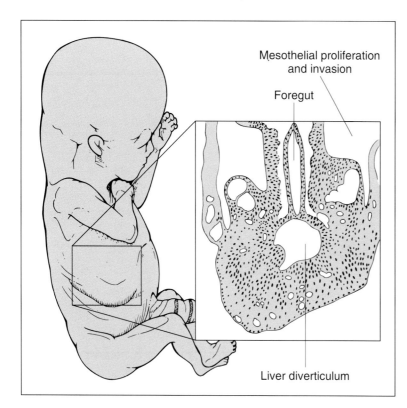

FIGURE 11-1.

FIGURE 11-1.

Embryologic development of the liver. The human liver is derived from the liver diverticulum and the septum transversum. The liver diverticulum, formed from proliferation of endodermal cells at the cranioventral junction of the yolk sac with the foregut, penetrates the septum transversum in a cranioventral direction. The septum transversum is composed of mesenchymal cells and a capillary plexus formed by the branches of the two vitelline veins and transversed by the umbilical vein. Between the third and fourth weeks of gestation, the diverticulum enlarges to form a double diverticulum and projects as an epithelial plug into the septum transversum. The solid cranial portion develops into the hepatic parenchyma forming cords of hepatocytes and intrahepatic bile ducts. The smaller cystic caudal portion forms through a process of elongation and recanalization of the primordium of the gallbladder, common bile duct, and cystic duct. The hepatocytes grow as thick sheets between branching channels of the vitelline veins to form a network of interdigitating hepatocytes and sinusoidal vessels (*Adapted from* Elias [1].)

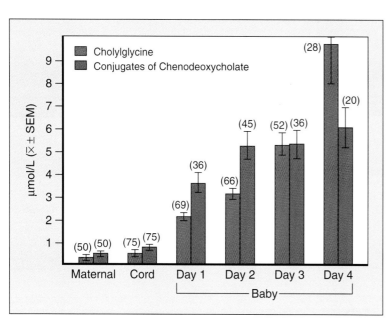

FIGURE 11-2.

Development of bile flow in the infant. Using serum bile acid concentrations as a measure of the efficiency of hepatic transport, during the first week of life, concentrations of primary bile acid conjugates increase progressively in the serum to levels even higher than seen in normal children or adults and comparable with levels observed in patients with cholestatic liver disease. A gradual decline to adult values occurs after 6 months of life. This period has been referred to as *physiologic cholestasis of the newborn*. (Numbers in parentheses indicate the number of subjects in each group.) (*From* Suchy [2]; with permission.)

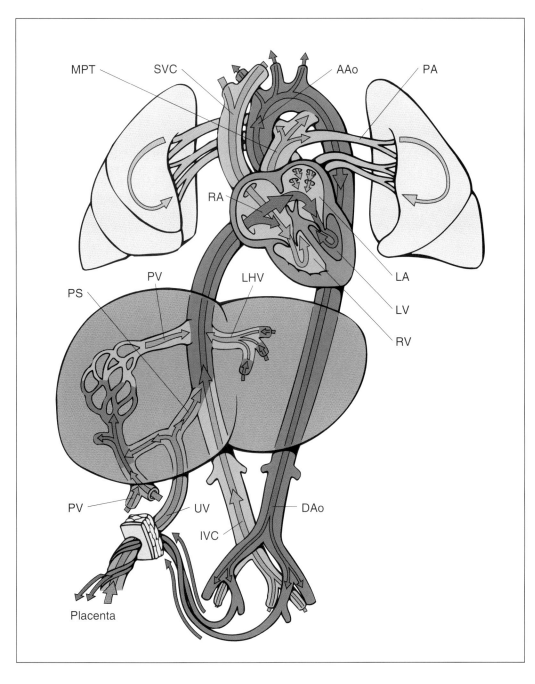

FIGURE 11-3.

Hepatic blood flow in the fetus. The fetus depends on the placenta for oxygenation. The fetal liver receives blood from the umbilical vein, hepatic arteries, and portal vein. The patterns of distribution of fetal hepatic blood flow have been described using microsphere techniques in near-term fetal lambs. Of the umbilical venous blood flow, half enters the liver and half bypasses the liver through the ductus venosus, which carries this relatively high-oxygen-content blood through the foramen ovale to the left atrium and ventricle to be delivered to the myocardium and brain. Of the total fetal liver blood supply, 75% is from the umbilical vein, 15% to 20% from the portal vein, and 5% to 10% from the hepatic arteries. Hepatic artery and umbilical venous blood flows are equally divided between the right and left liver lobes. Portal venous blood is diverted 90% to the right lobe, 10% to the ductus venosus, and none to the left lobe. The left lobe receives 95% of its blood supply from the umbilical vein and 5% from the hepatic artery. The right lobe receives 60% of its blood flow from the umbilical vein, 30% from the portal vein, and 10% from the hepatic artery. At birth, the placenta is eliminated and umbilical blood flow, the major source of fetal hepatic blood flow, abruptly ceases. Total portal blood flow increases significantly within hours after birth. AAo—ascending aorta; DAo—descending aorta; DV—ductus venosus; IVC—inferior vena cava; LA—left atrium; LHV—left hepatic vein; MPT—main pulmonary trunk; PA— pulmonary artery; PS—portal sinus; PV—portal vein; RA—right atrium; RHV—right hepatic vein; SVC—superior vena cava; UV—umbilical vein. (*Adapted from* Heymann [3].)

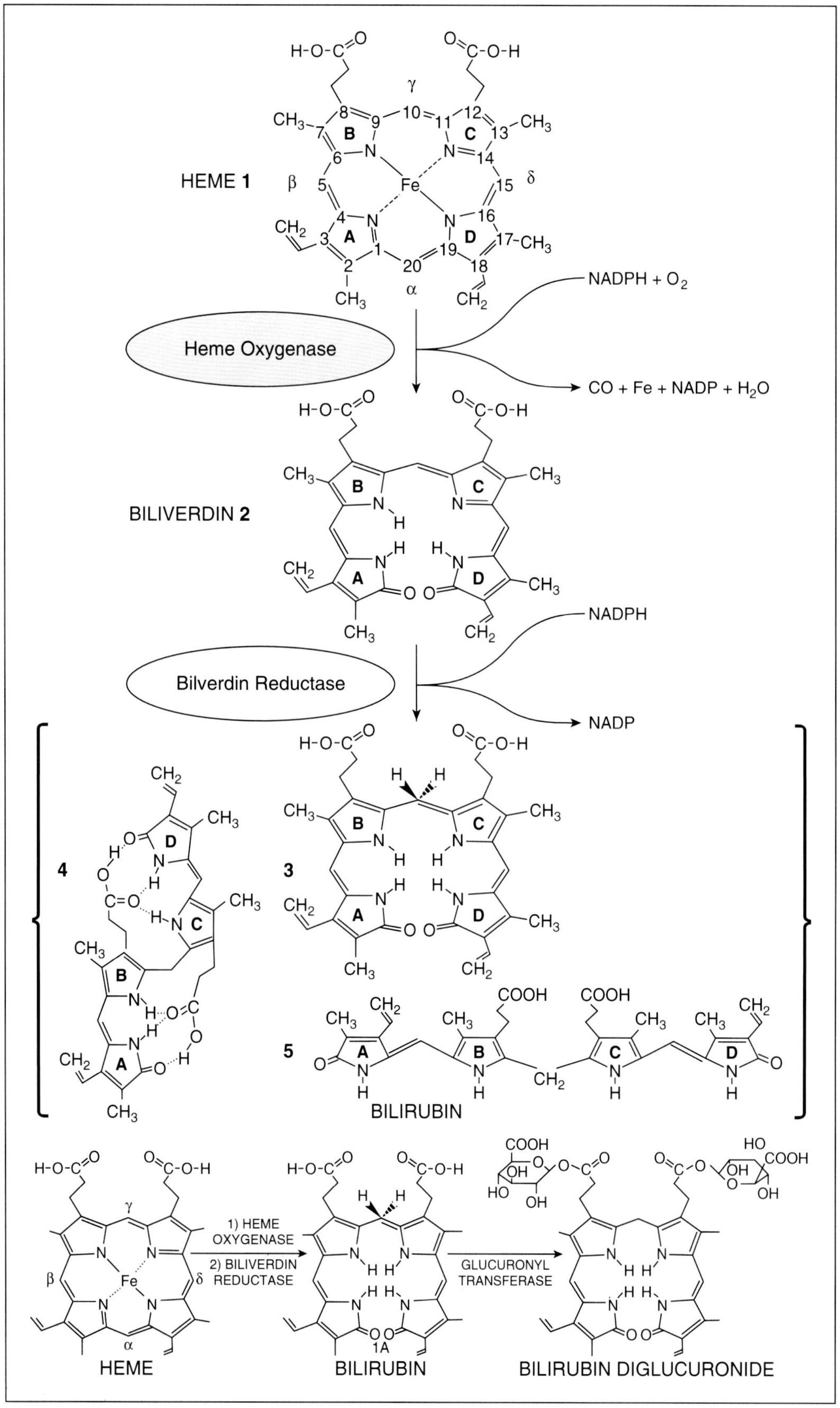

FIGURE 11-4.

Bilirubin synthetic pathway. Bilirubin is the end product of heme degradation. Heme oxygenase, the rate-limiting enzyme in the pathway, can be inhibited by the administration of various metalloporphyrins (Sn-protoporphyrin, Zn-mesoporphyrin) and has been used to reduce bilirubin production in human newborns. Unconjugated bilirubin is conjugated to form two bilirubin monoglucuronides (C-8 or C-12) or bilirubin diglucuronide. (*Adapted from* Suchy [4] and McDonagh *et al.* [5].)

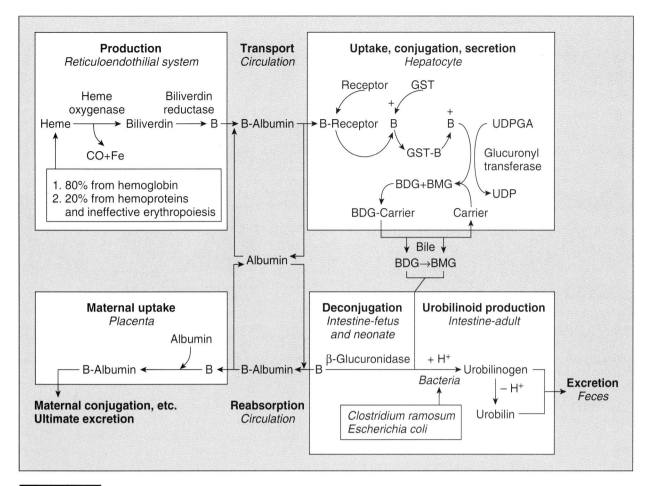

FIGURE 11-5.

An overview of bilirubin metabolism in the fetus, neonate, and adult. Fetal bilirubin is effectively eliminated by transplacental transport to the maternal circulation for conjugation and excretion. At birth, with interruption of the placenta, the newborn begins bilirubin conjugation corresponding to the period referred to as *physiologic jaundice* of the newborn during the first few days of life. Bilirubin conjugates secreted into the intestinal lumen in the newborn may be deconjugated to unconjugated bilirubin and reabsorbed through the enterohepatic circulation contributing to the increased serum bilirubin concentrations. Intestinal bacteria, not yet developed in the newborn but present in adults and older children, convert bilirubin conjugates to urobilinoids (urobilinogen, stercobilinogen) that are excreted in the stool. BDG—bilirubin diglucuronide; BMG—bilirubin monoglucuronide; GST—glutathione-S-transferase; UDP—uridine disphosphate; UDPGA—uridine disphosphate glucuronic acid. (*Adapted from* Gourley [5a]; with permission.)

■ NEONATAL CHOLANGIOPATHIES

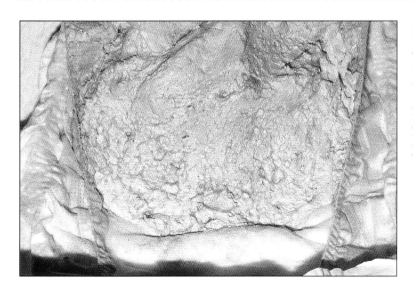

FIGURE 11-6.

Acholic stool. Stool specimen from an infant with obstruction to bile flow. Note the stool is white or acholic. Pigment in stools depends on bile flow and the presence of bilirubin conjugates secreted into the intestinal lumen wherein they may be converted to urobilinoids.

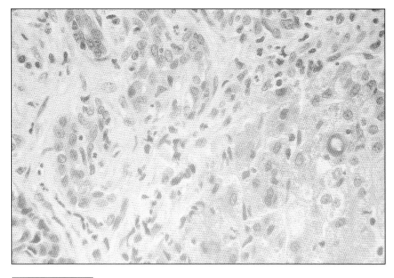

FIGURE 11-7.

Extrahepatic biliary atresia. Liver biopsy. This disorder is characterized by a necroinflammatory progressive destruction of the biliary tree including both the extrahepatic and intrahepatic bile ducts. In spite of numerous proposed mechanisms, its etiology and pathogenesis remain unknown. This slide shows the histologic characteristics of biliary atresia. There is cholestasis characterized by bilirubinostasis and bile plugs. Other findings include parenchymal giant cells (a nonspecific neonatal hepatocyte response to insult) and extramedullary hematopoiesis, ductular proliferation, and lymphocytic infiltration in the portal tracts and polymorphonuclear cells between the ductules. With continued cholestasis, portal and periportal fibrosis develop, proceeding to bridging fibrosis and cirrhosis if uncorrected. (Hematoxylin and eosin stain, original magnification × 450.)

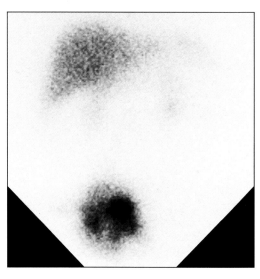

FIGURE 11-8.

Extrahepatic biliary atresia. Hepatobiliary scan of a 2-month-old child with conjugated hyperbilirubinemia and acholic stools. The scan demonstrates good uptake of tracer by the liver, but no excretion of isotope into the intestine. Instead, there is excretion of isotope through the kidneys into the urinary bladder. The evaluation of this child should proceed with a liver biopsy and an intraoperative cholangiogram to assess the patency of the extrahepatic biliary tree.

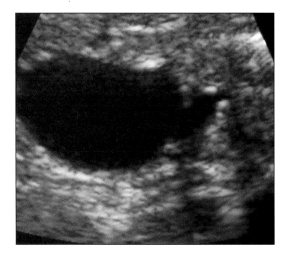

FIGURE 11-9.

Choledochal cyst. Ultrasonographic findings of a choledochal cyst in an infant who presented with direct hyperbilirubinemia and acholic stools. The incidence of choledochal cysts is between 1 in 13,000 to 1 in 2,000,000 live births with girls being affected 4 times more often than boys. The evaluation of this child should proceed with an intraoperative cholangiogram to confirm the diagnosis, to define the anatomy of the biliary tree, and to aid in determining the surgical approach for its removal. Because of the well-established potential for malignancy with choledochal cysts, the cyst should be completely excised if technically feasible. Reconstruction to allow for biliary drainage to the intestine can take several different avenues depending on the type of cyst encountered. Anastomoses include hepaticoduodenostomy, hepaticojejunostomy, or jejunal interposition.

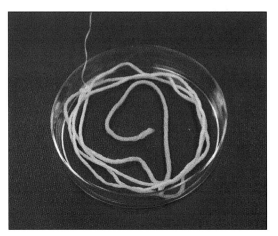

FIGURE 11-10.

Neonatal hepatitis. A string test used to collect duodenal bile from an infant with conjugated hyperbilirubinemia and a history of acholic stools. Note the yellow pigmented distal end of the string. Analysis of the fluid revealed bilirubin conjugates and bile acids confirming patency of the extrahepatic biliary tree.

TABLE 11-1. EVALUATION OF NEONATAL CONJUGATED HYPERBILIRUBINEMIA

Fractionate serum bilirubin

Serum AST, ALT, alkaline phosphatase, GGT, albumin, cholesterol

Prothrombin time

Examine stool color for pigment

Cultures (blood, urine, CSF)

Hepatitis A, B, and C screens, TORCH titers, VDRL test

Serum α-1-antitrypsin level, protease inhibitor typing

Metabolic screen: urine/serum amino acids, organic acids, urine for reducing substances

Thyroid screen

Ophthalmologic examination

Sweat chloride

Radiographs of skull, long bones, abdomen, and chest

Abdominal ultrasound

Duodenal fluid examination: color, bilirubin, bile acid analysis

Hepatobiliary scintigraphy

Percutaneous liver biopsy

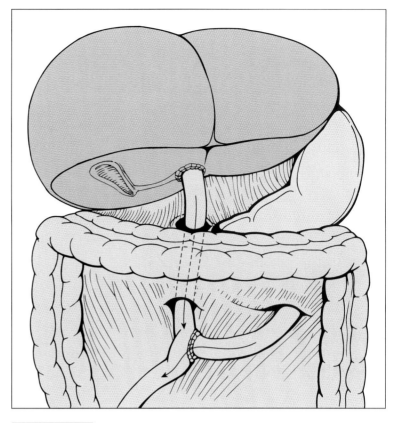

TABLE 11-1.

Evaluation of neonatal conjugated hyperbilirubinemia. These studies are suggested to aid in the evaluation of, and to determine the need for, surgical exploration. Physicians at each institution need to decide, based on the local expertise, the sequence of studies to be performed. Although no single test is capable of differentiating among the various etiologies, this systematic method of study allows efficient and cost-effective work-up. ALT—alanine aminotransferase; AST—aspartate aminotransferase; CSF—cerebrospinal fluid; GGT—γ-glutamyl transferase; TORCH—Toxoplasmosis, Other, Rubella, Cytomegalovirus, and Herpes simplex virus; VDRL—Venereal Disease Research Laboratory.

FIGURE 11-11.

Kasai portoenterostomy for extrahepatic biliary atresia. In this surgical procedure, there is excision of the extrahepatic biliary tree, identification of a ductal remnant at the porta hepatis, and anastomosis of a bowel segment to the ductal remnant in an attempt to re-establish bile flow. Success of the operation is dependent on age of the child at the time of surgery (< 60 days), degree of fibrosis and duct size at the porta hepatis, rate of bile flow following surgery, and the size, velocity, and direction of flow in the portal vein following the portoenterostomy. Cholangitis remains the most common and injurious complication of the surgery. Although many patients with a Kasai portoenterostomy eventually require liver transplantation, early portoenterostomy has a high success rate and can delay the need for hepatic transplantation until the child is a larger size, making transplantation less technically demanding, improving morbidity and mortality. For this reason portoenterostomy is primary therapy for extrahepatic biliary atresia. (*Adapted from* Altman [6].)

ALAGILLE'S SYNDROME

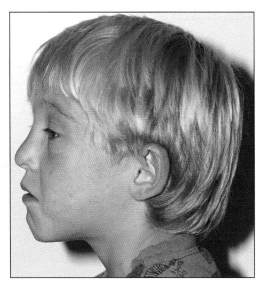

FIGURE 11-12.

Alagille's syndrome (arteriohepatic dysplasia). Typical facies associated with chronic cholestasis include frontal bossing, deep-set eyes, bulbous tip of nose, and a pointed chin. The classic syndrome includes chronic cholestasis usually presenting in infancy with significant pruritus, xanthomas, and hypercholesterolemia. Liver biopsy reveals a paucity of the interlobular bile ducts. The usual cardiac abnormality in Alagille's syndrome is peripheral pulmonic stenosis, though other cardiac anomalies, including tetralogy of Fallot and coarctation of the aorta, have been reported. The typical bone defect is *butterfly vertebrae*. Other bone defects reported include hemivertebrae, a lack of the normal progressive widening of the interpedicular distance down the lumbar spine, shortening of the distal phalanges, and an abnormally short ulna. Ophthalmologic findings in Alagille's syndrome include posterior embryotoxon (a thickening of Schwalbe's line) and retinal pigmentary changes. Recent reports suggest an association of Alagille's syndrome with small deletions on the short arm of chromosome 20 (*ie*, 20p deletion).

FAMILIAL INTRAHEPATIC CHOLESTASIS SYNDROMES

TABLE 11-2. DIFFERENTIAL DIAGNOSIS IN FAMILIAL INTRAHEPATIC CHOLESTASIS

HALLMARK	ALAGILLE'S	BYLER'S	NORWEGIAN	NAIC	GREENLAND	BRIC
Birth weight	↓	↔	↑	—	↔, ↓	—
Age at onset	< 3 mo	3–12 mo	< 3 mo	< 3 mo	< 3 mo	1–15 yr
Associated anomalies	Heart, eye, bones, kidney	None	Lymphedema	None	None	None
Chromosomal abnormalities	20p deletion	None	—	—	—	—
Attacks	—	+	+	—	—	—
Lab:						
GGTP	↑↑	↔	↑	↑	—	↔
Cholesterol	↑↑	↔	↑	↔	↔	↑
Biopsy	↓↓ Interlobular bile ducts	Centrizonal fibrosis	Portal fibrosis	Giant cells, cirrhosis	Centrizonal fibrosis	Cholestasis
Outcome	Cholestasis improves, prolonged survival	Death	Good	Death	Death	Good
Inheritance	Aut dom	Aut rec	Aut rec	Aut rec	Aut rec	?

TABLE 11-2.

Differential diagnosis. Key features that may help discriminate between these familial hepatic syndromes are shown. Cholestasis is common to these disorders; usually jaundice and pruritus are also present. Family history generally includes affected siblings or parents, consanguinity, or an inbred population. Hepatomegaly is often observed on physical examination during the early course of the disorder. Biochemical tests often reveal elevated bile acid and γ-glutamyl transpeptidase levels. Normal γ-glutamyl transpeptidase levels help to discriminate among the various types. Liver biopsy demonstrates cholestasis, a paucity of intrahepatic bile ducts when adequate portal areas are available for study, and giant cells. These disorders are characterized by persistent or recurrent bouts of cholestasis with concomitant fat malabsorption, failure to thrive, and bony abnormalities. These disorders can progress to hepatic insufficiency and portal hypertension and even occasionally hepatic malignancy. Therapy includes fat-soluble vitamin supplementation, drugs to stimulate bile flow (cholestyramine, phenobarbital, ursodeoxycholic acid), and surgery for biliary diversion or liver transplantation. Aut dom—autosomal dominant; Aut rec—autosomal recessive; BRIC—Benign Recurrent Intrahepatic Cholestasis; GGTP—γ-glutamyl transpeptidase; NAIC—North American Indian cholestasis. (*From* Riely [7]; with permission.)

TABLE 11-3. CONGENITAL HEPATIC FIBROSIS (CHF)

CHF—autosomal recessive
   polycystic kidney
   disease (infantile
   polycystic disease)

CHF—autosomal dominant
   polycystic kidney
   disease (adult
   polycystic disease)

CHF—malformation syndromes
   CHF—Meckel-Gruber syndrome
   CHF—Ivemark's syndrome
   CHF—vaginal atresia
   CHF—tuberous sclerosis
   CHF—Laurence-Moon-Biedl syndrome

CHF—no renal disease
CHF—choledochal cyst
CHF—Caroli's disease

TABLE 11-3.

Fibrocystic cholangiopathies. Congenital hepatic fibrosis and inheritable hepatorenal disorders. This table outlines the various associations of this hepatic disorder of portal fibrosis, hyperproliferation of interlobular bile ducts within the portal areas with various shapes and sizes of bile ducts and preserved lobular architecture. The hepatic abnormalities result from ductal plate malformations. Renal abnormalities accompany the hepatic disease and often manifest as renal cysts. Clinical presentation depends on the age of the patient and the extent of organ involvement. The hepatic disorder becomes clinically recognizable as the patient grows older. Nomenclature for these disorders has been confusing in the past primarily because of changes in classification of the renal cystic lesions. (*Adapted from* Suchy [4].)

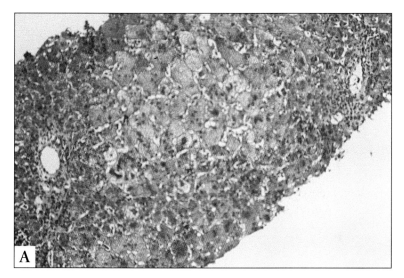 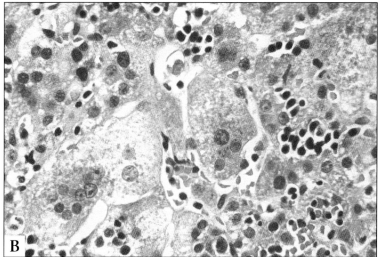

FIGURE 11-13.

Neonatal hepatitis. Needle liver biopsy from a 6-week-old infant who presented with jaundice and cholestasis. Extensive investigation, including infectious and metabolic causes, failed to reveal an etiology. At final diagnosis, neonatal hepatitis accounts for approximately 40% of all infants with cholestasis and is the most commonly encountered liver disorder in early infancy. Males predominate over females (2:1). Some familial cases have been reported suggesting either a maternal factor or autosomal recessive inheritance. **A**, Loss of lobular architecture with preservation of portal and central vein zonal distribution. **B**, Ballooning degeneration of hepatocytes and multinucleated giant cells are present. Abundant extramedullary hematopoiesis and variable amounts of inflammation may be present. (**A**, Hematoxylin and eosin stain, original magnification × 100; **B**, Hematoxylin and eosin stain, original magnification × 450.)

TABLE 11-4. FULMINANT HEPATIC FAILURE IN CHILDREN

DEFINITION

Hepatic failure within 8 weeks of onset of illness
Encephalopathy
Prolonged prothrombin time
Massive hepatic necrosis

TABLE 11-4.

Definition of fulminant hepatic failure in children. The generally accepted diagnosis of fulminant hepatic failure in a child depends on establishing the following criteria: clinical onset of liver disease within the past 8 weeks without evidence of chronic liver disease; hepatic encephalopathy; prolonged prothrombin time signifying hepatic injury and dysfunction; serum alanine aminotransferase and aspartate amino transferase levels are frequently markedly elevated; and massive hepatic necrosis or severe hepatocellular injury. This definition implies that recovery is possible if the child can be supported until the liver can regenerate itself and after the etiologic agent can be eliminated.

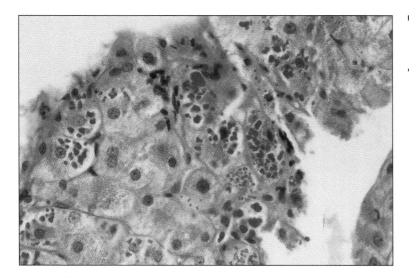

FIGURE 11-14.

Deficiency of α-1-antitrypsin. Liver biopsy. Distinctive periodic acid-Schiff-positive diastase-resistant globules in the endoplasmic reticulum of hepatocytes in a patient with α-1-antitrypsin deficiency. Homozygous protease inhibitor phenotype ZZ is a common gene disorder affecting between 1 in 1600 to 1 in 2000 live births in North America and Northern Europe. Deficient α-1-antitrypsin is the most common genetic cause of liver disease in childhood and the most common genetic disorder requiring liver transplantation in children. It is an autosomal recessive disorder that causes an 85% reduction in the circulating levels of α-1-antitrypsin in serum, premature emphysema, chronic liver disease progressing to cirrhosis and portal hypertension, and even hepatocellular carcinoma. Liver involvement is usually recognized in the first 2 months of life as persistent jaundice. Serum transaminases are elevated and hepatomegaly may be appreciated. Diagnosis is made by determining the α-1-antitrypsin phenotype. Serum α-1-antitrypsin levels may be useful but on occasion may be misleading because they may increase in response to inflammation. Liver transplantation has been successfully undertaken in children with significant liver disease resulting from α-1-antitrypsin deficiency. The recipient assumes the α-1-antitrypsin phenotype of the donor liver. Whether the pulmonary disease or recurrence of hepatic disease can occur in transplanted children awaits long-term follow-up of these individuals. (Periodic acid-Schiff stain with diastase, original magnification × 100.)

TABLE 11-5. LIVER AND BILIARY TRACT COMPLICATIONS IN CYSTIC FIBROSIS

LOCATION	COMPLICATION	INCIDENCE, %
Liver	Steatosis	20–66
	Focal biliary cirrhosis	10–72
	Multilobular biliary cirrhosis	<1–24
	Portal hypertension	<5–28
Gallbladder	Nonvisualized gallbladder	12–40
	Microgallbladder	30
	Distended gallbladder	3–20
	Atretic cystic duct	16
	Cholelithiasis	0–33
Common bile duct	Distal stenosis	10–33
	Sclerosing cholangitis	1
	Cholangiocarcinoma	Rare

TABLE 11-5.

Hepatobiliary disorders associated with cystic fibrosis (CF) in childhood. Various complications are observed in the liver and biliary tract of children with CF. With improved management of the respiratory, pancreatic, and nutritional complications, an increasing incidence of hepatobiliary disorders in CF has been seen. CF is an autosomal recessive disorder affecting 1 in 2500 live births in the white population. It is characterized by thick, tenacious secretions that obstruct the pulmonary, pancreatic, intestinal, and biliary systems. The presence of an elevated sweat chloride concentration aids in diagnosis. The CF gene encodes a protein, the CF transmembrane conductance regulator (CFTR), which is a cyclic adenosine monophosphate–dependent chloride channel. In the liver, CFTR has been localized to biliary epithelial cells but not to hepatocytes. Although over 100 mutations of the gene have been recognized, Δ F508 is a frequently encountered mutation. (*Adapted from* Suchy [4].)

TABLE 11-6. INHERITED DISORDERS OF INTRAMITOCHONDRIAL FATTY ACID OXIDATION

Deficiency	Fasting Coma	Hepatic Steatosis	Cardiomyopathy	Myopathy	Rhabdomyolysis*	Others†
MCAD	+	+				
LCAD	+	+	+	+	+	
SCAD	+	+		+	+	
HMG-CoA lyase	+	+				Profound acidosis
ETF (mild)	+	+		+		Failure to thrive, extrapyramidal movement disorder
ETF (severe)	+	+	+	+		
ETF-DH	+	+	+	+		Dysmorphic facies, polycystic kidneys, rocker-bottom feet
LCHAD	+	+	+	+	+	Lactic acidosis, retinitis pigmentosa, peripheral neuropathy
CPT II (mild)				+	+	
CPT II (severe)	+	+	+	+		
CPT I	+	+				Malignant hyperthermia
CT	+	+	+	+		

*Occurrence in late childhood, adolescence, or young adulthood.
†Described in some cases.

TABLE 11-6.

Inherited disorders of intramitochondrial fatty acid oxidation. This table lists the defects in mitochondrial β-oxidation and their common presentations. These disorders often manifest in early life with hepatomegaly, elevated serum transaminase levels, and lethargy or coma following an overnight fast or illness that results in decreased appetite and poor oral intake. Treatment for acute metabolic decompensation in these disorders includes prompt intravenous dextrose and supportive therapy (correcting electrolyte and clotting abnormalities). Chronic prophylactic therapy may include avoidance of prolonged fasts, high carbohydrate and low-fat diets, overnight feedings, or feedings with starch. CPT—carnitine palmitoyl transferase; CT—carnitine transport; ETF—electron transport flavoprotein; ETF-DH—electron transport flavoprotein-dehydrogenase; HMG—hydroxymethylglutaryl; LCAD—long-chain acyl-CoA dehydrogenase; LCHAD—long-chain 3-hydroxyacyl-CoA dehydrogenase; MCAD—medium-chain acyl-CoA dehydrogenase; SCAD—short-chain acyl-CoA dehydrogenase. (*Adapted from* Suchy [4].)

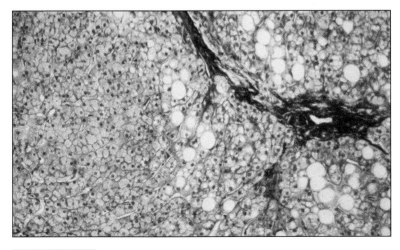

FIGURE 11-15.

Hereditary fructose intolerance. Liver biopsy findings in a 9-month-old child with failure to thrive, poor feeding, vomiting, and hepatomegaly. Note the diffuse fat droplets, scattered hepatocyte necrosis, and intralobular and periportal fibrosis. This child was being fed a soy-based formula containing sucrose. Hereditary fructose intolerance is an autosomal recessive trait affecting 1 in 20,000 people. The disorder results from a deficiency in aldolase B in the liver, kidney, and small intestine. This enzyme converts fructose-1-phosphate to d-glyceraldehyde and dihydroxyacetone phosphate. The gene for aldolase B has been localized to chromosome 9. Diagnosis involves assay of fructose-1-phosphate aldolase activity in liver or small intestinal tissue. Recent work with DNA amplification has demonstrated diagnosis of hereditary fructose intolerance based on genetic analysis of chromosome 9. Treatment requires removal of fructose and sucrose (disaccharide composed of glucose and fructose) from the diet. This is no easy task because of the wide distribution of fructose and sucrose as sweetening agents in available commercial foods and drugs. Additionally, sorbitol must be removed from the diet because it is converted to fructose. (Hematoxylin and eosin stain, original magnification × 100.)

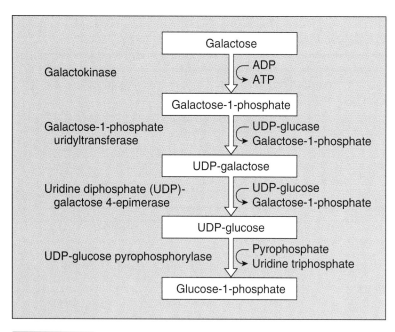

FIGURE 11-16.

Galactosemia. Galactose metabolic pathway. Reactions responsible for galactose metabolism to glucose. Galactose is a monosaccharide derived from the hydrolysis of milk sugar or lactose (disaccharide composed of glucose and galactose). Three distinct disorders of galactose metabolism with their own clinical presentation have been recognized: (1) transferase deficiency galactosemia, the classic form of the disease, char-

acterized by malnutrition, failure to thrive, cataracts, progressive hepatic disease, mental retardation, and ovarian failure; (2) galactokinase deficiency galactosemia characterized by cataract formation; and (3) epimerase deficiency galactosemia in which the defect in most cases is limited to erythrocytes and leukocytes and affected individuals display no clinical manifestations of galactosemia.

These defects are acquired by autosomal recessive inheritance. Classic galactosemia affects 1 in 50,000 live births. In classic galactosemia, newborns present with abdominal distention, vomiting, diarrhea, anorexia, and hypoglycemia after milk feeding. Jaundice and hepatomegaly develop within weeks and a persistent conjugated hyperbilirubinemia often exaggerated by severe hemolysis is observed. Continued galactose feedings result in significant hepatic damage, cirrhosis, and the development of ascites within several more weeks. Diagnosis can be suspected in an infant being fed lactose-containing milk who has positive reducing substances in urine that are negative with glucose oxidase urinary dipstick reagents. Many states that include galactosemia in their mandated newborn screen use a test that assesses erythrocyte uridine diphosphate (UDP)–glucose consumption. Treatment consists of elimination of dietary galactose found predominantly in milk and dairy products. Galactose in grains, fruits, and vegetables may, however, contribute to suboptimal improvement and may also require severe restriction. Nutritional therapy may reverse acute symptoms and biochemical abnormalities and also allow for normal growth and normalization of liver function. Neurologic disorders, mental retardation, growth retardation, and ovarian failure may, however, continue to pose problems in survivors. (*From* Suchy [4]; with permission.)

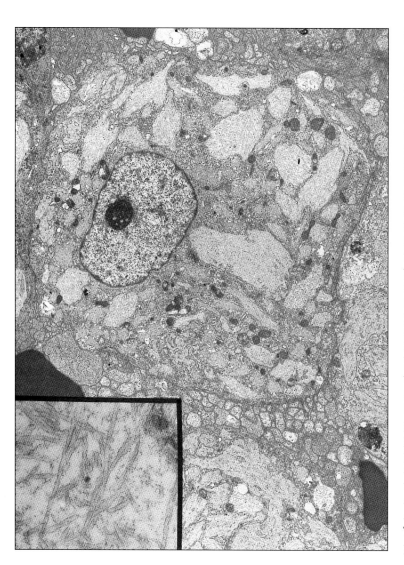

FIGURE 11-17.

Gaucher's disease. Electron photomicrograph of a Gaucher cell with stored cerebroside. Gaucher's disease is an autosomal recessive disorder resulting from a deficiency of the enzyme glucocerebrosidase (β-glucosidase), which degrades sphingolipids with terminal glucosyl residues in a β linkage. The reticuloendothelial cells in which the abnormal glycolipids accumulate produced the characteristic Gaucher cell depicted here. On electron microscopy, lysosomes filled with tubular structures are observed. The liver is involved in all forms of Gaucher's disease and massive hepatosplenomegaly is seen. Type I (adult non-neuropathic form) is most common and frequently occurs in Ashkenazi Jewish populations. Hepatomegaly and abnormal liver function are present but progression to cirrhosis and liver failure are uncommon. Type II is the severe neuropathic form, which is often fatal to patients by 2 years of age. Hepatosplenomegaly and progressive neurologic deterioration are observed. Type III has a later onset of neurologic symptoms and a more prolonged course than type II with many patients surviving into adulthood. Hepatosplenomegaly occurs in childhood and precedes the neurologic disease. Diagnosis of Gaucher's disease is confirmed by determination of β-glucocerebrosidase activity in leukocytes or cultured fibroblasts. Treatment was previously limited to symptomatic care. Recently, enzyme replacement using synthetic enzymes has shown some success but its expense makes any routine use unlikely. Bone marrow transplantation has been used successfully and gene transfer also offers potential therapy for Gaucher's disease. Orthotopic liver transplantation for the chronic adult form has been successful in several patients but the long-term success of this procedure is unclear. Lipid analysis of the transplanted organs has demonstrated reaccumulation of glucocerebroside. This figure demonstrates the classic accumulation of cerebroside in phagolysosomes. The lower left insert depicts the tubular structures seen within the phagolysosomes. (Original magnification × 7800; Inset, × 25,000.)

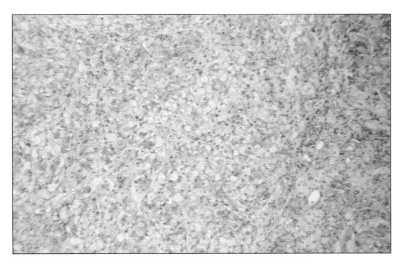

FIGURE 11-18.

Glycogen storage disease. Liver biopsy from a child with glycogen storage disease type IV. In type IV disease the periodic acid–Schiff positive material is only partially digested by diastase. Glycogen is the primary carbohydrate storage compound. Its formation and degradation are highly regulated by at least eight enzymes. Deficiencies of each enzyme have been recognized and 12 forms of glycogen storage disease are appreciated. Types I, III, and IV primarily involve the liver. Type I (glucose-6-phosphatase deficiency) is typically noted for growth failure, severe hepatomegaly, and profound hypoglycemia following short periods of fasting. Although hepatic biochemical abnormalities may be mild, hepatic adenomas and even hepatocellular carcinomas develop over the course of time. Type III (amylo-1, 6-glucosidase deficiency) is characterized by failure to grow and hepatomegaly. Fasting hypoglycemia is not as severe as in type I patients. Hepatic fibrosis may progress to cirrhosis and liver failure in some patients with type III glycogen storage disease. Muscle symptoms appear in adulthood and present as weakness and muscle wasting. Type IV (1,4, glucan-6-glycosyltransferase deficiency) is characterized by failure to thrive, hepatosplenomegaly, and abdominal distention. Shown here are hepatocytes whose cytoplasm is distended by clear, amorphous material. Progressive liver dysfunction, cirrhosis, and development of hepatic adenoma have been observed. Abnormal neuromuscular and cardiac function have been reported. Diagnosis of glycogen storage disease requires enzyme analysis, often of hepatic tissue. Dietary regimens including continuous drip feeds or starch to avoid prolonged periods of fasting have been used successfully. Orthotopic liver transplantation has been performed in type I and IV glycogen storage diseases for individuals with advanced liver disease. Improvement of cardiac glycogen deposition has been reported in type IV following liver transplantation. (Hematoxylin and eosin stain, original magnification $\times$ 100.)

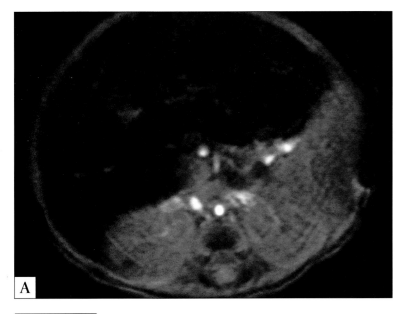

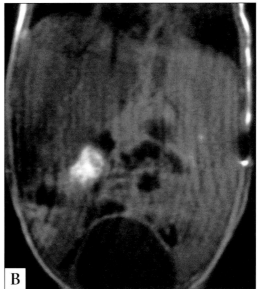

FIGURE 11-19.

Neonatal hemochromatosis. **A,** This is an axial gradient recalled echographic image of an infant with congenital hemochromatosis. The liver appears black as a result of the iron deposition. **B,** The liver is better visualized on the coronal T_1-weighted image. These infants present with fulminant hepatic failure hours after birth and have siderosis in extrahepatic sites but lack increased iron in the reticuloendothelial cells of the spleen, bone marrow, and lymph nodes. A history of recurrence in siblings may exist.

Hypoglycemia, hypoalbuminemia, edema, ascites, hemorrhagic diathesis, thrombocytopenia, and anemia may be seen in these newborns. The liver is small and bile stained. Microscopic examination reveals hepatocellular loss, collapsed stroma, and various degrees of regeneration. Hepatocytes show marked siderosis whereas Kupffer's cells are spared. Diagnosis by liver biopsy, although helpful, may be dangerous in severely ill infants with bleeding abnormalities. Magnetic resonance imaging to determine the distribution of siderosis in tissues has been useful in some patients. Neonatal hemochromatosis is distinct from adult onset hereditary hemochromatosis. Treatment has included orthotopic liver transplantation to control the symptoms of hepatic insufficiency with some success. A "cocktail" of antioxidants (n-acetylcysteine, α-tocopherol polyethylene glycol succinate, and selenium) combined with aggressive iron depletion may offer a useful and less invasive therapy.

TABLE 11-7. HEME BIOSYNTHETIC PATHWAY WITH ENZYME DEFECTS RESPONSIBLE FOR THE PORPHYRIAS

	Enzyme	Porphyria
Glycine + succinyl CoA		
↓	—	—
Delta-aminolevulinic Acid		
↓	ALA dehydrase	Acute intermittent porphyria variant (ALA dehydrase deficiency)
Porphobilinogen		
↓	Porphobilinogen deaminase	Acute intermittent porphyria
Hydroxymethylbilane		
↓	Uroporphyrinogen III cosynthase	Congenital erythropoietic porphyria
Uroporphyrinogen III		
↓	Uroporphyrinogen decarboxylase	Porphyria cutanea tarda
Coproporphyrinogen III		Hepatoerythropoietic porphyria
↓	Coproporphyrinogen oxidase	Hereditary coproporphyria
Protoporphyrinogen IX		
↓	Protophyrinogen oxidase	Variegate porphyria
Protoporphyrin IX Fe^{2+}		
↓	Ferrochelatase	Protoporphyria
Heme		

TABLE 11-7.

Heme biosynthetic pathway with enzyme defects responsible for the porphyrias. The porphyrias are a group of inherited disorders of heme biosynthesis that result in excess production of porphyrins and their precursors. Porphyrias are classified as hepatic or erythropoietic depending on the predominant site of involvement. This table depicts various enzyme deficiencies and types of porphyrias encountered.

Clinically, the porphyrias are recognized by their neurologic deficits and photocutaneous lesions. Defects in the initial portion of the heme biosynthetic pathway are associated with abdominal pain and neuropsychiatric complaints whereas more distal blocks are associated with dermatologic problems. ALA—Δ-aminolevulinic acid. (*From* Rosenthal and Thaler [8]; with permission.)

TABLE 11-8. INDIAN CHILDHOOD CIRRHOSIS

Significant cause of mortality in Indian children; some cases reported outside India

Liver biopsies show tremendous amounts of copper accumulation

Normal serum copper and ceruloplasmin levels in distinction to Wilson's disease

Association with boiled milk stored in brass or copper containers and water contaminated by copper pipes

Rapid progression from hepatomegaly and abdominal distention to cirrhosis, portal hypertension and encephalopathy in months

Treatment: D-penicillamine chelation

Prevention: Avoid contamination by copper

TABLE 11-8.

Indian childhood cirrhosis. Indian childhood cirrhosis is a significant disease contributing to mortality in India and surrounding areas in children 1 to 3 years of age. Cases outside of India have been described. An association of Indian childhood cirrhosis with the ingestion of boiled milk stored in brass containers has been observed. The copper found in these utensils is capable of binding to casein and thus perhaps exacerbates a genetic predilection to copper overload. Some cases of Indian childhood cirrhosis have been linked to copper overload as a result of contaminated water drawn from copper pipes. Similar to Wilson's disease, children with Indian childhood cirrhosis have tremendously large concentrations of hepatic copper. Unlike Wilson's disease, children with Indian childhood cirrhosis have normal or elevated serum copper and ceruloplasmin levels. Clinically, over the course of weeks to months, children with this disorder progress from hepatomegaly with abdominal distention and anorexia through jaundice, portal hypertension, and splenomegaly to ascites, cirrhosis, hepatic encephalopathy, and death. Diagnosis is considered in the appropriate clinical setting and confirmed by histologic tests and determination of the quantitative copper levels in the liver. Treatment has consisted of D-penicillamine copper chelation therapy. This has had moderate success if begun early in the course of the disease. Indian childhood cirrhosis was prevented by eliminating the practice of storing boiled milk in copper vessels.

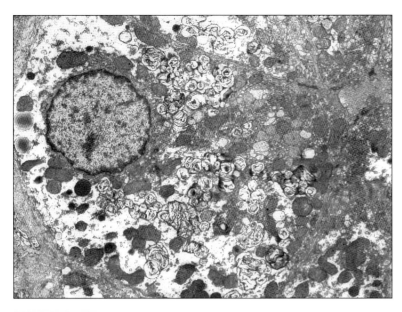

FIGURE 11-20.

Niemann-Pick disease. Electron photomicrograph from a patient with Niemann-Pick disease demonstrating whirled inclusions of sphingomyelin within lysosomes, the typical ultrastructural finding

in this disease. This disease is an autosomal recessive inherited group of disorders accompanied by hepatosplenomegaly and various amounts of sphingomyelin and cholesterol deposition in the reticuloendothelial system, viscera, and brain. Four subtypes (A,B,C, and D) are recognized based on either marked deficiency of sphingomyelinase activity (A,B) or mild or normal activity (C,D). Livers appear pale yellow as a result of fat accumulation caused by Niemann-Pick disease. Hepatocyte vacuolization and foam cells are seen throughout the parenchyma. In type C disease, cholestasis as well as a rapidly progressive form of hepatic dysfunction may be prominent in infancy. No established therapy exists for type C disease. In type A disease, neurologic deterioration may be rapidly progressive during the first years of life. This is the acute neuropathic form of the disease often affecting patients of Ashkenazi Jewish descent. Corneal opacifications may be present as may a cherry red spot in the macula. Death usually occurs by 4 years of age. Liver transplantation has been unsuccessful. Currently, there is no therapy for type A disease. Type B disease is the benign form of the disease. Many patients attain adulthood although some cases of fatal liver failure have been recorded in children. Bone marrow transplantation has been unsuccessful for type B disease. Although liver transplantation has been used in an adult with type B disease, its long-term effect remains unknown. (Original magnification $\times$ 7,500.)

TABLE 11-9. INBORN ERRORS OF BILE ACID SYNTHESIS

3β-Hydroxy-C_{27}-steroid dehydrogenase/isomerase deficiency

Δ^4–3-Oxosteroid 5β-reductase deficiency

Screening by FAB-MS

Familial, progressive infantile or pediatric cholestasis and hepatitis

Biochemistry: Elevated serum transaminase and bilirubin levels

Liver biopsy with neonatal hepatitis: Inflammation, giant cells, bile stasis, and canalicular plugs

Therapy: Oral primary bile acids

TABLE 11-9.

Inborn errors of bile acid synthesis. These recently described defects in bile acid metabolism awaited the application of a screening technique found in fast atom bombardment ionization-mass spectrometry (FAB-MS). This procedure permits rapid and direct analysis of bile acid conjugates in biologic fluids. Clinically, these defects present as familial and progressive infantile or pediatric cholestasis and hepatitis.

3β-hydroxy-C_{27}-steroid dehydrogenase/isomerase deficiency is associated with progressive jaundice, conjugated hyperbilirubinemia, and elevated serum transaminase levels but with a normal serum γ-glutamyltranspeptidase level. Hepatomegaly and fat and fat-soluble vitamin malabsorption are present. By routine methodology, serum bile acid concentrations are normal despite the severe cholestasis. Liver biopsy reveals findings characteristic of neonatal hepatitis with giant cells, inflammation, bile stasis, and canalicular plugs. Therapy consists of orally administered primary bile acids that downregulate bile acid synthesis, limit further production of potentially toxic bile acids, and stimulate bile flow. Using this approach, liver function has been normalized and jaundice resolved in several of these patients. Another recently described defect of bile acid synthesis that presents as progressive neonatal liver disease involves deficiency of the enzyme Δ^4-3-oxosteroid 5β-reductase, the fourth step in the pathway for bile acid synthesis from cholesterol. Normally seen as a familial disorder, biochemical abnormalities included elevated serum transaminase and γ-glutamyltranspeptidase levels, marked hyperbilirubinemia, and coagulopathy. Liver histology reveals giant cells and pseudoacinar formation, bile stasis, and extramedullary hematopoiesis. Treatment consists of primary bile acid (cholic acid) and ursodeoxycholic acid therapy. If initiated before significant liver damage has occurred, resolution of jaundice and normalization of liver function has been observed.

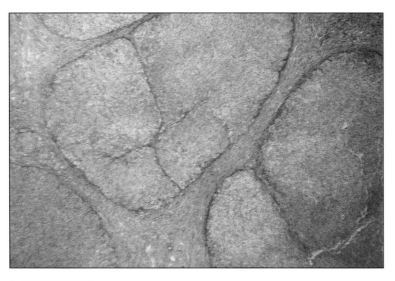

FIGURE 11-21.

Tyrosinemia. Liver biopsy specimen demonstrating micronodular cirrhosis, bile duct proliferation, and fibrotic septa. There is various steatosis and pseudoacinar formation. Tyrosinemia, an autosomal recessive trait, is caused by reduced levels of enzyme fumarylacetoacetate hydrolase, the last enzyme in the tyrosine degradation pathway.

Intermediary metabolites, maleylacetoacetate, and fumarylacetoacetate are believed responsible for the hepatic and renal symptoms observed and succinylacetone for the neurologic crises. Diagnosis of tyrosinemia should be considered in any infant with hepatocellular necrosis, cirrhosis, or impaired hepatic synthetic function. Elevated plasma tyrosine levels may suggest the disease but may also be present in other hepatic disorders. Succinylacetone in blood or urine should, however, strongly suggest the diagnosis. Enzyme assay in lymphocytes, erythrocytes, or liver tissue can confirm the diagnosis. Development of hepatocarcinoma can occur by 2 to 3 years of age. Although α-fetoprotein levels do not correlate with development of hepatocellular carcinoma in these children, a significant rise of α-fetoprotein should raise the suspicion of hepatocarcinoma. Therapy for these children has included the use of specialized formulas that restrict phenylalanine and tyrosine. Recently, treatment with NTBC [2-(2-nitro-4-trifluoro-methyl-benzoyl)-1,3-cyclohexanedione], an inhibitor of 4-hydroxyphenylpyruvate dioxygenase, has resulted in biochemical normalization of several patients with tyrosinemia. Whether the substantial risk for hepatocarcinoma is altered with NTBC remains to be learned, however. Currently, liver transplantation offers the only means of curing hepatic disease associated with tyrosinemia. Kidney transplantation may be required for some patients with advanced renal disease, the result of their tyrosinemia. (Hematoxylin and eosin stain, original magnification × 40.)

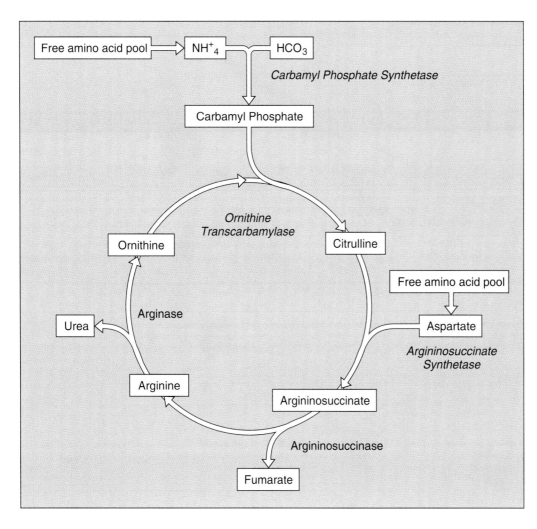

FIGURE 11-22.

Urea cycle defects. The urea cycle (Krebs-Henseleit cycle). Ammonia is detoxified to urea along this enzymatic pathway. Defects with severe hyperammonemia involving each enzyme in the cycle that can result in brain damage and death have been described. These disorders are inherited in an autosomal recessive manner except for ornithine transcarbamylase deficiency, which is X-linked. Clinically, these patients present with lethargy, irritability, and vomiting that progress to seizures, stupor, unresponsiveness, posturing, cerebral edema, increased intracranial pressure, and cerebral herniation. Patients may present in infancy, although presentation may be delayed. These patients may be erroneously mistaken for patients with fulminant liver failure and hepatic encephalopathy or with Reye's syndrome. Diagnosis is confirmed by measuring serum ammonia and plasma amino acid levels and making urinary orotic acid determinations. Occasionally, it may be necessary to obtain a liver biopsy for enzymatic analysis to confirm the diagnosis. Treatment in childhood includes dietary restrictions to allow adequate protein for growth and development. Further supplementation with citrulline or arginine, essential amino acids in these disorders, is helpful. Because dietary therapy alone is often not successful, drugs to promote waste nitrogen excretion have been used, such as sodium benzoate and sodium phenylacetate. More recently, however, sodium phenylbutyrate has been more favored.

TABLE 11-10. DIAGNOSTIC STUDIES FOR EVALUATING WILSON'S DISEASE

DIAGNOSTIC TEST	DIAGNOSTIC VALUES	CAUSES OF FALSE-POSITIVE	CAUSES OF FALSE-NEGATIVE
Serum ceruloplasmin	< 20 mg/dL	Kwashiorkor, nutritional copper deficiency, protein-losing state, fulminant hepatitis, hepatic failure, hereditary hypoceruloplasminemia, Wilson's disease heterozygote, Menkes' syndrome, normal neonate	Acute inflammation (hepatitis), malignancy, pregnancy, or estrogen therapy in Wilson's disease (5% of patients)
Hepatic copper concentration	> 250 µg/g dry wt	Primary biliary cirrhosis, Indian childhood cirrhosis, chronic cholestatic liver disease, primary sclerosing cholangitis, Alagille's syndrome, liver tumors, newborn liver	Copper chelation therapy in Wilson's disease
24-Hour urine copper excretion	> 100 µg/24 hr	Copper chelation therapy, chronic active hepatitis, chronic cholestatic liver diseases, primary biliary cirrhosis, primary sclerosing cholangitis, hepatic failure, nephrotic syndrome	Copper chelation therapy in Wilson's disease
Presence of Kayser-Fleischer rings	Present	Chronic cholestatic liver diseases, primary biliary cirrhosis, neonatal cholestasis	Early Wilson's disease
Incorporation of ^{64}Cu into ceruloplasmin	Low	Ceruloplasmin < 20 mg/dL, Wilson's disease heterozygote	Pregnancy, estrogens, inflammation, or malignancy in Wilson's disease

TABLE 11-10.

Wilson's disease (hepatolenticular degeneration). Evaluation for Wilson's disease. Wilson's disease is a recessive disorder localized to chromosome 13. Most patients present in childhood with a hepatic disorder although later presentation in adulthood with neurologic or psychiatric findings can occur. Although the primary defect remains unknown, excess accumulation of copper in the liver and subsequently in other organs is responsible for the clinical features of the disease. Clinical disease is rare in patients under 5 years of age because accumulation of copper must be significant enough to produce symptoms. Accumulation of copper first occurs in the liver and may cause acute hepatitis, fulminant hepatic failure, chronic hepatitis, cirrhosis, gallstones, or an unexplained elevation of serum transaminase levels. After the hepatic copper storage capacity is exhausted, copper begins to be distributed throughout the body, resulting in symptoms in the nervous, ocular, endocrine, and renal systems. Accumulation of copper in the cornea results in the Kayser-Fleischer ring, a green-brown ring at the periphery of the cornea best observed during a slit-lamp examination. Neurologic findings may include tremors, drooling, dysarthria, clumsiness, dystonia, ataxia, headache, and seizures. Renal abnormalities include renal tubular dysfunction, decreased glomerular filtration rate, and diminished renal plasma flow. Although a low ceruloplasmin level is suggestive of the disease, both false-positive and false-negative results can occur. A 24-hour urine copper determination and D-penicillamine challenge may aid in diagnosis. Determination of hepatic copper content on liver biopsy is essential in confirming the diagnosis. If the diagnosis has been established, then D-penicillamine therapy should be instituted and maintained indefinitely. This drug chelates copper and causes its excretion into the urine. Side effects of the drug include fever, rash, lymphadenopathy, and pancytopenia. Patients intolerant to D-penicillamine may benefit from trientine (triethylene tetramine dihydrochloride). Its side effects include bone marrow suppression, renal toxicity, and skin and mucosal lesions. It also chelates copper in the body. Zinc therapy, by inhibiting copper absorption from the intestine, may also be used in patients with Wilson's disease after adequate stabilization has been achieved. A diet low in copper is also advised. Orthotopic liver transplantation has been life-saving in patients with Wilson's disease who have fulminant liver failure or decompensated cirrhosis. Neurologic symptoms improve and Kayser-Fleischer rings disappear following liver transplantation. (*From* Suchy [4]; with permission.)

TABLE 11-11. WOLMAN'S DISEASE AND CHOLESTEROL ESTER STORAGE DISEASE

Autosomal recessive inheritance

Deficiency of lysosomal acid lipase

Wolman's disease clinically presents with hepatosplenomegaly, vomiting, diarrhea, malabsorption, and anemia with rapid neurologic deterioration

Cholesterol ester storage disease is more benign with hepatomegaly and hyperlipidemia

Wolman's disease with enlarged, calcified adrenal glands seen on radiographs

Liver transplantation is successful for cholesterol ester storage disease

TABLE 11-11.

Wolman's disease and cholesterol ester storage disease. Both disorders are inherited through an autosomal recessive gene and result from deficiency of the lysosomal enzyme acid lipase found on chromosome 10. Wolman's disease presents clinically with vomiting, diarrhea, malabsorption, hepatomegaly, splenomegaly, and anemia during infancy. Neurologic examination is initially normal but rapidly progresses with onset of abdominal distention. By 3 months of age, 50% of patients are dead and the great majority succumb by 6 months of age. Patients presenting with cholesterol ester storage disease are less severely ill with asymptomatic hepatomegaly and hyperlipidemia. Liver disease progresses to fibrosis, cirrhosis, and portal hypertension over many years. In Wolman's disease, laboratory studies reveal elevated levels of transaminases, anemia, normal serum cholesterol and triglycerides levels, and vacuolated lymphocytes. Cholesterol ester storage disease is indicated by elevated levels of serum cholesterol, triglycerides, and vacuolated lymphocytes. The liver in these disorders is often grossly enlarged, greasy, and yellow. Hepatocytes and Kupffer's cells contain birefringent cholesterol crystals. Triglyceride and cholesterol esters are increased several fold over control values in the liver. Typical of Wolman's disease is the presence of enlarged calcified adrenal glands on abdominal radiographs. Lipid accumulation in intestinal cells contributes to the malabsorption observed in Wolman's disease. Whereas clinical findings suggest the diagnosis, definitive diagnosis is confirmed by enzyme analysis of liver, fibroblasts, or leukocytes for acid lipase. Therapy in the past has been limited to supportive care and the use of lovastatin and cholestyramine to lower serum lipid levels. Orthotopic liver transplantation has been successfully employed in cholesterol ester storage disease, but not in Wolman's disease.

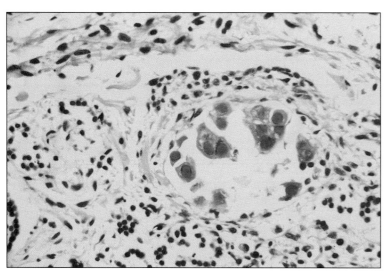

FIGURE 11-23.

Cytomegalovirus (CMV) hepatitis in the newborn. CMV may be acquired transplacentally, at delivery, from secretions (such as saliva or breast milk), or from blood transfusions in the nursery. Most congenitally acquired CMV infections are asymptomatic, but the 5% to 10% that are clinically apparent may manifest signs and symptoms, including low birth weight, microcephaly, periventricular cerebral calcifications, chorioretinitis, thrombocytopenia, purpura, deafness, and psychomotor retardation. On physical examination there may be hepatomegaly and splenomegaly secondary to extramedullary hematopoiesis. Elevated serum transaminases and conjugated hyperbilirubinemia are found on laboratory examination. Liver biopsy reveals giant cell transformation, large intranuclear inclusion bodies in bile duct epithelium, and intracytoplasmic inclusion bodies in hepatocytes. Bile stasis, inflammation, bile duct proliferation, and fibrosis may also be present. Diagnosis may be made by culture, serologic tests, and the use of electron microscopy and monoclonal antibody techniques on liver tissue. Treatment includes the use of the antiviral drug, ganciclovir, and specific CMV-immune globulin. Liver transplantation has been successfully used for severe hepatic disease that progressed to cirrhosis and portal hypertension. Prognosis remains poor for infants with neurologic sequelae and severe disease. Note CMV inclusions present in the bile duct in this slide. (Hematoxylin and eosin stain, original magnification × 450.)

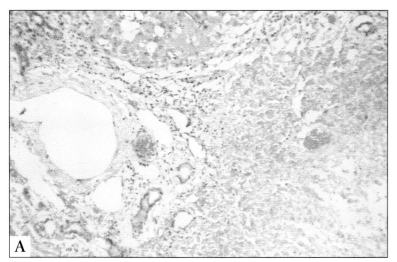 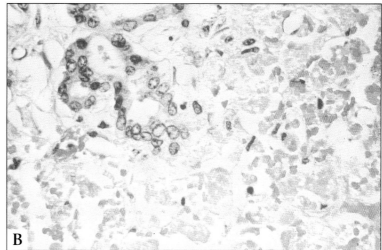

FIGURE 11-24.

Herpes hepatitis in the newborn. Herpes hepatitis may present as part of a systemic disease in the newborn. Symptoms may not appear until 4 to 8 days of age, corresponding to the incubation period for herpes. Congenital herpes may cause microcephaly and ulcerative, vesicular, or purpuric mucosal or skin lesions. Hepatic involvement results in jaundice, hepatomegaly, splenomegaly, and abnormal coagulation. Severely affected infants may have coagulopathy, gastrointestinal bleeding, encephalitis, and seizures. Diagnosis is suspected by the typical mucosal or skin lesions, antibody titers, or viral identification. Liver biopsy may reveal characteristic intra-nuclear acidophilic inclusions in hepatocytes, variable necrosis, and multinucleated giant cells. Liver tissue culture or, more preferably, immunohistochemical staining can be useful in confirming the presence of the virus. Treatment with the antiviral drug, acyclovir, has improved survival rates. The patient from whom these slides were taken had massive coagulative necrosis but lacked inclusions (**A** and **B**); herpes simplex was grown from a skin lesion and maternal decidual tissue stained positively for herpes. (**A**, Hematoxylin and eosin stain, original magnification × 100; **B**, Hematoxylin and eosin stain, original magnification × 450.)

TABLE 11-12. PEROXISOMAL LIVER DISORDERS

Genetic diseases with a general impairment of numerous peroxisomal functions and reduced or undetectable peroxisome numbers
  Cerebrohepatorenal (Zellweger) syndrome
  Infantile Refsum's disease
  Neonatal adrenoleukodystrophy
  Hyperpipecolic acidemia

Genetic diseases with a single enzyme defect and a normal number of peroxisomes
  X-linked adrenoleukodystrophy (VLCFA acyl-CoA ligase deficiency)
  Adult Refsum's disease
  Acatalasemia
  Pseudo-Zellweger syndrome (3-oxoacyl-CoA thiolase deficiency)
  Pseudoneonatal adrenoleukodystrophy (Acyl-CoA oxidase deficiency)
  Peroxisomal bifunctional enzyme deficiency

TABLE 11-12.

Peroxisomal liver disorders. Disorders of peroxisomes are associated with abnormalities in bile acid synthesis. Abnormal findings in liver function tests often result in referral of these children to a gastroenterologist. Peroxisomal disorders may be categorized into either those disorders where the number of peroxisomes is diminished or a group wherein the number of peroxisomes is sufficient but a single enzyme defect is present in the peroxisomes. If there is sufficient impairment in peroxisomal function, abnormalities in bile acid synthesis and metabolism and significant liver disease will exist. The same peroxisomal fatty acid oxidation system responsible for very-long-chain-fatty acids (VLCFA) is responsible for sidechain oxidation of 3α,7α-dihydroxy-5β-cholestanoic acid and 3α, 7α, 12α-trihydroxy-5β-cholestanoic acid. Elevations of these compounds are observed in the biologic fluids of Zellweger's syndrome, infantile Refsum's syndrome, neonatal adrenoleukodystrophy, and patients with pseudo-Zellweger syndrome. Treatment is largely supportive because there is multiorgan involvement with the peroxisomal abnormality. Oral primary bile acid therapy may aid the liver disease in some patients with peroxisomal disorders. (*From* Suchy [4]; with permission.)

TABLE 11-13. HEPATIC VENOUS OUTFLOW OBSTRUCTION

Level of obstruction
  Intrahepatic
  Hepatic veins
  Suprahepatic vena cava

Intrahepatic veno-occlusive disease (VOD)
  After bone-marrow transplantation
  After ingestion of herbal teas containing pyrrolizidine alkaloids

Budd-Chiari syndrome
  Noncardiac hepatic venous outflow obstruction
  Sudden onset of ascites and hepatomegaly

Suprahepatic vena cava
  Thin membrane at the vena cava or atrium is most common
    cause worldwide

Diagnosis: Doppler ultrasound and MRA

Therapy: Often surgical, transhepatic stent, liver transplantation
  in select cases

TABLE 11-13.

Hepatic venous outflow obstruction. The level of obstruction (intrahepatic, hepatic veins, suprahepatic vena cava) aids in differentiating the cause. Intrahepatic obstruction, referred to as veno-occlusive disease (VOD), is most commonly seen in children following bone marrow transplantation. Reports of VOD occurring in children who frequently drink herbal teas containing pyrrolizidine alkaloids have also been described. Budd-Chiari syndrome refers to a noncardiac hepatic venous outflow obstruction that causes sudden onset of ascites and hepatomegaly accompanied with abdominal pain, distention, and splenomegaly. Collateral blood flow causes abdominal and chest wall vessel enlargement. Biochemical changes may reveal only minimal elevations in serum bilirubin and transaminases. Suprahepatic vena cava obstruction resulting from a thin membrane, usually at the vena cava or atrium level, is the most common cause of hepatic venous outflow obstruction throughout the world. Though believed to be of congenital origin, symptoms often do not appear until adulthood. Diagnosis of hepatic venous outflow obstruction has been significantly aided by the use of Doppler ultrasound. Confirmation of the diagnosis may require magnetic resonance imaging with angiographic sequencing (MRA). Therapy focuses on treatment of the underlying predisposing cause of obstruction. Surgery is directed at removal of the obstruction or portosystemic decompression. In selected patients, percutaneous transhepatic venous stent placement can be helpful. For patients with progressive liver disease, orthotopic liver transplantation should be considered.

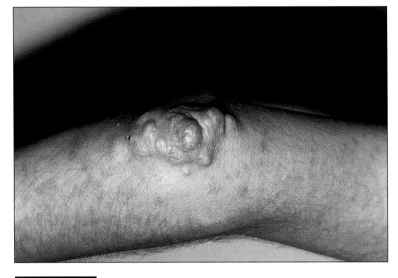

FIGURE 11-25.

Xanthomas. This slide depicts severe cutaneous xanthomas in a 7-year-old boy with Alagille's syndrome whose serum cholesterol level is approximately 1 g/dL. Severe intrahepatic cholestasis is associated with hypercholesterolemia, the deposition of cholesterol in skin, mucous membranes and arteries, and the development of xanthomas.

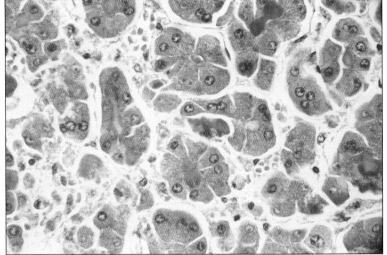

FIGURE 11-26.

Total parenteral nutrition (TPN)–associated cholestasis. Significant cholestasis, inflammation, and fibrosis in the liver of a premature infant who developed necrotizing enterocolitis and received total parenteral nutrition for 3 months before this biopsy specimen was taken. Cholestatic liver disease associated with the administration of TPN in preterm infants is a well-recognized clinical entity that occurs much more frequently in infants than adults. Despite numerous efforts to establish its mechanism, the origin of TPN–associated cholestasis remains undefined and no specific therapy exists. Continuation of TPN may further exacerbate the cholestasis and result in significant hepatocellular injury with the development of fibrosis and cirrhosis, but cessation of TPN in an infant with a dysfunctional gastrointestinal tract may itself result in starvation, malnutrition, and death. (Hematoxylin and eosin stain, original magnification × 450.)

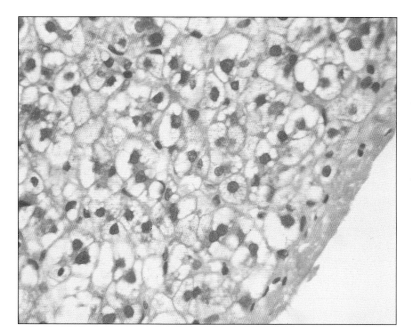

FIGURE 11-27.

Reye's syndrome. Liver biopsy findings of a child with Reye's syndrome. Hematoxylin and eosin (H&E)–stained section of a needle liver biopsy in Reye's syndrome reveals a cytoplasm with a foamy appearance caused by accumulated triglycerides with a centrally placed (owl's eye) nucleus. The microvesicular fat droplets characteristic of Reye's syndrome are best seen with a fat stain, such as Sudan red or Sudan black. Reye's syndrome is a severe systemic metabolic disorder with an acute noninflammatory encephalopathy and hepatitis. Classically, vomiting usually occurs within a few days following a viral syndrome, such as influenza or varicella. This can progress to alterations in consciousness, obtundation, and a brief period of agitated delirium followed by coma. For those who recover, the process usually takes 5 to 10 days. Laboratory studies reveal elevated serum transaminases (up to 20–30 times the upper limit of normal), prolonged prothrombin time, elevated concentrations of ammonium concentrations in the blood, and usually an initial normal serum bilirubin concentration. Hypoglycemia, especially in infants, may be severe. Intravenous infusions of glucose are frequently required, and if given early in the course, may be beneficial in preventing the disease's progression. (Original magnification $\times$ 450.)

■ QUANTITATIVE LIVER FUNCTION TESTS IN CHILDREN

TABLE 11-14. QUANTITATIVE LIVER FUNCTION TESTS IN CHILDREN

Indocyanine green clearance test
Galactose elimination test
Caffeine clearance test
Aminopyrine breath test
Lidocaine metabolism test (MEGX)

TABLE 11-14.

Commonly performed tests assess liver function in children. The processing of drugs by the liver depends on their rates of uptake, metabolism, and excretion. Indocyanine green is an anionic dye that is eliminated by the liver and is metabolically inert. Administered intravenously as a low-dose bolus (0.5 mg/kg) with blood sampling over 20 minutes, it is an excellent measure of hepatic blood flow.

The galactose elimination test measures the transformation of galactose to galactose-1-phosphate by galactokinase present in the hepatocytes. Elimination of galactose depends on liver cell mass.

Galactose (0.5 mg/kg) in a 20% solution is infused intravenously over 5 minutes. Blood is taken every 10 minutes for 1 hour to determine galactose clearance over time. This is an excellent test to assess for cirrhosis and to monitor liver function serially.

The caffeine elimination test assesses the hepatic mixed function oxidase system. After orally administered caffeine (2 mg/kg) is given, blood or saliva samples are taken at 4, 16, and 24 hours to obtain clearance values. Saliva collection, although noninvasive, is not easily done in small children.

The aminopyrine breath test assesses demethylation by the cytochrome P-450 system in the liver. Orally or intravenously administered aminopyrine with either C^{13}- or C^{14}-labeled methyl group is converted to labeled CO_2, which is detected and an estimate of the amount excreted per unit is made. It is an excellent test of liver dysfunction and correlates with the severity of cirrhosis. The test may be adversely affected by cholestasis or the concomitant use of other drugs which may alter the cytochrome P-450 system.

The lidocaine metabolism test assesses demethylation of lidocaine to its metabolite monoethylglycinexylidide (MEGX). Intravenous lidocaine is administered and the serum MEGX level is measured at 15 and 30 minutes following injection. The test has been useful for assessing liver donor quality, liver graft function following transplantation, and for recognizing hepatic dysfunction.

LIVER TRANSPLANTATION IN CHILDREN

TABLE 11-15. LIVER TRANSPLANTATION IN CHILDREN

Indications	Contraindications
End-stage liver disease	Systemic sepsis
Acute liver failure	Extrahepatic malignancy
Nonresectable hepatic malignancy	Anatomic contraindications
Correctable inborn error of metabolism	Severe irreversible extrahepatic organ failure
	AIDS

TABLE 11-15.

Indications and contraindications. Any child with end-stage liver disease, acute liver failure, a nonresectable hepatic malignancy localized to the liver, or a correctable inborn error of metabolism is a potential candidate for liver transplantation. Contraindications to liver transplantation include systemic sepsis, extrahepatic malignancy, anatomic contraindications that do not allow for vascular connection of the donor organ, severe irreversible extrahepatic organ failure, and acquired immune deficiency syndrome. Extrahepatic biliary atresia remains the leading etiology for liver transplantation in children. Among the metabolic causes of liver transplantation in children, α-1-antitrypsin deficiency is the most frequent.

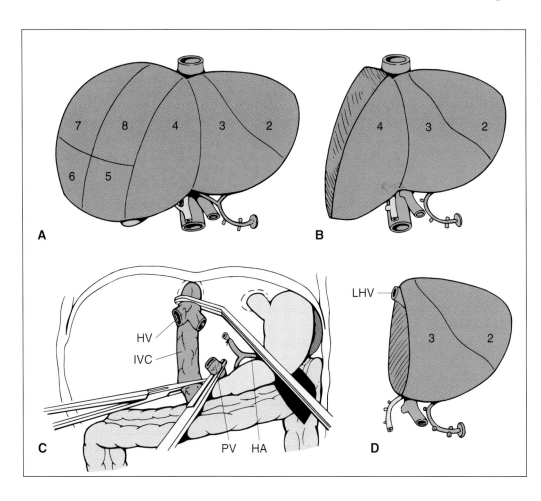

FIGURE 11-28.

Surgical techniques. Livers for transplantation are matched by blood type and size. There are problems due to the disparity between the size of donor organs (which most frequently come from older children and adolescents) and the size of most pediatric recipients (who are under 2 years of age). Reduced-size grafts, split liver transplants, and living-related liver transplants have evolved. The left lateral liver segment is the most frequently used technique for the child recipient. This figure demonstrates the liver segments utilized in various reduced-size grafts. **A,** Whole donor liver ready for transplantation. Numbering of segments according to Couinaud. **B,** Reduced liver graft, with the right lobe removed. **C,** Recipient liver removed, leaving the inferior vena cava *in situ.* **D,** Reduced liver graft, segments 2 and 3 without the vena cava. CBD—common bile duct; IVC—inferior vena cava; PV—portal vein; HA—hepatic artery; HV—confluence of hepatic veins; LHV—left hepatic vein. (*From* Calne *et al.* [10]; with permission.)

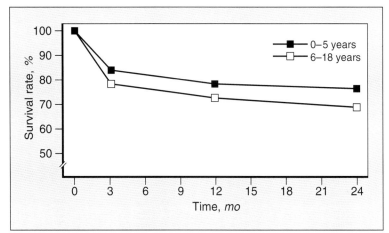

FIGURE 11-29.

Results. Survival statistics for children who have undergone liver transplants in the United States, based on data supplied by the United Network for Organ Sharing (UNOS) for 1988 to 1991. Compared with adults, children have better overall survival rates. Children less than 1 year old do not do as well as older children because the small size of their vessels are subject to thrombosis. (*Data from* the 1993 Annual report of the U.S. Scientific Registry for Transplant Recipients and the Organ Procurement and Transplantation Network [11].)

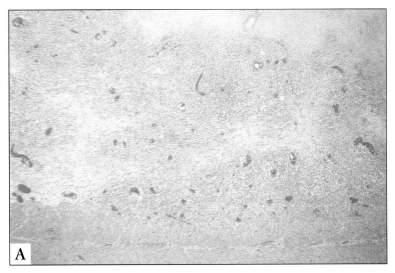

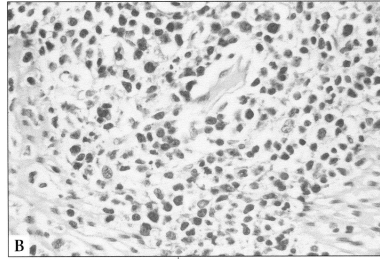

FIGURE 11-30.

Complications. Post-transplant lymphoproliferative disease (PTLD). PTLD is an often fatal complication of immunosuppression. PTLD is associated with a wide range of abnormal proliferation of B lymphocytes, with Epstein-Barr virus (EBV) believed to play an important potentiating role. The disease may present as a benign B-cell hyperplasia or as a progressive and fatal lymphoproliferation. Because children are often seronegative for EBV at the time of transplantation, children are at greater risk to be exposed to EBV after transplantation; thus, PTLD is more common in children than in adults. These children may present with fever, lymphadenopathy, tonsillar enlargement, splenomegaly, abdominal pain, or difficulty in breathing. Diagnostic evaluation includes a computed tomographic survey of the abdomen and chest for the presence of tumors or lymph node enlargement. Confirmation of the diagnosis is made by serology and biopsy of tonsillar or lymph node tissue or tumor. Biopsy tissue should be specifically analyzed for EBV nuclear antigens and EBV DNA. There should be an assessment to determine the clonality of the B-cell proliferation (benign polyclonal or malignant monoclonal). No specific therapy has been demonstrated to be effective in the treatment of PTLD. Reduced immunosuppression and intravenous acyclovir therapy, however, appear to be helpful at the current time. These images demonstrate a low-power view (**A**) and a high-power view (**B**) of a high-grade PTLD in the intestine of a child 2 years after liver transplantation who was receiving tacrolimus and prednisone immunosuppression when he developed a primary infection caused by EBV. (**A**, Hematoxylin and eosin stain, original magnification × 40; **B**, Hematoxylin and eosin stain, original magnification × 450.)

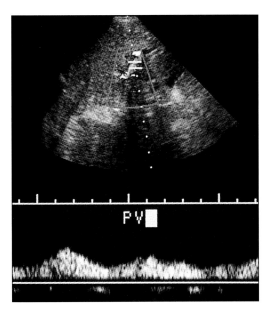

FIGURE 11-31.

Doppler ultrasound study to assess patency of the portal vein after liver transplantation. Doppler ultrasound signal observed in a patent portal vein following orthotopic liver transplantation in a child. The small caliber of the vessels in children predisposes the pediatric recipient of a donor liver to thrombosis. Doppler ultrasound affords a noninvasive, rapid, and relatively inexpensive means of assessing vessel patency.

PEDIATRIC LIVER TUMORS

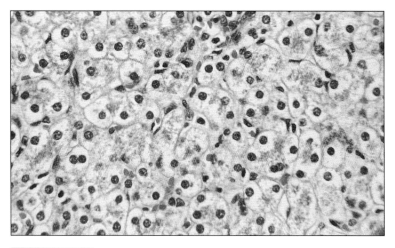

FIGURE 11-32.

Hepatoblastoma. Hepatoblastoma is the most frequently encountered liver tumor in children. It usually presents as an abdominal mass in a child less than 2 years of age and is more common in boys. A variety of malformations have been described in association with hepatoblastoma, including renal abnormalities, hemihypertrophy, and precocious puberty. In patients with hepatoblastoma, α-fetoprotein levels may be significantly elevated (100,000–1,000,000 ng/mL range) in patients with hepatoblastoma. Hepatoblastoma is classified into various types depending on histologic results. There is an epithelial type and also a mixed epithelial and mesenchymal type. This slide depicts the biopsy of a hepatoblastoma from a 2-year-old boy with the fetal epithelial tumor. Note the small, round, uniform cells with abundant cytoplasm and distinct membranes. The cells are arranged in thin trabeculae. Prognosis depends on the resectability of the tumor. For incompletely resected or inoperable tumors, various chemotherapeutic regimens have been used by the Children's Cancer Study Group. Orthotopic liver transplantation has been successfully used for some cases of nonresectable hepatoblastoma. (Hematoxylin and eosin stain, original magnification × 450.)

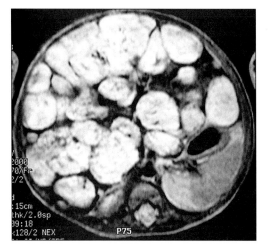

FIGURE 11-33.

Infantile hepatic hemangioendothelioma. Infantile hepatic hemangioendothelioma is the most common benign hepatic tumor encountered in children and the most common liver tumor observed in children less than 1 year old. Presentation may include congestive heart failure, abdominal mass, failure to thrive, jaundice, respiratory distress or the presence of skin hemangiomas. The tumor is more common in girls. Diagnostic imaging is useful in the evaluation of these tumors. Shown is a magnetic resonance image of infantile hepatic hemangioendothelioma. The tumors are bright signal intensity on this T_2-weighted image. Treatment for this tumor has included steroid administration, radiation therapy, surgical excision, hepatic artery ligation or embolization, cytoxan administration, and more recently, interferon therapy. A poor prognosis is suggested by congestive heart failure, jaundice, and the presence of multiple tumor nodules.

PRIMARY SCLEROSING CHOLANGITIS

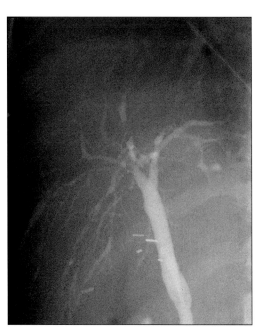

FIGURE 11-34.

Primary sclerosing cholangitis (PSC) in childhood. Improvements in the performance of hepatobiliary imaging studies in children and recognition of the entity occurring in the pediatric group has led to an increased diagnosis of this disorder in childhood. *Sclerosing cholangitis* is defined as a chronic hepatobiliary disorder with inflammation of the intra- or extrahepatic bile ducts resulting in focal dilatation, strictures, narrowing, or even obliteration accompanied by periductular fibrosis. PSC is the most common liver disorder associated with inflammatory bowel disease. Of note, liver disease may be clinically apparent long before the symptoms of the intestinal disorder become recognizable. Unlike adults, children with PSC may present with growth failure or delayed puberty. When diagnosis is suspected, it can be confirmed by endoscopic retrograde cholangiopancreatography (ERCP). This image depicts the findings from an ERCP performed in a 13-year-old boy with chronic liver disease, cirrhosis, and massive splenomegaly who presented for liver transplant evaluation. Note the irregularity of the intrahepatic bile ducts and areas of stenosis and dilatation. Intestinal symptoms of inflammatory bowel disease were not present at the time of this study but developed later in the course of therapy.

HEPATITIS PROPHYLAXIS

TABLE 11-16. ROUTINE HEPATITIS B IMMUNIZATION SCHEDULES

MATERNAL HBsAg	DOSE	AGE
Negative	1	Birth–2 days
	2	1–2 mo
	3	6–18 mo
Positive	1	Birth (in 12 hrs)*
	2	1 mo
	3	6 mo
Unknown	1	Birth (in 12 hrs)
	2	1–2 mo
	3	6 mo

*Also HBIG therapy.

TABLE 11-16.

Hepatitis B. Recommendations for universal hepatitis B immunization among newborns. Both the American Academy of Pediatrics and the Centers for Disease Control have made public recommendations for the immunization of all infants against hepatitis B. These recommendations resulted from the inability of previous strategies, such as selective immunization of high-risk populations and screening of all pregnant women for hepatitis B in order to control hepatitis B infection. Universal infant immunization for hepatitis B was determined to be the most effective means to combat hepatitis B in the United States because it will eventually reach all individuals, the cost of vaccinating an infant is lower than an adult, and immunization of infants is easier to accomplish and can be readily incorporated into the existing childhood immunization schedule.

Currently, two licensed recombinant hepatitis B vaccines are commercially available. This table lists several of the recommended hepatitis B routine immunization schedules. Note that the schedules are based on the hepatitis B status of the mother. For infants born to mothers who are hepatitis B surface antigen (HBsAg)-positive, hepatitis B immune globulin (HBIG) should also be administered to the infant shortly after birth.

ACKNOWLEDGMENTS

I wish to thank Dr. Sheila Moore for the radiologic slides, and Dr. Linda Ferrell and Dr. Samuel H. Pepkowitz for the histologic slides.

REFERENCES

1. Elias H: The early embryology of the liver of vertebrates. *Anat Anz* 1955, 101:153–167.

2. Suchy FJ, Balistreri WF, Heubi JE, *et al.* Physiologic cholestasis: Elevation of the primary serum bile acid concentrations in normal infants. *Gastroenterology* 1981, 80:1037–1041.

3. Heymann MA: Fetal cardiovascular physiology. In *Maternal-Fetal Medicine: Principles and Practice.* Edited by Creasy RK, Resnick R. Philadelphia: WB Saunders; 1984.

4. Suchy FJ: *Liver Disease in Children.* St. Louis: CV Mosby: 1994.

5. McDonagh AF, Lightner DA: "Like a shriveled blood orange"—bilirubin, jaundice, and phototherapy. *Pediatrics* 1985, 85:443–455.

5a. Gourley GR: Jaundice. In *Pediatric Gastrointestinal Disease: Pathophysiology, Diagnosis, Management.* Edited by Wyllie R, Hyams JS. Philadelphia: WB Saunders; 1993:293–308.

6. Altman RP: Recent developments in hepatobiliary surgery. *Pediatr Ann* 1977, 6:87–97.

7. Riely CA: Familial intrahepatic cholestatic syndrome. *Semin Liver Dis* 1987, 7:119–133.

8. Rosenthal P, Thaler MM: Porphyrias. In *Rudolph's Pediatrics*, edn 19. Edited by Rudolph AM, Hoffman JIE, Rudolph CD. East Norwalk, CT: Appleton & Lange; 1991: 382.

9. Scheinberg IH, Sternlieb I: *Wilson's Disease.* Philadelphia: WB Saunders; 1984.

10. Calne RY, Friend PJ, Johnston PS, Jamieson NV: Surgical Aspects of Liver Transplantation. In *Wright's Liver and Biliary Disease*, edn 3. Edited by Millward-Sadler, Wright, and Arthur. London: Harcourt, Brace; 1992:1452.

11. 1993 Annual Report of the U.S. Scientific Registry for Transplant Recipients and the Organ Procurement and Transplantation Network-Transplant Data: 1988–1991. Richmond, VA: UNOS and Bethesda: Division of Organ Transplantation, Bureau of Health Resources Department, Health Resources and Services Administration, U.S. Department of Health and Human Services; 1993.

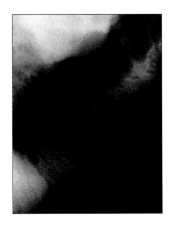

Index

Page numbers followed by *t* or *f* indicate tables or figures, respectively.